W9-DAM-247

Stem Cell Therapy
A Rising Tide

How Stem Cells are Disrupting Medicine and Transforming Lives

Neil H. Riordan

Stem Cell Therapy: A Rising Tide
How Stem Cells are Disrupting Medicine and Transforming Lives

www.cellmedicine.com
info@neilriordanbooks.com

This book is not intended as a substitute for the medical advice of physicians. The information provided in this book is designed solely to provide helpful information on the subjects discussed. The reader should regularly consult a physician in matters relating to their health and particularly with respect to any symptoms that may require diagnosis or medical attention. While all the stories in this book are true, some names and identifying details have been changed to protect the privacy of the people involved.

Layout design by www.iPublicidades.com

Illustrations by
Blake Swanson – Innercyte: Medical Art Studios
Steve Lewis – Blausen Medical
Stem Cell Institute & Riordan Medical Institute

Cover art design by n23art

Printed in the United States of America.
First Printing: 2017
ISBN: 978-0-9990453-0-5

TABLE OF CONTENTS

Foreword

As I read this book, I became very emotional. I had to go back about 28 years ago when my wife and I sat in a doctor's office and listened to a neurologist list in grim detail how our beautiful three-year-old son Ryan would spend his next 20 years. The doctor told us there was nothing that they could do at that time. He suggested that we do everything we could to keep Ryan active in order to maintain the strength he had as long as possible. And hopefully in the next 20 years they might find a cure for muscular dystrophy. The prognosis changed our lives forever. It was a very painful time for all of us.

As I continued to read about all of the patients who have been treated by Dr. Riordan, I realized that we all had one thing in common: traditional medicine had given up on us. There was nothing that could be done. Our own government, founded on the premise of life, liberty, and the pursuit of happiness, had evolved into overreaching bureaucracy that would attempt to prevent us from seeking lifesaving alternative treatments.

But once again, we all had something else in common. We found a man who was willing to do everything in his power to offer us options and give us hope for the future of our loved ones. Dr. Riordan has truly dedicated himself to his profession as a medical pioneer. He has sacrificed everything he has to give those who have been told there are no options a fighting chance and real hope for the future.

Dr. Riordan has never wavered in the face of scrutiny. It takes true courage to stand up to the often judgmental "traditional" medical community—those who act offended when you suggest that there might be a different way.

Fortunately for all of us, Dr. Riordan had the foresight to look beyond the walls of traditional medicine and fight the fight for us. I encourage you to read this book, and not just the chapters related to your condition. As a whole, the book lays out Dr. Riordan's courageous and successful journey through his stories and the stories of his patients.

Thank you, Dr. Riordan, for all that you have done for us and our families. You truly are a hero!

George Benton, Ryan's father

Introduction
BY ARNOLD CAPLAN, PHD

Neil Riordan, PhD, PA is a pioneer of the highest order, in some ways like John Glenn or Neil Armstrong. Neil has ventured where the routes were uncharted and the dangers huge. His rocket of cell therapy was launched on a rickety platform filled with hopes and dreams, and powered by an engine of money. This pioneer has hacked his way through the jungle of naysayers and has produced miracles of enormous proportions. He has taken our scientific dreams and translated them into a high-caliber medical facility that does good by offering exposure to cell therapy treatments that we working scientists only dream about.

Although there are those in my professional realm who would say that Neil is a medical "cowboy" who "experiments" with human subjects, I would say that he is providing access to therapies that are no more experimental than one sees every single day in the surgical suites of major medical centers. In such situations, the surgeon is "forced" to improvise because of the complexity of the wound field. Such improvisation sometimes involves using materials that are not approved but that the surgeon "feels" will work well in the situation he faces. For example, human decellularized skin from dead people was approved for topical applications for ulcerated wounds in diabetic patients. But these "membranes" are fabulous for closing abdominal surgical wounds in hernia repair operations and have changed the way such closures are done. This surgical improvision, originally performed by a "cowboy" surgeon, is now the standard of care. We move forward in medicine by the skill and insightful work of pioneers—some with IRB approval and some not. Riordan's procedures with MSCs currently have IRB approvals.

In a sense of transparency, let me say that I have accepted honoraria from Neil Riordan and gifts of hotel rooms, meals, and, indeed, infusions of MSCs. These all have monetary value, but none influences my opinion. The monetary success of Neil's enterprises evoke jealousy in some entrepreneurs, but Neil's continual reinvestment of money into his next medically successful enterprise displays his true motives—the advancement of a medically necessary science despite great obstacles. The key to his success is in the enormously high quality of his facilities; the people, doctors, nurses, receptionist, PR team, etc. are *all* highly principled and care about the patients they serve. These people care about what they do because Neil recruits them for their skills and attitude. He does not discuss this in this book, but they are present on every page. He talks about Dr. Paz, but he does not tell you of his long medical experience and his reputation in the United States and in Panama for caring and experienced medical judgements. In all of Neil's clinics, quality control labs, hotels for patients, and restaurants where they eat, the staff behind the scenes are dedicated to providing the highest quality medical care possible. Some clinics and hospitals in the United States could take lessons from the Riordan gang. That said, the cell-based therapies Neil's clinics provide have not all been approved and tested by double-blind, placebo control and rigorously monitored clinical trials, although such trials are currently underway. But, like innovative surgeons, these open-label uses have proven effective, as hopefully we will see in published peer-reviewed reports of his studies.

Each chapter of this book recounts the personal stories of how Neil's unwavering confidence that cell-based therapies with MSC preparations from fat, marrow, or umbilical cords can make a medical difference. Neil made medical tourism work, and what he has done is highly laudable, not only because of the patients he has helped, but because of the laws that have been written to support cell-based therapies in Panama. This book is not what I pleaded with Neil to write, however. I have, for many years, begged him to give us outcome reports of his many patients: what they have as clinical problems, what they walk in with, and the longitudinal outcomes after the cell infusions. Hopefully these will be forthcoming, but they are not in this book. What is here in these pages is, none-the-less, amazing.

I first learned about Neil's clinic in Costa Rica and thought his procedures and therapies were brilliant. And these were crude compared to those currently underway in Panama. The Panama GMP-production facilities, his offices and treatment rooms, and the products including MSCs from umbilical tissue are of the highest quality. These are the vehicles and the platform that allow him to write this treatise of the therapies they provide. It is a shame that we have to fly to Panama to have access to these therapies instead of having them available in the United States. How long will it take for such therapies to be available to the patients covered by Medicaid or Medicare instead of those from Beverly Hills or Long Island who can afford to travel to Panama?

Almost daily I receive emails from people who want access to "stem cell" treatments. I tell them that I am just a PhD researcher and cannot suggest an avenue of treatment for medical issues. If you have this book in hand, read the chapters. They are honest, open, and spellbinding. While Neil is not a medical doctor, his clinical experience as a physician assistant along with his research background have prepared him for the serious medical issues for which Neil has organized cell therapy treatments, often with quite significant outcomes. Neil is certainly a student of the medical arts and an expert using innovative treatments. I have talked to patients of Neil's clinics and their family members about their treatments; the stories told in this book are just the tip of the iceberg. This is an interesting book and an interesting and gutsy journey of Neil Riordan. His physician father would be proud to recognize Neil's passion and medical achievements.

Arnold I. Caplan, PhD

Skeletal Research Center

Department of Biology

Case Western Reserve University

10600 Euclid Avenue

Cleveland, Ohio 44106

January 15, 2017

Chapter One

THE SEED IS PLANTED—HOPE FOR MUSCULAR DYSTROPHY

George Benton and I had been classmates since elementary school in Wichita, Kansas, but we didn't get really close until we became dads. My Chloe was born a week before the Bentons' Ryan. We lived only a few blocks from each other in the same neighborhood.

Our families ended up spending so much time together that Chloe and Ryan fast became playmates. Around the age of three, Ryan's physical development started to lag behind Chloe's. We noticed he had trouble getting up from the floor. He didn't just jump up like the other kids. For him, standing up was a three-point movement that required him to steady his hand on his knees to maneuver himself upright. And he couldn't simply dash up the stairs—Ryan had to take them one at a time.

At first we thought Ryan was just a little clumsy, or maybe he wasn't going to be very physically active. But the Bentons' friend, who was doing a residency in orthopedics, told them Ryan had classic signs of muscular dystrophy. When his diagnosis was confirmed, we all went into mourning. The diagnosis meant, at best, Ryan would live into his early twenties. It was inconceivable to me, feeling how much I loved Chloe and all the hopes I had for her, that a life so tender and promising could be snapped off just as it was beginning to blossom.

There is no cure for muscular dystrophy, of which Duchenne, the type Ryan has, is the worst form. People with Duchenne do not produce enough dystrophin, a protein that helps maintain the integrity of the muscles. Without it, the skeletal muscles break down first, and then, year by year, other muscles and tissues begin to die off. Ryan's body would eventually collapse on itself. It broke everyone's heart to realize that this boy, with such a great spirit and a huge appetite for life, probably wouldn't be able to walk by the time he was twelve, and that by the time he reached his twenties he'd most likely need a respirator. All I could think was, why can't someone help Ryan? Although I didn't realize it at the time, a seed was planted in my mind that would later grow into a strong passion for finding answers to some of medicine's toughest questions.

The Bentons handled this tragedy bravely. They became very involved in the Muscular Dystrophy Association (MDA)—Ryan was even a poster child for a while. Ryan traveled all over the state speaking to groups about his condition and raising money for research for a cure, which his doctors told Ryan's parents would be realized within his lifetime. At home, the Bentons tried to give Ryan as normal a life as possible. He was in Boy Scouts, and they even signed him up for tee-ball. He'd hit and another teammate would run the bases for him. Ryan's friends were the kind of young people who give you hope for the future: kind, caring, loyal, and true friends to Ryan no matter what kind of a day he was having.

Ryan was a brave boy, and he hid his condition well. In fact, until he was seven, he didn't even think he was different than his peers. But by that time the effects of the disease became undeniable. His frailty began to show. One day Chloe flirtatiously shoved him while playing hoops, and he went flying across the yard. She didn't realize how far her playful gesture would launch her friend. I'll always remember the look of shock on her face.

By the time he was eight, Ryan wore leg braces. Kids with Duchenne tend to walk on their toes to get better balance, but that shortens the muscles in their ankles. The Bentons were on a mission to keep Ryan ambulatory as long as possible. He complained about having to wear long, uncomfortable leg braces when he went to sleep at night. They'd often find the braces removed and by the side of the bed in the morning. All the exercise—the swimming, physical therapy, and time on the treadmill—couldn't postpone the inevitable. By the time Ryan and Chloe were thirteen, when my family and I moved to Arizona, Ryan was in a wheelchair full time. After our last visit with Ryan as we were departing Wichita, I wondered what shape I'd find him in when we saw him again.

In all of my later travels, which eventually led to working with adult stem cell therapies, Ryan was never far from my mind. When I marveled at the beautiful, independent young lady Chloe was becoming, I'd think of the Bentons and how different their life with Ryan was. After we left Wichita, George and his wife Sandra divorced and each remarried. I kept in touch with George. Every time I saw medical research about any slim advance in the treatment of muscular dystrophy, I'd forward it to him. When I visited Wichita, we'd see each other, and inevitably we'd talk about Ryan's condition and how it was deteriorating. "Dad, I remember you told me they'd have a cure," Ryan said, referring to what the doctors told his dad when Ryan was first diagnosed.

"How do you answer that?" his dad pleaded with me.

It wasn't until I lived in Costa Rica, where I had established a medical laboratory and clinic treating patients with stem cells, that I could finally bear fruit from the seed planted in my mind so many years before. My colleague at the Stem Cell Institute, Fabio Solano, MD, said he wanted to treat a patient from Ireland who had muscular dystrophy.

Our Irish patient had a less severe form of the disease, Becker's muscular dystrophy, which doesn't appear until later in life. With Becker's, the body produces some, but not enough, dystrophin. Data from our own research, and that of other scientists from around the world, showed that when adult stem cells are injected into muscle, they become part of the muscle and persist there for a period of time. No one is certain exactly how long the stem cells remain viable, but for at least a few months, some of the cells survive. Our theory was that if the cells were from a healthy donor, they would produce some dystrophin. Even a little dystrophin could help.

I had read of one case of a child diagnosed with Duchenne when he was fourteen, more than a decade past the average onset of the condition. When he was much younger, he'd received a bone marrow transplant for another malady, so his immune system and blood-forming system was essentially that of someone else. The cells from that bone marrow cycled through his body and seeded the other cells, which helped to combat the onset of his Duchenne. In fact, when he was diagnosed, he had one of the mildest cases of Duchenne his doctors had ever seen. I thought some of the cells from his bone marrow transplant must have produced muscle-fortifying dystrophin. After considering our Irish patient's chances carefully, we decided to proceed with treatment.

As Dr. Solano and I reviewed the literature and talked about our Becker's case, I thought, of course, of Ryan. Maybe we could do something with adult stem cells for him. If treatment went well with our Irish patient, perhaps the Bentons would be willing to take a chance on treating Ryan.

When our Irish patient came into the clinic, he reminded me of Gollum, J.R.R. Tolkien's fictional character who lived underground, hunched over from years of obsessing over the precious golden ring he coveted. Our patient was only in his thirties, but he was bent over and used a cane with a four-pronged base to walk. Dr. Solano and I decided to concentrate treatment on his core muscles because he could barely hold himself upright. In order to treat our Irish patient effectively, Dr. Solano injected thirty-five vials into this man's muscles even though he was charged much less for the treatment. I told Fabio, "Man, we're going to go out of business!" This was very early on in our work, when each vial of stem cells cost us thousands of dollars to produce. I'm thankful that technological advances since then have greatly reduced that cost.

A few months later our Irish patient walked fully upright into the clinic and said in a strong, clear voice, "I want to see Dr. Solano." I couldn't have been happier. And I thought, what good news this could be for Ryan.

At first, I didn't know how to approach the Bentons to suggest that they try this unconventional treatment. I didn't want him to think I was pressuring him or that I was trying to use our friendship to get business for my clinic. I genuinely believed this treatment could help Ryan. A good friend of ours talked to him about it and reported back that George was enthusiastic.

At that point Ryan was twenty-two. His Duchenne muscular dystrophy had followed the normal trajectory and Ryan's body was falling apart. He had metal rods holding up his spine so his body weight wouldn't crush his internal organs. They'd built a ramp at the front of the house so he could get in and out on his own in his wheelchair, but when he took the down slope too fast, his head would often flop onto his chest. He'd have to wait until someone came along to pick up his head for him. The most worrisome for George and Sandra were his lung infections. Four times a year he'd get bronchitis, which would always turn into pneumonia, and Ryan would end up in the hospital. At that point he weighed only 70 pounds. Sadly, his parents knew it was only a matter of months before Ryan would die.

The next time I was in Wichita I met with George, Sandra, and Sandra's second husband Curt to discuss the treatment. Sandra was very concerned about using donor stem cells to treat Ryan. Where would those stem cells come from? I told her that we would use stem cells from donated umbilical cords that underwent extensive testing, but she was still very uneasy. For many years researchers felt similarly—injecting cells from someone else's body would surely trigger immediate rejection, they thought. But with umbilical cord cells, which are a type of immature cell that the immune system doesn't recognize as foreign, this is simply not true. After considerable discussion, we decided to use stem cells cultured from Ryan's sister Lauren's menstrual blood. From that, we grew a culture of 200 million cells. Three months later George and Ryan, along with Ryan's best friend Clint, flew to Costa Rica for the first treatment.

When they brought Ryan in for his shots, I was stunned by how much his condition had deteriorated. His skeleton frame had almost no muscle fibers.

George and Clint transferred him from his wheelchair to the treatment bed, but one of them alone could have picked him up.

We injected cells in sites throughout Ryan's body with a strong concentration in his neck. Dr. Solano knew that we had to proceed slowly because the injections were painful. When Dr. Solano inserted the needle, he was splitting muscle fibers. Ryan didn't have that many of those, so his treatment was limited by his ability to tolerate pain. Each day we gave him ten shots until a total of thirty-five vials had been injected into his muscles. Then he returned to Wichita, and we waited. I told them that it might be two weeks to a month before Ryan felt any different.

I watched my email every day for a message from George. Three weeks after the treatment, he reported that Ryan had been at the swimming pool where he takes physical therapy, and suddenly he could sit up on his own. A week later, one of the physical therapists playfully tried to push him over, but he resisted the shove. George tried pressing the back of Ryan's head, and he couldn't get it to move. Ryan suddenly had strength in his neck, the kind of strength he'd lost years ago. And he was gaining weight.

I knew these gains wouldn't last. We had treated patients with other genetic and chronic degenerative diseases, and the benefit was usually temporary. Eventually the number of active stem cells would decline. After a few months, the cells become recognizable to the immune system and are cleared by the body. It was difficult to assess how many of them would persist and continue to produce dystrophin. Yet for Ryan, the impact was overwhelming. He had hope for the first time in his life. "There was so much movement in my legs that I hadn't felt in so long," he said. "I was gaining, and I'd never felt that gain before. All I knew was loss."

Ryan had been down for treatment six times (one more in Costa Rica, and the rest in Panama), and each time he got a little better, plateaued and then declined a bit. His overall health, stamina, physical strength, and ability to breathe improved each time and then began to decline again. After about four treatments using injections directly into his muscles, I came upon a study that showed intravenous injection of stem cells without immune suppression was possible, and effective, in an animal model of Duchenne.[1] We added intravenous injection of stem cells for his last two treatments in

Panama. The effects of adding IV stem cells were apparent. "Wow! Whatever you did this time is leaps and bounds above what I had before," Ryan told me. We knew we were on the right track.

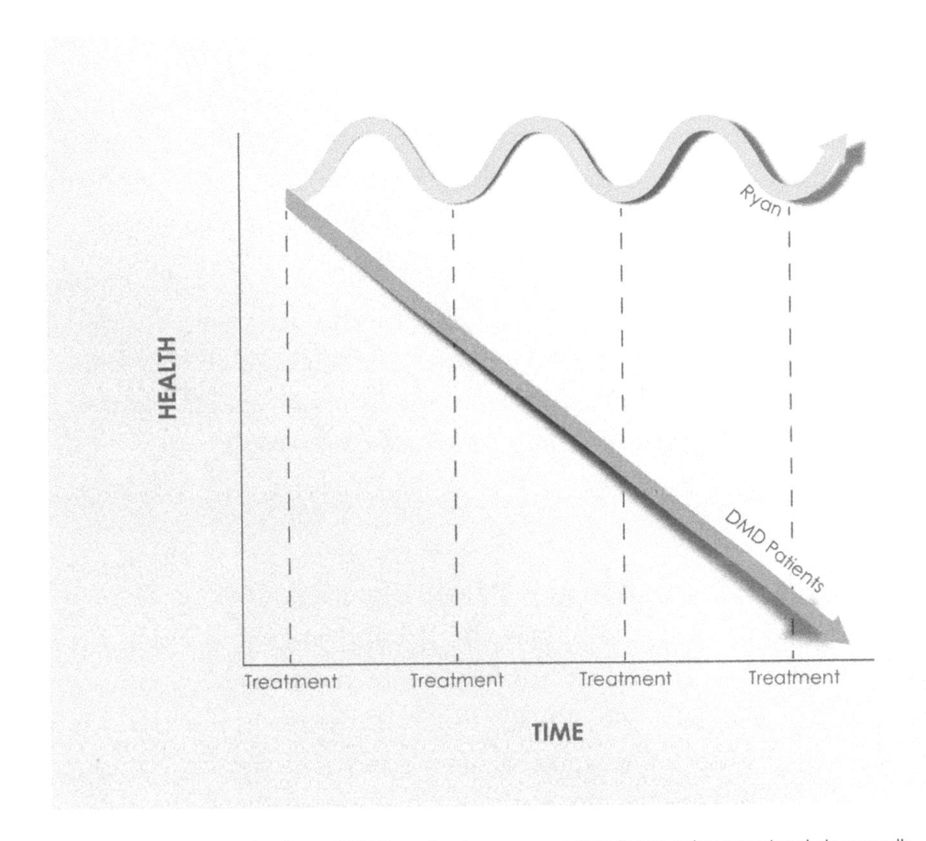

Average decline of DMD patients compared to Ryan, who received stem cells.

The effort necessary to come to Central America for treatment was tough on him, but the improvements he experienced made it worth it. Since that initial treatment with his sister's stem cells, with consent from his parents we augmented his regimen to include stem cells from donor umbilical cords injected both into the muscle and into the vein. Younger cells, as found in umbilical cords, are more energetic in the system and hence have a better chance of persisting and being more effective. Since his first treatment in 2008, Ryan has continued to improve. He's gained more than twenty pounds, and he no longer suffers through terrible lung infections. "It's a miracle," George said. "For the first time since he was three, we've all got hope." Ryan is the most optimistic of all, but he's realistic too.

Stem Cell Treatment for Duchenne Muscular Dystrophy

Duchenne muscular dystrophy (DMD) is a degenerative disorder in which muscles progressively become weaker. Genetic abnormalities cause problems in the production of dystrophin, a protein responsible for maintaining muscular tissue.[2] When muscle cells (myofibers) begin to die and do not have an efficient way of regeneration, fibrous and fatty connective tissues take over the muscle.[3] This inevitably leads to muscle wasting, complete paralysis, and eventually death by cardiac or respiratory failure.

The use of pharmacological agents to treat DMD has not produced favorable results in clinical trials.[4] Only corticosteroids manage to delay the progression of the disease[5] but come with many adverse effects.[6] It may be possible to modify the genetic regions responsible for the dystrophin deficiency with gene therapy, but this is still under development.[7]

Given the stresses of traveling to Panama for treatment, in 2014 we applied for and received a compassionate use investigational new drug approval from the FDA. This allows for Ryan to be treated in his hometown by his physician, Maurice Van Strickland, MD, with stem cells from Panama. He was first approved to be treated every six months, but since January, 2016, has approval to be treated every four months to try to stay ahead of any declines he experiences. He is the first Duchenne muscular dystrophy patient granted approval for this form of medical therapy inside the United States.

Ryan recently celebrated his 30th birthday, a rare event for Duchenne patients. "How could I complain?" Ryan said recently when I asked him how he felt about this. "Ever since growing up I remember asking all the time, 'If there's not a cure, is there something to stop the decline?' Dealing with the effects of muscular dystrophy is hard enough, but knowing it's going to get worse is so depressing. I spent the whole first year of treatment going to funerals of the kids I knew from MD summer camp. I haven't really declined since treatment. I want more, and I will always push for more, but I can't imagine what I would be if you hadn't treated me."

Cell therapy focuses on aiding the regeneration process of the muscle cells. The regenerative and anti-inflammatory properties of mesenchymal stem cells (MSCs)[8,9,10] make them a viable treatment option for DMD. Additionally, MSCs have immunomodulatory properties via their secretions that allow engrafting into the damaged muscle tissue to help in the regeneration process.[11,12] MSC treatment has been applied to animal models, particularly in Golden Retriever dogs as they are affected by a muscular disorder known as Golden Retriever muscular dystrophy (GRMD) with remarkable similarities to human DMD. A recent study where GRMD dogs were treated with MSCs showed that it was a safe procedure and no long-term adverse events were reported;[13] MSCs were able to reach, engraft, and express human dystrophin in the dogs' damaged muscles up to six months after treatment.[14] Studies in mice models have also shown expression of dystrophin after MSC administration.[15] We have reported positive results for MSC treatment on a DMD patient[16] and several clinical trials are approved and recruiting to demonstrate the safety and efficacy of MSCs for this condition.[17,18,19,20,21]

I agree with Ryan about that aspect of the human character that always pushes for more. I think about how many more kids with muscular dystrophy and other diseases could be helped with stem cell therapy, if only the laws of the United States would permit me to conduct my work there more broadly. The doctors at the Stem Cell Institute also treated a young boy of three and a half years in Panama who had just been diagnosed with Duchenne. After one treatment, the little boy was symptom free and remained so for nearly a year, running and jumping with his friends without any weakness or hesitation. After receiving five treatments without any side effects of consequence, like Ryan, this boy has also received permission from the FDA for stem cell treatment as a compassionate use investigational new drug at age six. His first treatment in the United States began in January, 2016. If the laws permitted it, we could set up clinics all over the United States to treat children in the early stages of muscular dystrophy with stem cells and continue this treatment throughout their lives. If our early results treating this six-year-old boy are any indication, we could relieve the suffering of thousands of families and give these children normal lives.

Yet there are significant barriers to advancing this life-saving and life-extending therapy. I wrote this book to explain how important this work is and the potential it holds for alleviating the pain and suffering of millions of people around the world diagnosed with a wide range of diseases. In the next chapters, I will describe how I got involved in this research, the science that supports these breakthroughs, and the legal and economic barriers that prevent these therapies from widespread use.

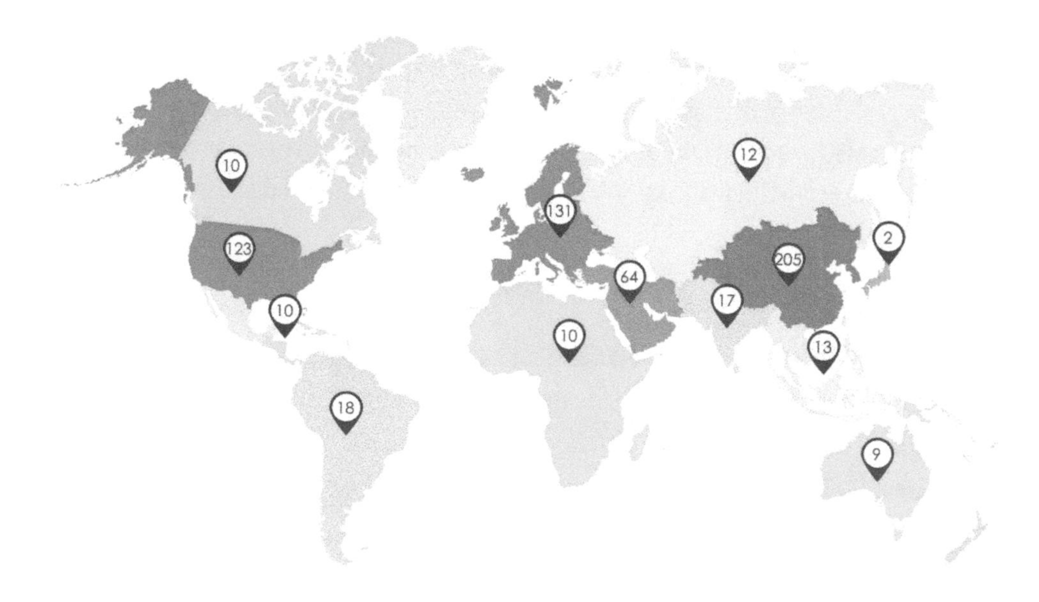

Number of studies using mesenchymal stem cells worldwide registered on Clinicaltrials.gov as of May 2017.

Chapter Two

THE BODY'S INNATE HEALING ABILITY—CANCER SPELLED BACKWARDS

My dad, Hugh Riordan, MD, was as formidable a figure in the world of natural medicine as he was to his children. His outsized presence was powerful, partially because of the way he looked, but mostly because you knew that he was a guy who didn't give a damn what anyone thought of the way he lived his life.

My dad was a maverick doctor who believed that in many cases the best thing he could do for a sick patient wasn't to load him or her down with prescription medicines, but to refocus the body's natural healing powers to encourage it to cure itself. He'd started his career working with vitamin deficiencies. As a medical student, he worked with rats that were deprived of a key nutrient: selenium. He observed how the selenium-deprived rats gradually lost vigor and how the sheen of their coats dulled. Yet shortly after he reintroduced selenium to the rats' diet, all of these effects reversed. Later, after he became a psychiatrist, he explored how tailoring the right balance of nutrients to each individual's needs could produce profound improvements in the lives of mentally ill patients, particularly schizophrenics.

By the time I was in high school in the 1970s, he had expanded this research to conditions outside of mental health. He was treating cancer patients with high doses of vitamin C at his Center for the Improvement of Human Functioning (now named The Riordan Clinic). The Center took a lot of criticism from the medical establishment for this unconventional treatment—many called him a quack, and worse. But my dad had a way of laughing at the forces that conspired against him. He knew what was working for his patients.

As a teenager, I spent a lot of time at my friend Joel's house. I thought of his mom Esther as a second mom. By the time I was in my first year as a business major at Wichita State University, coursework I considered dull and not relevant to the real world, Esther got cancer.

She had squamous cell cancer that started at the base of the tongue and metastasized throughout her body. It seemed so unfair that this woman, who didn't smoke or drink, or even cuss, should get this aggressive and hard-to-treat disease. In my 18 years I had never seen anyone treated so poorly as Esther was by the medical establishment. The chemotherapy ravaged her body, and by the time she passed, she weighed only seventy pounds. She died a miserable death in the hospital, lying in her own feces. Her poor treatment left a strong impression on me that makes me shudder to this day. She was the first person I loved who died.

For a while, the world didn't make sense to me. I was angry and full of sorrow, and unsure of how to deal with it. I didn't know what to do with my life at the time, but I knew that I wanted to get out of Wichita. My dad told me about a job working as a diver in the oil fields in the Gulf of Mexico, so I moved to Louisiana and took it.

As it turned out, I had the perfect set of skills to be a diver, and the work was interesting. A year later I enrolled in diving school in California and, after I graduated, I got a job diving in the oil fields of Dubai. After a few years there I met Shirley, my beautiful English wife, who was working at a bar in a Dubai hotel. We fell in love and got married. Just before we were about to take off for our honeymoon, I got a fantastic gig—one that all the other divers in the area wanted. I would be in a diving chamber underwater with a partner for 30 days, but we'd be making a thousand dollars a day. Shirley was pregnant with our first child, our daughter Chloe, so it seemed like a great opportunity to bank some money for our family's future. What happened there changed the course of all of our lives and made an abrupt turn in my career.

When my partner and I came up from our 30 days underwater, we had been in the deepest nitrogen/oxygen saturation dive ever to take place to date, so there was no decompression table to guide our company on how to bring us back up. They had a hypothesis about how do to it, but they got it wrong at the end.

The closer the divers are to the surface when they are in the decompression chamber, the more care you have to take, because the bubbles inside the divers' bodies grow at the greatest rate. We had been brought up very slowly over the course of two days, but right in the last ten minutes, they rushed it. They figured we'd been in there long enough, right at the moment when we were at our greatest vulnerability. The minute they broke the seal on the chamber, I felt my hands and legs go numb.

The guys who were bringing me up immediately put me in another decompression chamber and recompressed me to 60 feet and put me on pure oxygen. I felt pretty good right then, and my symptoms cleared up. When they started bringing me up again, I got another bubble and all the symptoms returned. I couldn't feel my hands and feet and I started going numb. Here I was with a new wife and a baby on the way and suddenly I couldn't stand up.

The company kept me in Dubai for a while trying to figure out how to solve this problem. Then they sent me to the University of Dundee, Scotland where Philip James, MD, a world-renowned diving doctor, had been working with hyperbaric oxygen. Dr. James made a strong impression on me. He was the only doctor, other than my father, who thought outside the box and didn't care what "the establishment" thought about his work. He was pursuing research into the effects of hyperbaric oxygen therapy for patients with multiple sclerosis, a therapy no one else was exploring at the time. He became a major influence on me and later took on the role of mentor.

The next stop was back in the United States where I sat in a big hyperbaric oxygen chamber (the only known treatment at the time for decompression sickness, or the bends) for 30 days in a row alongside people who had non-healing wounds, radiation poisoning, and other maladies. That was incredibly depressing. Many of the people there were suffering the effects of an overdose brought on by cancer treatment. One lady who sat next to me had been so mis-dosed with radiation, I could see right through her neck when she turned her head at a certain angle. Seeing the barbaric effects of those treatments reminded me of what had happened to Esther when she got sick.

Eventually the weakness in my legs was resolved, although I still have hand and foot numbness, particularly on my fingertips. I knew I'd never be able to dive again. I went from being a very successful diver with a promising career to again feeling a little lost. Shirley and I moved to Wichita where I went to work in my father's research lab. I also went back to school and eventually decided to enroll in a program to become a physician's assistant. I graduated from the Wichita State University program summa cum laude.

During my residency period, prior to graduating with my degree, I discovered that my real interest was in research and finding cures that can help thousands of people. At my father's lab, he was supervising a groundbreaking program using high-dose vitamin C to stop the growth of cancerous tumors. Within a year of working in the lab I was overseeing all of the research projects.

In 1986 my father had a patient named George Williams who had stage IV kidney cancer with multiple metastases that had spread to his lymph nodes. This is a cancer that doesn't respond to chemotherapy. In fact, it was at that time considered malpractice to prescribe chemotherapy for it. He'd tried a number of therapies, but nothing worked. His doctor suggested that he get his affairs in order because he didn't have long to live.

George had heard about the work Linus Pauling and some Scottish doctors were doing with mega doses of vitamin C to treat cancer. My dad agreed to treat him with 30 grams of vitamin C delivered intravenously twice a week for six weeks. Within six weeks, his tumors had shrunk significantly and by six months they just melted away like butter in the sun. My dad started treating him when he was 70 years old, and he lived to be 84, receiving vitamin C drips every few months. When he died, he had no evidence of cancer. He died of congestive heart failure, which is too bad because we could have probably helped him with that too knowing what we know now about stem cells.

In 1989, the center received a $13 million grant from the Garvey Foundation of Wichita to advance this work on treating cancer with vitamin C. Bob Page, the head of the foundation, was very specific about what he wanted from us. He said he'd give us ten years, and ten years only, to look for nontoxic therapies that were clinically applicable for cancer patients. He said he didn't want us to make a career of this or to spend a lot of time looking for a small molecule that is not found in nature that would take ten years of animal testing before we could even try it in a human. He wanted us to come up with something that was clinically applicable now.

We called it the RECNAC project, which is "cancer" spelled backwards. We weren't taking the conventional medical approach of poisoning the entire body to weaken the cancer. We wanted to strengthen the immune system to enable it to battle the tumors more effectively. The body has an innate ability to heal itself under the right conditions. My work has always centered around this premise. The first place we looked was nutrition. We had data on vitamin C and its selective toxicity, or how it kills tumor cells and leaves normal cells alone. We started our work there.

I'm thankful that I was working with my dad, a guy who was used to swimming against the tide. We were up against data from a 1979 Mayo Clinic study discrediting the use of vitamin C to treat cancer.[1] Clinical tests conducted there found that treatment with vitamin C didn't alter the course of the disease, and the paper recommended that it be abandoned as a course of treatment.

We found several flaws with the Mayo Clinic's methods and conclusions based on our research. We'd been giving our patients vitamin C intravenously and treating them over a long period of time. The Mayo Clinic delivered their vitamin C doses to the patient orally via pills, a method that our research showed did not deliver the vitamin in high enough doses to be toxic to the tumors. Two articles later published in the *Canadian Medical Association Journal* suggested the Mayo research was flawed and the scientists were biased against the use of "alternative" cancer treatments.[2,3] John Hoffer, MD, PhD, a professor of medicine at McGill University, said, "In 1971, even saying that vitamin C could be useful was so outlandish that a conversation would stop between scientists and physicians." But the tables have turned. The Mayo Clinic is now interested in doing a clinical trial on the use of IV ascorbic acid for the treatment of cancer.

When I first began studying intravenous vitamin C treatment for cancer, it was considered by many to be pure quackery, but just a few months ago I was invited by the Marcus Foundation to evaluate grant proposals by Thomas Jefferson University, Johns Hopkins, the National Institutes of Health, and Mayo Clinic for the use of intravenous vitamin C for cancer. Prestigious medical organizations throughout the world are now studying the effects of this natural treatment. Yet since 1997, I hold the U.S. patent, along with my dad, for the use of intravenous vitamin C as a tumor cytotoxic chemotherapeutic agent.[4] I also hold the U.S. patent, along with Joseph Casciari, PhD, for the use of intravenous vitamin C along with lipoic acid for the treatment of cancer.[5]

We had started in a different place than the treatment devised by most oncologists. Because our starting point was to bolster the immune system, we wanted to know if our patients had any vitamin deficiencies. The immune system can't work properly without vitamins. In some studies, up to 30 percent of cancer patients have the equivalent of scurvy—a significant deficiency in vitamin C.[6] The white blood cells that engulf cancer cells and other foreign organisms, called phagocytes, don't work well if there's not enough vitamin C in the system. One of our first tests was to see if the patients' phagocytes would gobble up foreign particles, such as yeast. We found that with cancer patients, sometimes as little as one or two percent of the phagocytes engulfed the yeast, whereas in a healthy individual that number would be between 40 and 70 percent. These numbers went up in cancer patients treated with vitamin C, which demonstrates a bolstered immune response to the vitamin. In one study of patients with stage IV pancreatic cancer, intravenous vitamin

C added to the standard chemotherapy drug increased survival by over ten months when compared to the chemotherapy drug alone.[7]

We also looked into the stress the patients were experiencing in their lives. Some studies have shown that stressful life events are associated with an increased risk of cancer in the following years.[8] When the adrenal glands are working overtime, as they do during stressful episodes, the body uses up a tremendous amount of vitamin C to synthesize the stress hormones. The book *Molecules of Emotion*, by Candace Pert, PhD, describes the link between mental wellness and immune dysfunction. Basically, your macrophages, or white blood cells, almost immediately get a message from your brain of whatever you are thinking. Most of my cancer patients had been through a severely acute stressful period prior to their diagnosis.

What convinced me about the immune system's role in fighting cancer was a study of 77 women with breast cancer that was published in the *Annals of the New York Academy of Sciences* by James McCoy, PhD.[9] When these women underwent surgery, the surgeon took tumor tissue and co-cultured it with some of the patients' white blood cells. In some women, the white cells didn't react to the tissue, but in others they were stimulated to proliferate. In other words, the women's immune systems responded to the cancer. Researchers followed the women for twelve more years. Of the women whose immune systems didn't respond, 47 percent were dead twelve years later. But of the women whose immune systems were aroused by the cancer, 95 percent were still alive.

The immune systems of the women who died had developed immune tolerance, meaning that they had tolerated the growth of the cancer. The goal of our work was to break the immune tolerance and transform it into immune competence, or the ability to produce a normal immune response to foreign invaders—in this case, to cancer. We worked with a number of different techniques to get the immune system to recognize and attack tumors so that the body could heal itself of cancer without needing chemotherapy or radiation, or just minimal doses, which would prevent the destructive side effects I'd seen in Esther and in those people I shared the hyperbaric oxygen chamber with in Texas.

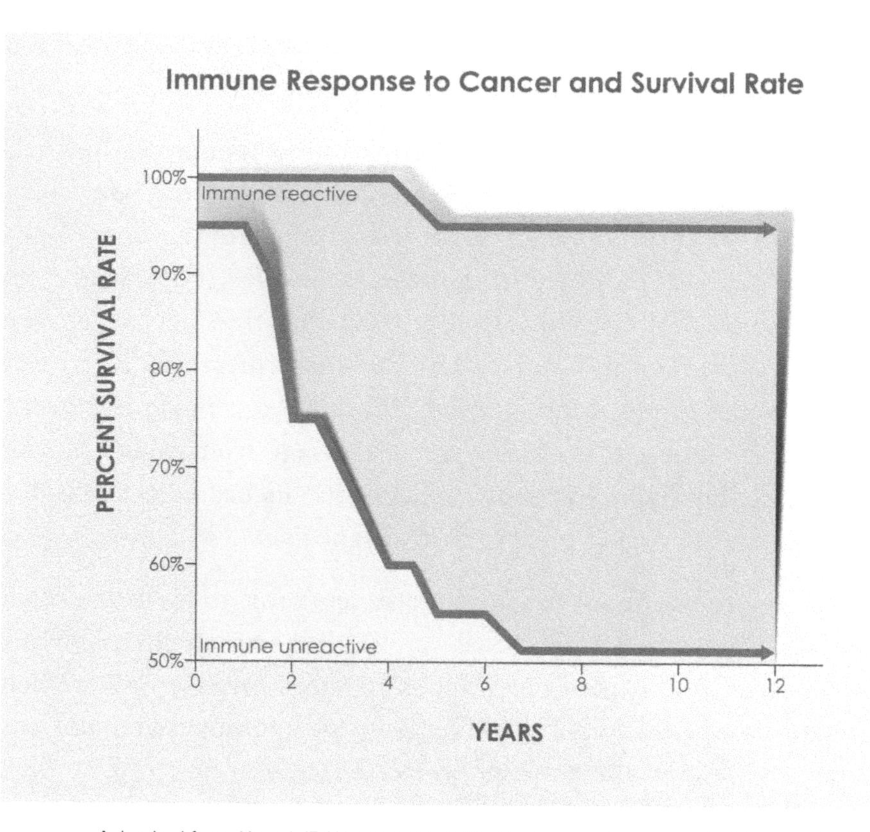

Adapted from Head JF, Wang F, Elliott RL, McCoy JL. Assessment of immunologic competence and host reactivity against tumor antigens in breast cancer patients. Prognostic value and rationale of immunotherapy development. Ann N Y Acad Sci. 1993;690:340-2.

We had been successful in finding a nontoxic way to fight cancer. Toward the end of the RECNAC decade, we had results, and I pushed hard to find a place to publish our findings.[10] But I found something else when I was reviewing all the data for all the patients we'd treated over that ten-year period. Some of these patients, even the miracle cures like George Williams, hadn't received high enough doses of vitamin C to have a toxic level in the blood. Something else we were doing to stimulate the body's natural defenses against disease, along with the high doses of vitamin C, was killing the cancer.

It was then that I started to think of cancer as a non-healing wound. This is very different from the conventional explanation for cancer, which states that environmental factors or a genetic predisposition to a type of cancer causes the cells to mutate in such a way that they continue to divide and become a tumor mass. There had been a study in South Korea that demonstrated my idea. Scientists inserted metal plates into the stomachs of rabbits, and in response the rabbits always developed a cancer around the plates. But if the researchers perforated the plates, the rabbits didn't develop tumors. My theory was that when the plates were a solid mass, the tissues were never able to communicate that the wound had healed, so it continued to grow the tumor around the chronic irritation.

There was another great study of veterans who came back from the war with wounds. There's a high incidence of tumors forming right at the wound site, the site of the chronic irritation. Lung cancer is a great example of this. Smoking is chronic irritation to the lungs, and it increases lung cancer rates. So this is my hypothesis: Most or all tumors form as a last ditch effort to heal a non-healing wound.

The body has a number of acutely responsive reactions that rush to heal an insult or a wound. There are cells that activate when the body detects an imbalance, a wound, or inflammation, and rush to the site of the problem

Cancer as a Last-Ditch Effort to Heal a Non-Healing Wound

A beautiful study that supports my cancer theory was conducted by JeanMarie Houghton, MD, PhD and published in *Science* magazine.[11] In a mouse model of stomach carcinoma, which begins with an ulcer-inducing *H. pylori* infection, she showed that transplanted bone marrow cells from another animal grew into stomach cancer cells. This turns the conventional cancer model—that the body's own cells undergo a three-step transformation process that leads to cancer—on its head. None of the cancer cells were from the animal itself—they all came from the donor animal as a last-ditch effort to heal the non-healing wound, in this case, the ulcer. So it's not the local tissue undergoing initiation, promotion, and transformation, as the conventional model of cancer suggests. Rather, it's the local tissue being depleted of the capacity to repair. I believe that a local deficiency in MSCs led to the failure to heal, which led to the release of bone marrow stem cells that proliferated in an attempt to heal the wound, but grew into cancer.

to begin the healing process. In our research, we discovered that vitamin C was incredibly useful in stimulating the immune system to attack these problems. I believed this was just the beginning of what we could discover if we went deeper into the healing mechanisms and researched ways to deploy these natural forces to combat disease.

By the end of the RECNAC decade, I knew it was time for my father and me to part ways. I had learned so much from him during that time and will be forever grateful for the guidance and support he gave me while I honed my skills as a researcher and a scientist. I was excited at the opportunities that I could create on my own using the knowledge of the body's self-soothing powers. It was time for me to make my own way as a true maverick is destined to do.

Chapter Three

REDIRECTING THE IMMUNE SYSTEM—CANCER EXPOSED

When I left my father's lab in 1999, I wanted to do different research than was allowed in his clinic. I'd been inspired by a treatment we performed in 1998 on a woman—I'll call her Patty—who got the same kind of cancer as my friend's mom Esther. We tried something different with her. When her cancer had progressed to her lymph nodes and the prognosis wasn't looking good, we explained to her what we wanted to try, and she agreed. I didn't want her to die the way Esther had.

I was interested in testing a different way of harnessing and targeting the body's immune system to cure chronic diseases. It was clear to me that our work on vitamin C and cancer was groundbreaking, and it set the foundation for my understanding of how natural substances could help bolster the body's healing forces to attack diseases for which the pharmaceutical industry had no effective solution. Yes, they had drugs, but most of those drugs were astronomically expensive and many damaged the body in order to treat the illness. What we'd seen in the work we did on cancer and vitamin C was that when we delivered high doses of the vitamin directly to the tumor site, other elements of the body's protective healing forces were stimulated. I wanted to find a way to work directly with those immune system cells. The place I started my work was with dendritic cells, which laid the foundation for my later work with stem cells.

The body has three layers of defense against disease. The first is the way the skin—the outer skin that covers the body and inner "skin" that lines our digestive and respiratory tracts—rejects foreign particles that are trying to enter the body. If the foreign substances are able to penetrate those barriers, the second defense—the inflammatory response—kicks in, moving blood plasma and white blood cells to the area of irritation to heal the wound. The third line of defense is the immune system response, which can be, and in many cases is, pre-primed specifically to battle a particular irritant.

The white blood cells that are aroused by the presence of an irritant to the system come in four forms: neutrophils, eosinophils, monocytes, and lymphocytes. Each of these has a separate function in the battle against disease. The neutrophils are the first to arrive at the site of an infection. Their job is to attack the infection. Eosinophils are special purpose cells most useful in fighting allergies and asthma. Monocytes are scavenger cells that scour the body for substances that don't belong there. For example, when a monocyte finds a tumor cell, it engulfs it, chewing off a piece of it for disposal. The lymphocytes, which mature in the thymus gland, produce antibodies that kill off disease and tumor cells.

There is innate, or pre-primed immunity towards tumor cells in which monocytes, neutrophils, and certain subsets of lymphocytes can and do have the ability to recognize and destroy tumor cells. In the clinical cancer patient that system is at least partially broken.

What interested me more at the time is another way the body recognizes and destroys tumor cells. Monocytes can become shape-shifters in the presence of cancer. A monocyte that is in the tissue is called a *macrophage*, which means "super eater." When the macrophage adheres to a cancer cell, it takes a bite out of it. Inside the macrophage are little enzyme packets that act like stomach acid to break down the tumor cell into smaller and smaller bits. After consuming the tumor cell, the macrophage knows it needs to alert

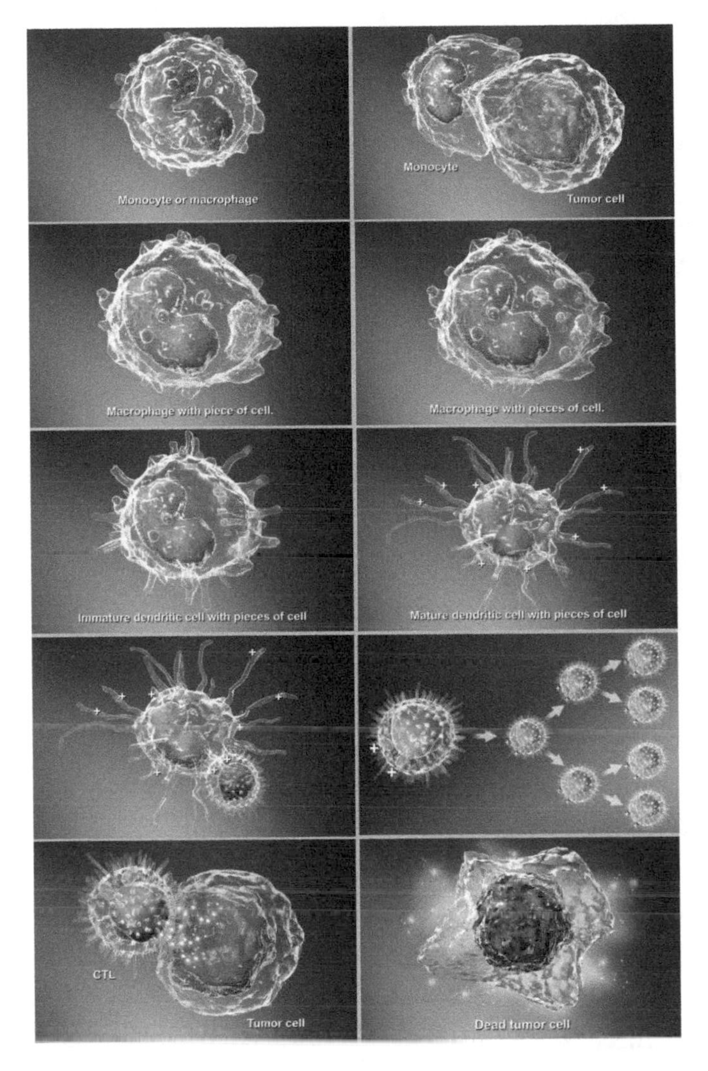

the rest of the body to the presence of this dangerous intruder. In many instances, the macrophage next transforms itself into a dendritic cell, which is a highly effective messenger to the body warning it that it must immediately begin a powerful immune system response to battle the tumor.

The dendritic monocytes take the little digested packets of tumor cell to the immune system, presenting information about the tumor to the lymphatic system (home of the immune system) so that it can rouse its forces to respond to the threat. When we're sick with an infection, we've all felt how the lymph nodes in our necks swell up as they rise up to battle the disease. There are also clusters of lymph nodes in the armpits and groin, as well as smaller clusters that reside close to the skin.

When the mature dendritic cell arrives at the lymph node, the node responds to the information it carries there by cloning an army of little soldiers that are specifically designed to attack that disease. These soldiers travel back to the offending cells and adhere, poking tiny holes in the cell membrane. Perforated in this fashion, the disease-inducing cell (in the case of cancer, the cancer cell) spills its guts and dies.

Dendritic Cell Treatment for Cancer

Jose Ignacio Mayordomo, MD, PhD led a team at the University of Pittsburgh that inoculated mice with different types of cancer and allowed the tumors to develop for one to two weeks.[1] The scientists isolated the dendritic cells, cultured them with some growth factors, and exposed them to tumor peptides (amino acids that carry information about the tumor cell membranes), in effect priming them to carry information about the tumor to the immune system. Then they injected these primed dendritic cells back into the tumor-bearing mice every four to seven days. Within seven to ten days after the first injection, the tumors stopped growing. Using this treatment, 80 percent of the mice with Lewis lung carcinoma and 90 percent of the mice with sarcoma were cured.

M. Krishnan Nair, MD, founding director of the Regional Cancer Center at Trivandrum, India, led a similar study.[2] Dr. Nair and his team induced malignant melanoma lung metastases

What I just described are the normal processes of the immune system when it is working as it is supposed to do. This powerful, subtle, and flexible system operates continuously every day in response to the millions of germs and viruses that enter our systems intending to cause us harm. When we discover that we have cancer, it means the immune system has failed to respond—the insult to the body has not been answered effectively. Cancer researchers have been studying what prevents the immune system from attacking effectively. They discovered that usually there are dendritic cells around a tumor, but most of them do not mature. The reasons why they don't mature are still a mystery. Is it that the macrophage doesn't recognize the foreign cell? For whatever reason, the dendritic cells don't properly present the information about the tumor to the lymphocytes, so the tumor cells are essentially ignored by the immune system.

The question that interested me was, how could we encourage the dendritic cells to mature and complete the process of stimulating the immune system to engage in the fight? I wanted to try to find a way to create the optimal circumstances to allow the dendritic cells to do their work and thereby attack the cancer without having to use toxic poisons to attack the body the way chemotherapy does.

(new tumors that spread from the first tumor) in mice, and then surgically removed the primary tumor. The mice were then treated with dendritic cells that had been primed in a manner similar to the Mayordomo study. Of the seven treated animals, four had no visible lung tumors, two had fewer than five remaining tumor nodules, and one mouse had fifteen nodules. The number of nodules in the control mice, those that did not receive dendritic cell therapy, were too many to count but comprised approximately three-quarters of the lung by weight.

At Stanford University, Frank J. Hsu, MD and his colleagues pioneered the use of dendritic cell therapy on cancer in humans.[3] They purified dendritic cells from the circulating blood of four patients with B-cell lymphoma who had previously been treated with chemotherapy. The dendritic cells were cultured and treated with tumor antigen (tumor cell membrane information) derived from the patients' tumors. The researchers injected the dendritic cells intravenously on four occasions. Two weeks after each dendritic cell injection, they also

Part of what stimulated my thinking in this area was research into kidney cancer, the cancer that is most likely to have a spontaneous remission. If you cut up a piece of tumor from kidney cancer, or renal cell carcinoma, and look at it under the microscope, you'll find millions of dendritic cells, many more than in any other type of tumor. As you'd expect, the majority of these dendritic cells are immature. What I believe happens when someone has a spontaneous remission of renal cell carcinoma is that the conditions in and around the tumor change enough to allow at least some of the dendritic cells to mature and activate the body's natural immune system. What if we could find a way to do that for other cancers?

Some scientists were pursuing the same line of thinking as I was. Both animal and human trials using dendritic cells showed some promising results and pointed in a direction I was eager to explore.

Given all of this compelling evidence that dendritic cells may hold a key position in effective, non-toxic treatments for cancer, we began studying them, and ways to help them mature.

Our lab had a leukapheresis machine, the same machine that the American Red Cross uses to harvest blood products when you donate blood.

injected the patients under the skin with tumor antigen, along with a protein that helps stimulate an immune response. All of the patients developed measurable T cell immune responses after one or two vaccinations. The treatment's success was measurable—there was one partial response, one minor response, disease stabilization in three patients with progressive measurable disease, and a complete response in a patient with minimal detectable disease. All of the patients remained progression-free when followed up two years later.

Gerald P. Murphy, MD and his team at Northwest Hospital's Pacific Northwest Cancer Foundation in Seattle have been testing the use of dendritic cells in patients with advanced prostate cancer.[4] All of the patients in the study had advanced prostate cancer and were unresponsive to conventional therapies, including hormone treatment. They cultured the patients' monocytes (macrophages) with growth factors and small pieces of protein found on the surface of prostate tumor cells. After priming the dendritic cells, the researchers

The procedure is time consuming, but it's relatively simple. We connected a needle and tube to each of Patty's arms and ran her blood through the machine to separate out the white blood cells, returning the rest of the blood to her. The procedure took about two hours.

After separating the white blood cells, we brought them to the laboratory where we immersed them in a special broth we'd devised that helped them transform into dendritic cells. This broth contained a highly concentrated mixture of growth hormones that are naturally found in the body. We also cultured her cytokines—the proteins that immune cells use to communicate with each other—and grew them in an incubator for two days. This cytokine mixture created a rich medium in which the macrophagic monocytes could transform into dendritic cells. Although I didn't know it at the time, I would later use a similar process to grow stem cells.

While the cells were changing over, we took a piece of Patty's tumor and made an extract. Once the dendritic cells matured, we introduced the tumor extract into the mix and let the cells mature for a few more days so they could respond to the information provided by the tumor extract. When the process was complete, we tested the cells for maturity and purity. After we reinfused the patients with the cells through an intravenous drip. They performed two studies. More than 27 percent of study patients who participated in both clinical trials showed some improvement, and the disease was stable in another 33 percent.

In addition to lymphoma and prostate cancer, the deadly skin cancer malignant melanoma has been treated successfully using dendritic cell therapy. In a recent human study led by Frank O. Nestle, MD at the University of Zurich, Switzerland, dendritic cells were used to treat 16 patients with advanced metastatic melanoma.[5] Objective responses were seen in five of the sixteen patients. There were two complete responses and three partial responses with regression of metastases in several organs, including skin, lung, and pancreas. Researchers followed their patients for fifteen months and found no cases of autoimmunity, a potential side effect of the therapy, in any of the patients. The authors concluded that vaccination with dendritic cells derived from the patient's own body is a safe and promising approach in the treatment of metastatic melanoma.

were certain the cells were strong and safe, we froze them in liquid nitrogen so they would be ready for use when we needed them.

We treated Patty with a combination of IV vitamin C and the specially manufactured dendritic cell vaccine. Her cancer basically disappeared. We were all amazed at how quickly her body started to respond to this vaccine and how powerful and long lasting the response was. Nine years later she was still cancer free. I remember thinking of Esther then and wishing I had been working in this field when she got sick. I don't know if I could have saved her, but I sure would have tried. More than ten years after we treated Patty, the first dendritic cell treatment for prostate cancer was approved by the FDA.

How many other Esthers were there out there who could benefit from this unique treatment, one that could be specifically tailored to the individual who was suffering and would have no toxic side effects? Unlike chemotherapy, this treatment would not weaken the body and ruin the immune system. In fact, it bolstered the patient's immunity, making them stronger and better able to fight disease than they were before. We wanted to set up a clinical trial for these cancer vaccines using dendritic cells, but we had a hard time getting a hospital in Wichita to allow us to use their facilities. Frustrated by the hospital bureaucracy, I decided to do what other scientists I respected did when faced with similar stubbornness by hospital review boards. I decided we should do our clinical trial overseas. This is how I got to know Dr. Fabio Solano, who was a big fan of my father and his work, and who operated a clinic in Costa Rica. We did a successful clinical trial on the dendritic cell vaccines and formed a strong friendship and partnership that was instrumental in my eventual move to Costa Rica.

When I left my father's lab, I set up a clinic in Arizona, which has a separate medical board and a distinct set of rules for naturopathic doctors and medical doctors who want to practice nutritional and integrative medicine. In this clinic, we treated hundreds of cancer patients with specially tailored dendritic cell vaccines.

Our first patient was there before we even opened the doors of the clinic. She had heard about our work and wanted us to treat her stage IIIC ovarian cancer. Following the same process we used with Patty, we treated her over the course of several years. While she never became cancer free—her bloodwork still showed the tumor marker for ovarian cancer—her body showed no more tumors. Shortly after that, we treated a businessman from Montana who had renal cell carcinoma. We isolated the tumor antigens by collecting his urine and running it through a sieve that would collect the molecules with a high molecular weight, as the tumor antigens are. Using these as a primer for the dendritic cells, we developed a vaccine for his cancer, which disappeared completely in twelve weeks. He hadn't told us that he also had melanoma at the time, but the vaccine we developed had such a powerful effect on his immune system that the melanoma on his back dried up and disappeared as well.

We had great luck with the cancer patients who came to us early—with stage I or II our treatment success rate was 85 percent. If the patient had progressed to stage IV, the numbers were much lower—our success rate slipped to 24 percent.

In 2014 I received a letter from the niece of one of the clinical trial patients we had treated in the past. She had stage IV metastatic lung cancer. In addition to radiation treatments, she underwent our dendritic cell and IV vitamin C therapy in 1999. Fifteen years later she is 76 years old and cancer free, living in Costa Rica with her husband, her niece reported. I had the pleasure of speaking with her and her husband last year.

I also recently heard from another patient, Cindy Brinkerhoff, who we treated at our clinic in the Bahamas. At the time, she had widely metastatic melanoma, Clark's level five, which means that the tumor has grown down into the fat under the skin. In 2000 she had had a tumor in her leg removed along with lymph nodes in her pelvic area, performed at the John Wayne Cancer Research Center in Santa Monica. After the surgery, she decided to forgo chemotherapy. By 2004, after a stressful period in her life, her leg tumors reappeared. She decided to undergo hyperthermic isolated limb perfusion, a procedure that involves blocking off the leg with a tourniquet and heating it up via blood vessels to kill off the tumors in her leg. The profusion removed the tumors, but they returned a few months later. At that time, in 2005, Cindy heard about our treatment in the Bahamas. She came down and we treated her with a tumor antigen vaccine derived from her urine, which eradicated all of her tumors except two in the popliteal lymph nodes behind her knee. We then removed one of those tumors and created an antigen vaccine against that tumor. After injecting her with the vaccine, the last tumor disappeared. She continued the vaccine injections, along with vitamin C injections, monthly for a couple years. She sent me a message the other day to let me know that she is alive and well thanks to this innovative therapy. Her PET CT scans no longer show glucose uptake, an indicator of tumor activity. "I'm still clear and thriving. I'm just so thankful I chose to do the vaccine therapy, because it saved my life. Nothing else seemed to be the magic bullet but those vaccines," Cindy said.

"I'm still clear and thriving. I'm just so thankful I chose to do the vaccine therapy, because it saved my life. Nothing else seemed to be the magic bullet but those vaccines," Cindy said.

With the great results we were getting using these unconventional treatments, I began to wonder whether more astonishing results might be close at hand if we kept working to strengthen and direct the natural power of the body's immune system. This is how my research moved from dendritic cells to adult stem cells and beyond.

Chapter Four

GETTING STARTED WITH STEM CELLS

In 2003, I sold my clinic in Arizona to fulfill a promise I'd made to my wife when we moved to Arizona that we would live in her home country, the United Kingdom, for a year to expose our children to that culture. Unfortunately, living in England was not the best fit for me. Not having any research to do was boring me to tears and I felt my mind wasting away. I wanted continue the work I'd been doing in Arizona, so I spent a lot of time traveling and not very much time at home with my family. Shirley and I reached a compromise in 2004 when I set up a laboratory in the Bahamas, and we moved the family there. I could continue pursuing cancer therapies in the Bahamas without having to be away from my family.

It was there that I started working with stem cells as an extension of working with dendritic cell vaccines. The process I'd developed in Arizona was a very efficient method of converting monocytes into dendritic cells. In the Bahamas, I wanted to see if we could do something similar with stem cells.

My aha moment regarding the reparative effects of stem cells occurred when a cancer patient who happened to also have a bad knee was undergoing treatment. In order to stimulate the release of CD34+ stem cells from bone marrow, our cancer patients received granulocyte-colony stimulating factor (GCSF), which mobilized these cells from their bone marrow. This patient experienced knee pain relief simply from the mobilization of the bone marrow stem cells, which led me to hypothesize that chronic injuries might be due to a lack of repair cells available to repair the injury. The mobilized stem cells likely homed in to the site of injury—in this case, the knee—repairing the chronic injury. The treatment of chronic injuries with autologous CD34+ hematopoietic cells, which could be mobilized using the drug mentioned above or pulled out of the bone marrow mechanically, has since been researched and found to have beneficial effects in the treatment of liver[1] and kidney disease,[2] spinal cord injury,[3,4] and a multitude of orthopedic conditions (see Chapter 12 for more on orthopedics).[5,6,7]

Working in the stem cell research field can be frustrating because there are so many misconceptions about these cells and their potential uses. When most people hear the words *stem cell*, they automatically assume that we're talking about embryonic stem cells, which have been at the center of so much controversy in the United States for more than a decade.

The perception is that all stem cells come from the unborn and that in order to harvest the life-saving properties of these cells, a scientist must sacrifice a yet-to-be-born child. The whole idea of taking life from one being to give it to another makes many people uncomfortable and raises moral

Autologous Bone Marrow Studies

Mesenchymal stem cells (MSCs) used for treatment may come from the patient (autologous, or self-derived) or from a donor (allogeneic). MSCs can be obtained from many tissues in the body, including fat, bone marrow, and umbilical cord. Bone marrow contains cells that are useful for regeneration, including MSCs and CD34+ cells. Bone marrow MSCs are usually extracted from the hip or the knee. In many cases, it is useful to concentrate the extracted cells that will be the most helpful—this is known as bone marrow aspirate concentrate (BMAC). Bone marrow MSCs have been used to safely treat various conditions with positive results (see Table 1).

and ethical questions. It makes me very uncomfortable too, for additional reasons. First, I believe the best stem cells—the ones with the best healing and regenerative power as well as the fewest complications—are adult stem cells, which can be obtained from donated umbilical cord blood; umbilical cord tissue from healthy, live births; or from a patient's own body—from the bone marrow or fat tissue, for example. Adult stem cells are not mired in controversy. In fact, the Baptist church endorses research with adult stem cells and the Catholic church has been funding adult stem cell research.

Table 1. Conditions treated with autologous bone marrow mesenchymal stem cells.

Condition	References
Multiple sclerosis	8,9,10,11
Duchenne muscular dystrophy	12
Spinal cord injury	13,14,15,16,17,18,19
Osteoarthritis	20,21,22,23
Heart failure	24,25,26,27,28,29
Wound healing	30,31,32
Autism spectrum disorders	33
Orthopedics	34
Cartilage repair	35,36
Tendon injuries	37,38
Arthroscopy enhancement	39,40,41
Bone healing and non-union	42,43,44
Myocardial infarction	45,46,47,48
Liver failure	49,50,51
Parkinson's disease	52,53
Diabetes	54,55,56
Ophthalmology	57,58
Amyotrophic lateral sclerosis	59
Crohn's disease	60,61

Second, I believe the public perception of embryonic stem cells and their usefulness is off the mark too. Embryonic stem cells have been touted as a potential miracle treatment for just about any disease, but the research has shown otherwise. When a zygote is fertilized, it starts as just two cells—the ovum and the sperm. These cells combine and start to divide and differentiate. These early cells are *pluripotent*—they have the ability to become, or differentiate into, any cell in the human body. Some cells become the fetus' heart, some the liver, some the skin, etc., until from those two initial cells develops a very diverse organism—the human body—with hundreds of different specialized functions performed by many different iterations of those first two cells.

With this idea as the starting point, it's easy to see how those unfamiliar with stem cell therapy research might think of embryonic stem cells, taken from a four- or five-day-old embryo, called a blastocyst, before it has been implanted in a woman's womb, as a form of magic seeds. If they can potentially differentiate into any kind of cell, by placing them in a sick person, they could transform into whatever tissue is needed to heal that person's illness. Stem cells injected into the brain might become brain cells and set about healing a brain malfunction, or those injected into the heart might become heart tissue and repair compromised arteries. Those who are suffering from Parkinson's disease, which is caused when the brain cells

Adult Stem Cell Therapy Endorsed by the Vatican

A symposium was organized in 2006 by the Vatican to address the use of stem cells. Pope Benedict XVI declared that adult stem cell research deserved "approval and encouragement" so long as it remained ethical.[62] This line of thought was expanded in the 2008 church document "Dignitas Personae," in which it was stated that research on adult stem cells should be "encouraged and supported."[63] Pope Benedict XVI restated this position of encouragement in 2011, qualifying adult stem cell-based therapies as a "significant step forward in medical science."[64] Also in 2011, the Vatican signed a one million dollar deal with a United States-based stem cell company to fund research and education on adult stem cells.[65]

that produce dopamine no longer function, have long held out hope that embryonic stem cells can be adapted to renew this function in the brain. Yet this therapy has never been successful.

Its ability to differentiate into any cell is the embryonic stem cell's double-edged sword. This potential to divide and differentiate indefinitely means that if even one embryonic stem cell contaminates a culture of differentiated cells, it will become a teratoma—a tumor mass, with tissue or organ components, that is trying to become a baby but can't. In experiments with rats, when researchers have introduced embryonic stem cells into the rat to help heal a cancer or some other disease, the rat always develops benign tumors. As a result, the tumorigenic risk of embryonic stem cell therapy has greatly inhibited its use. In addition, the costs associated with making darn sure there are no truly embryonic (and tumorigenic) stem cells left in the final product are very high. This was one of the reasons the biopharmaceutical company Geron pulled the plug on their much touted spinal cord injury trial using embryonic stem cells. When they pulled out, my colleagues and I wrote an article entitle "The King is Dead, Long Live the King,"[66] which described why we believe the Geron project failed. Incidentally, Stem Cells Incorporated recently pulled the plug on their fetal stem cell clinical trials as well, so it appears all of the hype will finally come to a halt, and the reality that adult stem cells are the only way to go will set in.

Not to mention, embryonic stem cells, once differentiated into new tissue cells, are antigenic, which means that the immune system recognizes the tissue as foreign and mounts an attack against it. Immune-suppressive drugs must be administered alongside treatment with embryonic stem cells, and can lead to complications. For all these reasons, there has not been a successful clinical trial using embryonic stem cells to date.

> ***There has not been a successful clinical trial using embryonic stem cells to date.***

I was interested in working with adult stem cells because they are easier to obtain, potentially as useful, not shrouded in controversy, and, unlike embryonic stem cells, when using postnatal or adult stem cells in the naïve state, meaning they haven't been manipulated genetically or chemically, none have ever produced secondary tumors in the patient. The cells are also immune privileged, meaning the immune system of the recipient does not recognize them as foreign, or "not self," when they are first administered. In addition, unlike embryonic stem cells, these cells do not want to become babies! Instead, their normal function is to support homeostasis (the healthy status quo) by responding to and decreasing inflammation and stimulating regeneration in tissue in need of it.

The best adult stem cell attribute of all is that when the cells start to become the tissue, also called the niche, in which they have taken up residence, they will begin to differentiate into that tissue type—a process known as maturing. When the cells get to a certain point of maturation they lose their "stemness," and molecules that say, "We are not you." start popping up on their surface. In response, the cells are gently cleared from the body by the immune system of the recipient. Ergo, no tumor formation.

Any stem cells that don't come from embryos or fetal tissue are known as adult stem cells. This includes those taken from umbilical cord blood and umbilical cord tissue donated from healthy, live births—one of the richest sources of highly potent stem cells. The potency of these cells comes from their ability to multiply, or double, in a short period of time as well as the enhanced quality of their secretome, or the range of bioactive molecules that they secrete.

Even though a newborn baby may seem the furthest thing from a grown-up, the stem cells taken from an infant's umbilical cord are still considered adult stem cells to make a clear distinction between them and the cells that are harvested from embryos or fetuses. For further clarification, I will also refer to umbilical cord stem cells as postnatal stem cells.

Stem Cell Type	Stem Cell Origin
Embryonic stem cells	Early development stage embryo (blastocyst)
Fetal stem cells	Fetus
Amniotic stem cells	Amniotic fluid during routine amniocentesis procedure
Postnatal stem cells	Umbilical cord blood or tissue from a healthy, live birth
Adult stem cells	Living human (postnatal stem cells are also considered adult stem cells)

Within the body, adult stem cells are undifferentiated cells that reside in tissues and organs alongside differentiated cells. Differentiated cells are those that have become specialized—no longer stem cells, they become a specific type of cell, such as a bone, muscle, or blood cell. Stem cells can renew themselves and, under certain conditions, can differentiate into specialized cell types. When the adult stem cell begins to divide, it produces one daughter cell—another identical stem cell—and one precursor cell that can differentiate into whatever kind of cell is needed. Mainly, stem cells repair the tissues where they are found. Back in the 1950s when scientists first started studying stem cells, they found two kinds in bone marrow. The first are known as hematopoietic stem cells, which form the various elements of blood. The others are bone marrow stromal stem cells (also called mesenchymal stem cells) that can repair bone, cartilage, and fat, and support the formation of fibrous connective tissue. Since then, researchers have found stem cells in many organs and tissues including the brain, blood vessels, skeletal muscles, skin, teeth, heart, gut, and liver. In fact, stem cells are found throughout the entire body. They live in a specific area of each tissue, a place called the stem cell niche, where they remain dormant for long periods of time until disease or injury activates them to begin to repair tissue.

Mesenchymal stem cells (MSCs) exist in many tissues as a dormant cell form known as a *pericyte* (*peri* means "around" and *cyte* means "cell"). Pericytes hold tight to capillaries, the smallest of blood vessels that exist throughout the body at the ends of arteries. When the body signals an injury or inflammation, pericytes are recruited to help heal tissues, at which point they become activated as MSCs.

Pericytes

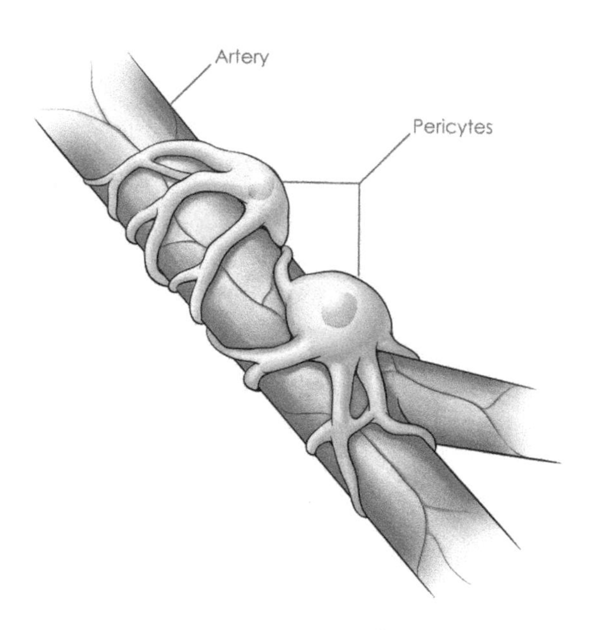

Mesenchymal stem cells are *multipotent*, meaning they are capable of differentiating into more than one type of new tissue. While multipotent cells have the ability to become more than once cell type, they are not to be confused with pluripotent cells (embryonic stem cells), which can become *any* cell type. Mesenchymal stem cells are considered multipotent because, by definition, they can become at least three different tissues—bone, cartilage, or fat. This is done all of the time in the laboratory. As you will find out later, however, this differentiation rarely happens in the body, and even when it does, has very little to do with the beneficial effects of the cells.

Despite being found throughout the body, there are only a small number of stem cells in each tissue. When I first began working with stem cells, research at the time had shown that they had a limited capacity to divide. My feeling was that if we could advance the technology we had used in our cancer research to induce stem cells to make more precursor cells for preparing dendritic cell vaccines, we might be able to culture stem cells similarly and deploy them to fix what ailed our patients.

In the Bahamas, we gave patients a drug that would stimulate the bone marrow to release hematopoietic (blood cell-forming) stem cells into the blood. We hooked them up to the leukapheresis machine to filter out the white blood cells and the stem cells and returned the rest of the blood to the patients, a process similar to dialysis for kidney disease patients. Then we cultured the stem cells in a cocktail of cell growth hormones, which encouraged the cells to divide.

This was very exciting work to be involved with, something that put us on the cutting edge of treating cancer because of the three different treatments we pioneered. We had the matured dendritic cells that consumed tumor tissue and presented information to the immune system so that it could attack the cancer. We had also developed an extract from a plant known as bindweed that undercut the tumor's infrastructure by preventing it from growing new blood cells to support its expansion. Now, with the army of stem cells we were able to release into the bloodstream, we had soldiers who were ready and able to initiate tissue repair. It was a useful trifecta.

By starting with stem cells and growing (expanding) them in the laboratory and then converting them into monocytes and then dendritic cells, we were able to make more potent vaccines than we had been able to produce in our clinic in Arizona. We successfully treated several patients with stage IV melanoma who remain cancer free today because of the vaccines we developed with their stem cells. The clinic also had excellent success with mesothelioma—a cancer caused by asbestos exposure for which there is currently no effective treatment. There are more mesothelioma patients alive and well from their treatment at our center in the Bahamas than from any other treatment center in the world.

Word of our advances in culturing stem cells and converting monocytes to dendritic cells started to spread throughout the medical community. A doctor approached the lab asking us if we could culture hematopoietic

CD34+ stem cells from the umbilical cord. The doctor hoped that if we could culture enough CD34+ cells, he would be able to use them to treat a little boy who was profoundly affected by cerebral palsy. Cerebral palsy is the result of a brain injury, usually before birth, that affects muscle tone and movement and delays overall development. People with cerebral palsy often have other conditions such as intellectual disabilities, vision and hearing problems, or seizures. People with cerebral palsy are deprived of oxygen at birth and as a result have decreased blood flow to the brain during a crucial time in development. What was hoped for was that the CD34+ cells, which are potently angiogenic, meaning they induce new blood vessel growth, and home to areas of low oxygen, or damaged areas of the brain, would increase blood flow to starved areas of the brain and could potentially allow for a "catching up" of the development of those parts of the brain.

A lot of this rationale was demonstrated by Paul Sanberg, PhD, DSc and his colleagues at the University of South Florida. They had already done pioneering work using umbilical cord cells to treat heart attacks and strokes in rats. He was my hero, actually, because of his experiments in which he induced heart attacks in rats and then gave one group stem cells.[67] Guess what? The hearts of the rats that received stem cells got better. The scarring on their hearts was a third of what it was in the untreated animals. He did the same thing with rats experiencing strokes.[68] He induced strokes in the rats and gave one group stem cells; their brains got much better when compared to those rats that didn't get stem cells.

We had refined the technology to produce these cells, and we had a doctor and a family who were willing to try a new kind of therapy for the first time in a human being. We cultured umbilical cord cells in our lab, and the doctor injected the cells into the boy with cerebral palsy, who at three years old was blind, deaf, dumb, and confined to a wheelchair. Then we waited.

Three months after he received the cells, the boy's father noticed his son's eyes tracking a ball that his brother was bouncing. Suddenly the boy could see! There had been nothing wrong with his eyes. Instead, his blindness was caused by damage to his cerebral cortex. After several more treatments, the boy started to hear and talk, and could eventually walk with the aid of a walker. His parents were ecstatic.

What I believe happened with our cultured cells is that they moved through the bloodstream to the damaged area, homing in on the site of the injury. Once there, the cells stimulated the formation of new blood vessels and secreted trophic factors, or bioactive molecules that encouraged new cell growth. Because the boy was so young and his system was so responsive, when blood started to flow to these areas, it jumpstarted his neural development and stimulated it to continue on a normal path, repairing some of the functions that had been damaged by his cerebral palsy.

Treatment of this patient opened up an entirely new area of healing for us. The notion that cultured umbilical cord stem cells could be used to regenerate damaged tissue was the fulfillment of a hope—the promise of using postnatal stem cells to treat chronic diseases—even if a full cure was surely decades away. Even more exciting, our initial work indicated that these umbilical cord stem cells were not as difficult to work with as bone marrow cells and did not stimulate any of the side effects that preliminary treatments with embryonic stem cells had shown. There was plenty of evidence regarding both the reparative effects of umbilical cord stem cells and the ability to transplant them without negative effects.

When a doctor treats a cancer patient with chemotherapy, the treatment also destroys the patient's bone marrow, and therefore the ability to make new blood cells. In order to compensate for this, the doctor also does a bone marrow transplant. The donor cells must be carefully matched or the body will reject them. The body recognizes the new bone marrow cells as foreign and the immune system attacks them. This phenomenon is known as a host versus graft reaction and will result in immediate destruction of the transplanted cells, rendering them ineffective. A more serious, and oftentimes fatal, complication of a bone marrow transplant is the engraftment of the bone marrow into the recipient's bone marrow after the bone marrow stem cells are destroyed by chemotherapy and/or radiation. With an empty T cell compartment, the donor bone marrow will start producing T cells that recognize the recipient's tissues as foreign and begin destruction. This is why matching the cells is so important and the recipient receives lifelong immune-suppressive treatments to reduce the possibility of the disease.

Cord blood, unlike bone marrow, is immune privileged. The stem cells that come from cord blood are immunologically more immature so they do not set off an attack from the recipient's immune system. This meant that we could treat patients with cord blood cells without the expensive and time-consuming process of matching the cells to the patient or needing to use potentially harmful immune-suppressive drugs. In 2010, my colleague Tom Ichim and I wrote a book chapter on the immune privilege of umbilical cord stem cells.[69]

It is also known that umbilical cord stem cells can act the same as bone marrow in that they can repopulate the bone marrow of a patient who is in need of new bone marrow because of chemo and/or radiation. In fact, the U.S. FDA classifies umbilical cord blood and the stem cells it contains as bone marrow in some of its regulations. Unlike bone marrow stem cells, transplanted umbilical cord stem cells when used for repopulating bone marrow have a much lower risk to the patient of developing graft versus host disease due to their immaturity. Umbilical cord blood is being used more and more in bone marrow transplants because of these advantages over bone marrow.

I guess my excitement over the successes we were having with this new treatment overcame my good judgment about publicity. When a reporter from a local newspaper, The Bahama Journal, contacted our medical director, John Clement, MD, about doing an article featuring our work, I didn't think twice about the request.

I vividly remember a pretty young reporter with a Channel 7 microphone coming out of our Dr. Clement's office with a huge smile on her face. She was positively beaming. I asked Dr. Clement what that was all about. He said this news reporter was going to do a story about stem cells and how we were helping so many people who had no other good treatment options.

The next day's front page headline read, "Secret Surgeries Exposed." The entire front page was dedicated to our clinic and the topic of embryonic stem cells even though we were using non-embryonic umbilical cord stem cells that were donated from healthy, live births. The article discussed how research with embryonic stem cells was banned in the United States. Buried on page 17 was the fact that we were *not* using embryonic cells. This publication took advantage of the wide misperceptions people have about stem cell research. It was the first of 14 articles about us, none of them good.

The avalanche of inaccurate news reporting about our research made a big impact in the Bahamas. One month later, in July of 2004, we received a letter from the Bahamian Minister of Health prohibiting us from any further treatments using stem cells.

Having seen the benefits of the cells, I wasn't close to giving up. I knew the potential of the treatments and wasn't going to let a misinformed government stop me from progressing with what I knew was cutting-edge research that could help treat devastating chronic diseases. I jumped on a plane to look for another place where we could legally treat patients with stem cells. After carefully evaluating six options, I decided that we would move our clinic to Costa Rica.

I decided on Costa Rica for a couple of reasons. It is a popular tourist destination with twenty direct jet flights every day from the United States and Canada. It has a thriving middle class and a very well-educated population. I received legal counsel that the treatments could be done there under informed consent between the doctor and patient, as long as the treatments were not part of a clinical trial. I also had previous work experience there. I had been in Costa Rica in 1998 and 1999 to perform treatments with dendritic cells, working with Fabio Solano, MD, who agreed to become the medical director of our new Stem Cell Institute. So in 2004 and 2005, I traveled to Costa Rica for ten days each month to build the laboratory and clinic.

Chapter Five

STEM CELLS IN ACTION

I began my work with stem cells using CD34+ cells, but shortly after establishing the clinic in Costa Rica, we began using mesenchymal stem cells (MSCs). I was inspired by the work of Osiris Therapeutics, a company based on stem cell technology discovered by researchers at Case Western Reserve University led by Arnold Caplan, PhD. Osiris was the first company to ever treat a patient with an autologous (self-derived) stem cell product in 1998, and then the first to treat a patient with an allogeneic (donor) stem cell product two years later. By 2007, they had launched a phase III clinical trial with MSCs for patients suffering from graft versus host disease (GvHD), and successfully brought the world's first approved stem cell drug to market in Canada and New Zealand for the treatment of GvHD. They were doing great work that made me feel comfortable using MSCs with our patients.

Not a lot was known about MSCs before 2004, but since then there has been a meteoric rise in interest, a trend that doesn't appear to be slowing down any time soon. We began using MSCs in 2006, and by 2009 every patient was getting MSCs, either exclusively or in combination with CD34+ cells. Today, and for the past few years, we only use CD34+ cells for a few conditions, and always in conjunction with MSCs.

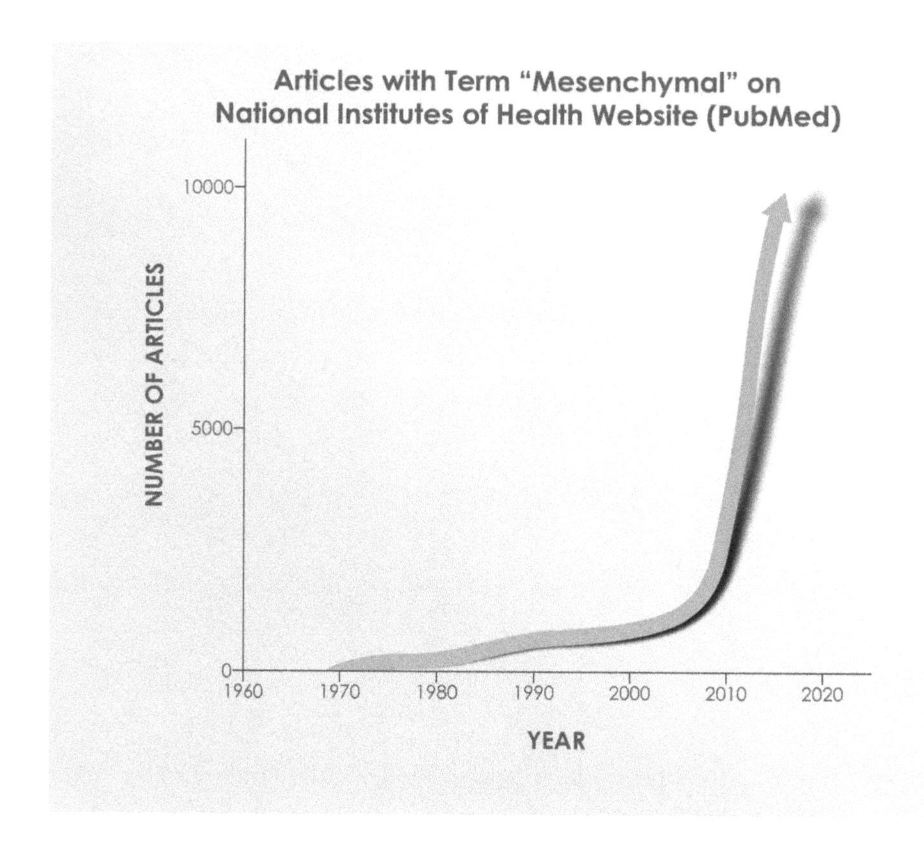

MSCs address immune imbalance and inflammation in ways that CD34+ cells cannot. CD34+ cells do not elicit a T cell response by the immune system, but MSCs take it one step further—they actually suppress immune response, an important safety factor when using cells from a donor. All doctors are taught in medical school that the presence of a foreign cell from another organism will always trigger a strong T cell immune response against the "invading" donor cell. But MSCs do not elicit this response. They are immunologically immature. In other words, MSCs are not antigenic, so they are tolerated by the immune system and do not require immune-suppressive drugs as part of their treatment. They are also non-tumorigenic because they do not differentiate into any cell, as do embryonic stem cells. Additionally, the safety profile of MSCs is excellent, making them the most-suited cell therapy for the conditions we treat.

Over time we have been able to carefully refine our cell selection and expansion process such that the cells we now use are more robust and effective than ever before. Most of all, we see equal or better treatment results in patients who receive MSCs as were seen using CD34+ cells. For all these reasons, MSCs are our cell therapy of choice.

Mesenchymal stem cells work in four main ways. They:

- Control inflammation
- Modulate the immune system
- Stimulate regeneration
- Reduce scarring

MSCs secrete a curtain of bioactive molecules, or trophic factors, that help to dampen inflammation where appropriate. At a site of injury, the cells release trophic factors that tell the immune system to stop overreacting to the injury, which is the immune system's natural response—to get to the site of injury and produce inflammatory molecules to help remove the damage. This inflammatory response often gets out of hand. MSCs don't completely shut down the body's inflammatory response, however. Rather, they shut it down when it appears to be excessive or inappropriate. More accurately, they work to modulate immune response, tuning it to an appropriate level.

MSCs tell the immune system to calm down while also sending the body signals to regenerate healthy tissue and heal. MSCs are masters of producing the right trophic factors at the right time and in the right place so that the body can restore its natural structure and function. As a result, less scar tissue is formed. If you have ever had a scar, you know that it looks and feels different than normal skin. Scars also form inside the body at sites of injury. Scar tissue is fibrotic and can get in the way of the normal functioning of the body. Patients in our clinics and I personally have experienced scar healing unrelated to the condition being treated with MSCs. Recently, a patient being treated for rheumatoid arthritis reported that her permanent makeup tattoos, which are made of scar tissue, disappeared. Similarly, I experienced the complete disappearance of a three-year-old burn scar on my arm after my first MSC injection.

Importantly, the ability of an MSC to regenerate tissue within the body lies not in the cell's capacity to replicate itself and create another cell but, rather, in its stimulatory effect on the body to naturally regenerate its *own*

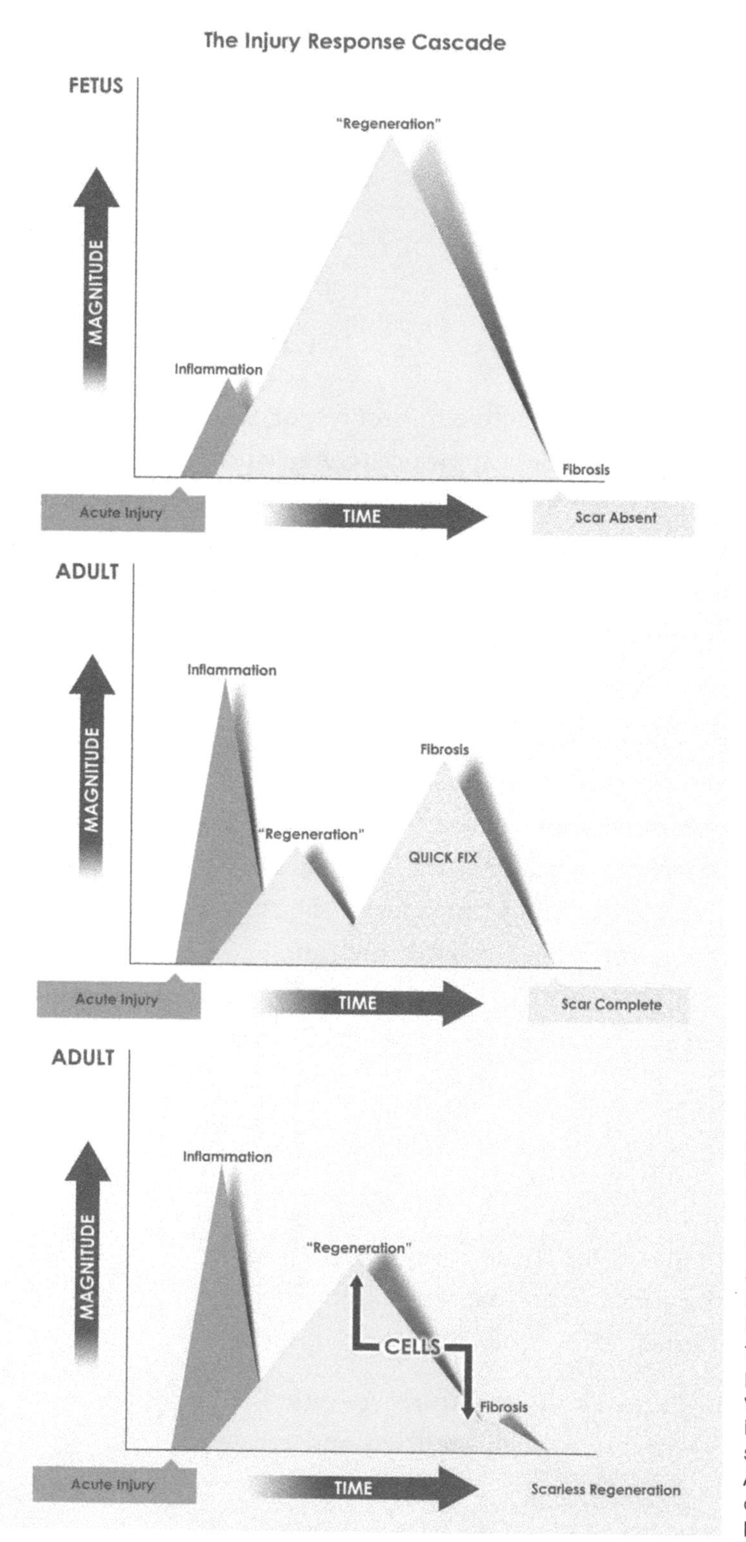

In a fetus, inflammation in response to injury is minimized while regeneration is maximized. Scar tissue is not formed.[1] In an adult, inflammation in response to injury is heightened, regeneration is stunted, and scar formation is emphasized. MSCs increase the regeneration phase of healing while decreasing inflammation and scar formation. Adapted from correspondence with Dr. Arnold Caplan.

cells. In study after study, MSCs do not become new cells themselves unless manipulated by a human to specifically do so. In fact, Arnold Caplan, considered the father of the MSC because he originally named it *mesenchymal stem cell*,[2] actually wants to rename the MSC as *medicinal signaling cell* because the most important functions of the MSC lie in its secretome, or the totality of secreted bioactive molecules from the cell, rather than in its ability to become another type of tissue.

"MSCs are multifactorial site-specific sensors with genetically wired molecular responses," states Caplan. "MSCs see a signal and they respond in a very controlled way. The management of innate regenerative potential is what they do. The MSC story will change the way medicine is practiced. Management of the patient's innate regenerative resources will be the new treatment."

Interview with Arnold Caplan, PhD, Professor of Biology and Director, Skeletal Research Center at Case Western Reserve University

Neil Riordan: I've known of Dr. Caplan's work for years. He named the mesenchymal stem cell, although he has some thoughts on changing that name. His work, patents, and intellectual property was the basis for the founding of Osiris, the second company in the world that was able to get a cell-based product approved in Canada and New Zealand for the treatment of acute graft-versus-host disease in children. Since then the product has also been approved for use in Japan. Can you talk a little bit about the regulatory landscape, your interpretation of the Japan law, and what that's led to?

Arnold Caplan: Japan passed legislation that simplified the clinical entry of cell-based products for a variety of conditions by requiring corporations or entities to show that the cell-based product was safe and that there was some reason to believe there was efficacy. The legislation allowed that the product could be provisionally approved. Within five years, enough clinical outcome information would be amassed by the company or investigators so that a proper review for efficacy could be entertained by the Japanese regulatory authority. At that time, the company or individual would petition for full approval of the product. If

In fact, MSCs only survive for about four to eight months in the body. They are initially tolerated by the immune system because they lack a molecule that says to the body, "I'm not you." But they eventually start producing that molecule, which triggers the immune system to engulf the cell and gently remove it from the body. This is a key point to their safety and a major differentiator between MSCs and other stem cells, particularly embryonic stem cells. They do not stick around, implanting in the body and growing into other tissue types or tumors.

So when you cut yourself, when you have a heart attack, or when you break your leg, the injury will mobilize these cells to repair it by secreting trophic factors that we also call cell survival molecules. They stimulate the molecules that are already there to repair the tissue. Essentially, MSCs help

there were adverse events, these would be immediately reported to the regulatory agency and the agency could withdraw provisional approval at any time.

This unique and game-changing legislation takes away the need for massive and hugely expensive phase III clinical trials, because provisional approval with paid products allows the company to conduct post-marketing analysis and provide substantial data to prove to the regulators that the product is efficacious. We don't have that provision in the United States and so very costly, time-consuming phase III trials must be entertained by every company. This further keeps these products out of clinical use until there is full approval, which can take two to four years past the phase II clinical trials. Many companies from the United States, Australia, and Europe have either out-licensed to Japanese companies or set up shop in Japan to take advantage of this new legislation. If a product is approved in Japan, it can make approval easier in Europe and the United States.

NR: What is the difference, in number of years and amount of money, between the current model in Japan and that in the United States to get a product moving down the road?

AC: The big difference is in the phase III trial, the submission of appropriate forms, and the deliberation of the FDA. Japan's model can save anywhere from two to five years and many tens of millions of dollars of investment money when compared to the process in the United States. At the time of this interview, there are current proponents of this accelerated pathway in the United States, and attempts by two or three groups to maintain the status quo in the body. My belief is that the vast majority of chronic diseases are due to a lack or dysfunction of mesenchymal stem cells, and to a lesser degree, other stem cells.

> ***My belief is that the vast majority of chronic diseases are due to a lack or dysfunction of mesenchymal stem cells, and to a lesser degree, other stem cells.***

One way in which MSCs stimulate regeneration is via angiogenesis, the process whereby new blood vessels are grown from the existing vascular network. In the case of injured or inflamed tissue, this newly formed blood supply facilitates the delivery of

provide such legislation through Congress. Certainly, in 2017 there will be legislative changes in the United States, but the exact content of those changes on the federal level are completely unknown. Meanwhile, as you well know, there are a number of lobbies attempting to get state legislators to pass laws that would make it easier for patients to get access to cell-based therapies. For example, the governor in California recently signed a bill for patients who are suffering from terminal disease, particularly cancer, on a compassionate use basis. These people can have access to life-saving drugs, even if they're still being tested in clinical trials.

NR: That's a right-to-try law?

AC: Yes, that's the short term for it. It lowers the liability risk considerably for pharmaceutical companies to provide these drugs to patients who are not on their clinical trial protocols.

NR: Switching from politics to science, one of the more compelling sets of slides in your talks is in the injury response cascade (see page 48). I was wondering if you could talk about how MSCs can affect the injury response and how that relates to chronic injuries and chronic inflammation?

AC: It turns out that MSCs exist in the body on every single blood vessel. When a blood vessel is broken, inflamed, or involved in a chronic wound, those perivascular (surrounding a blood vessel) cells come off and differentiate into what I call MSCs. An MSC in this context is a cell that makes drugs or molecules that are specific to the site where the injury has oxygen, nutrients, and molecules critical for the healing process. Without reestablishment of the blood supply after an injury, healing will not occur.

When you are born, you have a huge number of MSCs, and they are found everywhere in your body. As mentioned in Chapter 4, MSCs exist in dormant form as pericyte cells on capillaries throughout the body. The MSCs on your capillaries are your body's own pharmacy. Capillary density, or the amount of capillaries a person has, decreases as you get older. Therefore, your pharmacy disappears with age. Ask any surgeon if they would rather do surgery on a 24-year-old or an 84-year-old. They will all pick the younger patient. Complete wound healing requires revascularization, which is much easier to achieve with a higher capillary density and the higher number of MSCs housed on those capillaries, as found in younger

occurred. For example, the MSCs in brains of patients with stroke, or in hearts of patients with heart attack, though they're similar, will make different cascades of molecules. These cells naturally function to protect sites of injury from an over-aggressive immune system that is always trying to survey and interrogate injured tissues, looking for invasive components. And so, your natural immune response brings these very aggressive immune cells into the injury field. The MSCs slow them down and tell them to go away because they are not needed. They let the body know that the injury can take care of itself, and that it's not a huge infection.

These MSCs are sentinels for injury. Not only do they put up a local curtain on their front side, which stops these aggressive immune cells, but from the backside, these MSCs also produce molecules that allow the injured tissue to slowly heal without scarring. This is real tissue regeneration—not simply plugging the hole with a scar, but with more tissue, which takes time. The MSCs set up an environment in which real regeneration can take place.

The problem is that, as adults age, we lose blood vessels, and therefore we lose these very important regenerative cells. Very often, we need a booster shot of more MSCs. There are two ways to do that: You can isolate the MSCs from your own body and get them back to the injury site; or you can use cells from someone else. Because of the curtain of molecules produced by the MSCs, which is directed against immune cells, the MSC is sort of hidden from the immune system. Your MSCs in my body would temporarily not be seen by my individuals. When your capillary density decreases, the MSCs have nowhere to live, so they die. Even by the time you reach skeletal maturity, during the teenage years, 90 percent of your MSC bone marrow reserve, which is utilized for injury, is gone. That means that you are living on that 10 percent for the rest of your life.

Mesenchymal stem cells are intimately involved in the process of new blood vessel growth. The more vasculature or new blood vessel growth, the better the wound will heal and the stronger it will heal. The addition of MSCs along with their secretions to an injured site can speed up the healing. MSCs release secretions that promote angiogenesis, particularly vascular endothelial growth factor (VEGF). Endothelial precursor cells (EPC) and endothelial cells (EC) have CD34 and CD133 markers on their cellular

immune system. Some people call this immune-privileged, but that's not the case—the immune system eventually catches up with them. But for the short term, MSCs pour out molecules so the immune system can't see them. In essence, they are camouflaged. We call this immuno-evasion: MSCs evade the immune system.

In older people who don't have enough local MSCs, in particular for heart attack, you can inject MSCs from somebody else into the blood stream. The allogeneic MSCs will dock at the injury site and supplement the local MSCs, producing therapeutic effects. There's a gigantic number of clinical trials now in play using MSCs both from the patient and from an unrelated donor. So umbilical MSCs, which come from discarded tissue, are just as good as your own MSCs. In fact, when they are put in culture and caused to divide, they are actually more plentiful than your own MSCs as an adult.

There are a variety of ways in which you can propagate MSCs and get them to expand, and a variety of ways to get them to sites of injury. Direct to the injury site (e.g. into the knee cavity) is one way; and systemic delivery into the blood stream is another way to introduce MSCs from outside the body. MSCs put up this curtain of molecules, which protects the injured tissue from immune surveillance. In people who have a defective curtain, destruction of tissue by the immune system occurs. We call this autoimmune disease. Multiple sclerosis (MS) is an autoimmune disease in which the immune system attacks nerve coverings, destroying myelin. Therefore, the myelin insulation gets attacked by the immune system, short-circuiting those nerves. That's the basic clinical cause of MS. So even if you give surface and a receptor for VEGF.[3] When VEGF is present, signals are sent for EPC and EC to move to the area, and to start differentiating into tissue that will construct the new blood vessels.[4]

During treatment with MSCs, angiogenesis in the affected area helps the healing process. A recent review summarizes the substantial evidence of their role in blood vessel formation and their therapeutic effect for many different conditions, particularly for cardiovascular diseases (ischemia, myocardial infarction, etc.), diabetes ulcers, burns, and wound healing.[5]

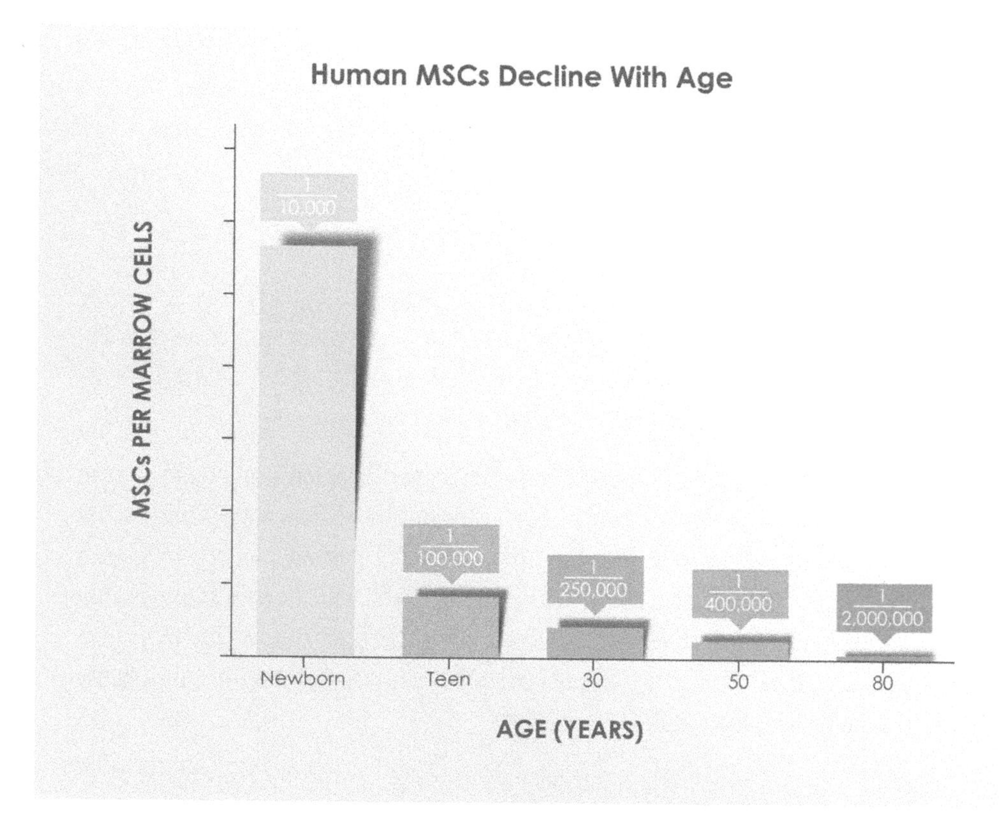

Adapted from data in Caplan AI. Why are MSCs therapeutic? New data: new insight.J Pathol. 2009;217(2):318-24.

Not only does the number of your MSCs decline with age,[6] but so does their robustness.[7] MSC robustness is determined by a few main factors: the rate at which the cells multiply, or double;[8] the amount of trophic factors they produce; and cell senescence, or deterioration.[9] MSCs in older individuals do not multiply, or double, as quickly, nor do they produce as many healing trophic factors as do the cells in younger individuals. This explains why umbilical cord MSCs are so potent—they come from a very young, healthy human being. We have found that umbilical cord MSCs are the most potent when compared to bone marrow, fat, and menstrual cell MSCs, all of which we have used and extensively tested.

somebody back their own MSCs, they may be defective. In people with autoimmune disease, it is probably better to deliver someone else's MSCs from normal, healthy donors who don't have autoimmune diseases. The choice between autologous (from yourself) versus allogeneic (someone else's) is a medical decision that needs to be made depending on the disease that these cells are introduced for treatment. This is subtlety. There is no question in my mind that some individuals will have MSCs with defects, and that's going to be the reason for certain autoimmune diseases.

NR: In the last couple years, Dr. Sun in Nanjing, China has done a bunch of work on lupus. He has identified the actual defect in the MSCs of people with lupus, and it's led to a lot of clinical trials, one very recently published.

AC: We are going to sponsor an investigator-initiated trial for rheumatoid arthritis (RA), which is quite similar to lupus in lots of ways. But the important aspect of the trial we're going to conduct here in Cleveland, is that we are going to use newly diagnosed rheumatoid patients. The FDA has allowed some companies to conduct clinical trials using MSCs in patients with refractory RA—patients who have tried every standard treatment but still continue to worsen. From our standpoint, a newly diagnosed patient would be perfect because all the downstream horrible effects of RA haven't happened yet. These patients' immune systems are overreacting to certain tissues at joints. We are going to take those allogeneic MSC preparations and optimize the cells for their response to these kinds of inflammatory situations at joints. We've developed an assay for picking a donor who will provide us with MSCs with the maximum response to inflammation, therefore having a better chance of curing the patients of their RA.

NR: That's a great idea. Like a surrogate assay?

AC: It's very simple. We have eight or nine donors from whom we've gotten bone marrow. We've isolated their MSCs and then exposed them to, for example IL-1. We pick a donor who gives us the best muting of that IL-1 response.

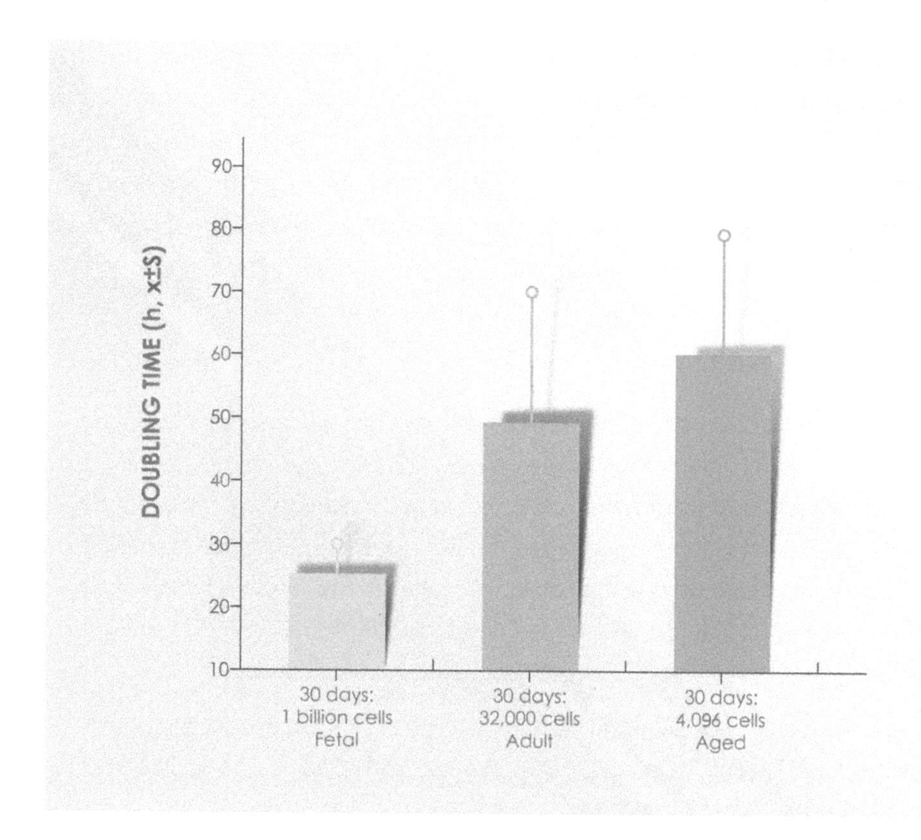

How long it takes for MSCs to duplicate in fetal, adult and aged bodies.
Adapted from data in Chang HX, Yang L, Li Z, Chen G, Dai G. Age-related biological characterization of mesenchymal progenitor cells in human articular cartilage. Orthopedics. 2011;34(8):e382-8.

NR: We're doing similar things. We take an immortalized monocyte line, expose it to lipopolysaccharide, co-culture it with the MSCs, and look at their secretions. We look for the maximum suppression of TNF-alpha and IL-6.

AC: Yeah, that's similar to what we are looking at. We've developed another potency assay for the ability of MSCs to make antibiotic proteins, and to optimize the immune system for taking care of massive infections. So for kids with cystic fibrosis, because of the secretion problems they have, they get massive lung infections. We will take kids 18 or older with cystic fibrosis, who have been through every antibiotic known to man to quell their lung infections, and we give them allogeneic MSCs, donor MSCs that have been put in culture with *Pseudomonas* or *Staphylococcus* bacteria. We've identified a donor spectacular in his

The MSCs we use in our Panama clinic have a similar doubling time as the cells from a fetus in the chart above: 20 to 24 hours. In an adult, the cell doubling time is roughly two days. In a 65-year-old, doubling time is only every 60 hours. This may appear to be a linear increase in doubling time, but with synchronous doubling, the difference in the total number of cells produced over time is exponential: in a fetus, 1 billion cells are grown from one cell in 30 days; in an adult, 32,000 cells are created in 30 days; in a 65-year-old, 200 cells are created in 30 days.

Why is cell robustness so important? We have found a high correlation between cell robustness and treatment effect at our clinics over the years. We became very aware of this when we were using MSCs derived from fat tissue. We were the first in the world to use MSCs from fat tissue in human beings, which we administered as stromal vascular fraction (SVF), a portion of fat tissue containing a mixture of pericytes, MSCs, and T-regulatory cells.[10] In a study we did with Indiana University, we found injection of SVF in the vein and joint to be safe and feasible for 13 rheumatoid arthritis patients

killing activity. We look at the immune response and the bacterial carcasses, which cause an endotoxin effect. We want a special macrophage to come in and clean them up. We have a donor who is particularly gifted at producing cells that carry away the carcasses. We want to specifically tune the cells to the disease state we're using them for.

NR: Wow, that's very interesting. It is mind blowing that these cells produce drugs that kill microbes. When was that discovered?

AC: We were partially responsible for discovering that. These molecules are called *defensins*, and they've been studied by dentists for twenty to thirty years. Defensins are naturally secreted in your mouth—it's how you control the bacteria loads that go to your gastrointestinal tract. These molecules have not only been studied as proteins, but their genes have been cloned. It turns out the MSCs have these same sequences in their genome, and if they bump into a bacterium, they produce defensins. If there are no bacteria around, these molecules have no adverse effects on any other cells. As a matter of fact, young women who have monthly bleeds never get sepsis. They have broken blood vessels, and when a pericyte comes off and differentiates into an MSC, if a bacterium is present and bumps into it, goodbye bacterium.

after one-, three-, six-, and 13-month follow-ups.[11,12] In the beginning, some patients did not respond as well to their own fat cell MSCs. When we tested their cells, we learned that their cells had a reduced robustness. There was a high correlation of MSC robustness and treatment effect. After learning this, we tested the robustness of the fat tissue-derived MSCs in all patients. For those patients with lackluster MSC robustness, we augmented their treatment with umbilical cord MSCs. Over time, the production of umbilical cord MSCs became so efficient, and the cell selection process so improved, that we discontinued using patient-derived fat cells altogether. As a result, we are able to treat our patients more efficiently. For example, we treat our multiple sclerosis patients in three days now compared to a two- to four-week treatment in the past.

NR: Can we visit the safety issue of using cells from another person—allogeneic MSCs? You mentioned that there are a lot of trials using allogeneic cells. Many people fear the use of stem cells for the treatment of cancer, because they are afraid of getting non-malignant tumors from MSCs. The fact that allogeneic umbilical cord MSCs have temporary immune privilege worries some people. Can you explain the mechanism by which allogeneic MSCs are allowed to be used clinically? And what is the mechanism in the body from the cells that makes them safe?

AC: These cells have been introduced into 30,000 to 50,000 people worldwide, and we don't know of any adverse events. The fear that these cells will cause cancer is a misnomer, and it's my fault because I named them *mesenchymal stem cells*. Everything I've just said about their abilities has nothing to do with a stem cell. If you have a heart attack, MSCs trigger the body's production of new cells, not new heart muscles. Calling them mesenchymal stem cells is inappropriate for what they do in the body, which is different than what they do in a petri dish. It's correct in that I can make MSCs "dance" on a petri dish, but back in the body they don't do that dance. They make drugs, naturally. I've written a paper to rename them to *medicinal signaling cells*—still *MSCs*. They make medicines that signal the tissue to regenerate itself. In a simplistic sense, they manage the patient's own capacity to regenerate tissues. We are always regenerating tissues, which is one of the most important aspects of life in general. In all of your tissues—every single tissue in your body—cells drop dead and are perfectly replaced. For example, every single second, 15 million blood cells drop dead and are perfectly replaced. They are perfectly replaced because in your bone marrow is a stem cell that gives its own stem cells. Your liver, heart, kidney, and skin also have their own stem cells. Every single day millions of cells are dropping dead and being replaced. That replacement is how we stay alive. If you can't regenerate that tissue, you won't be around very long.

That, indeed, is what the MSC manages. It manages your innate capacity to regenerate every single tissue of your body where the MSC resides—your liver, your fat, your skin, etc. The important aspect of MSCs put back in the body is to understand that they don't form tissues and so won't form cancers. One of the problems right from the beginning of MSC therapies is that cancers with a solid tumor in your body have what we call leaky blood vessels. If you put an MSC into your body and you already have a tumor growing, it will go to that tumor, see it as injured tissue, and pervert it to get larger. So there are experiments that are now being done where people are putting powerful suicide genes in MSCs and giving them to patients with tumors to trigger the tumor to commit suicide. But by themselves the MSCs will not form tumors. Again, 30,000 to 50,000 patients with no adverse events. When we have given MSCs to a couple million patients, we'll find complications, and we'll deal with them.

An important aspect missing from our regulatory process is transparency. We need a public website to register the clinical conditions of people who are getting MSCs. When they come for regular checkups, their conditions and outcome results can be monitored and put on the website. Those of us who are interested will see any problems immediately and be able to deal with them. To put this into modern context, consider the drug Vioxx, a non-steroidal anti-inflammatory drug that has since been taken off the market because it led to death in people with cardiac problems. If information from those patients had been on a publicly accessible, real time website, those deaths could have been prevented. We would have ranted and raved to stop the medication from being used in cardiac patients. [The manufacturer] Merck allowed a hundred people to die. Then to save their name, they withdrew the drug from the market, which is itself a crime because it's a useful drug. Transparency in reporting is one of the most important aspects of using new technologies.

MSCs produce these curtains of molecules that mute the response of the immune system, allowing the MSCs to evade the immune surveillance. Therefore, allogeneic MSCs can be used. In the end, this is one of the cheapest ways to provide suitable therapies for a large variety of diseases.

Safety

In May of 2016, the prominent *British Medical Journal* released a study that reported medical error to be the third leading cause of death in the United States.[13] That means you are more likely to die of a medical error made by your doctor or medical practitioner than you are of all but two other conditions—heart disease or cancer.

Before I started to use umbilical cord MSCs, there was only one published trial on their use. I had to have a high degree of comfort that the cells were safe. In addition to the work already done by Arnold Caplan and Osiris, I looked to microchimerism. When a woman has a baby, she will retain cells—some of which are MSCs—from that baby in her body for up

NR: I want to talk to you about vascular density with age. Do you have a reference for vascular density from skeletal maturity to old age? Is there a reference for that?

AC: They're not published, and no one's done a systematic study. It's hugely labor intensive to standardize the histological preparations for you to get quantitative information. But the best data available has to do with skin. If you take a skin biopsy from younger patients, you see variegations at the junction of the dermis and epidermis—they're called *rete ridges*. Underneath the dermis are huge loops of capillaries, which are what make baby skin the softest and most wonderful skin to touch—it's so highly vascularized because of these deep ridges. You can tell the age of somebody by these ridges. If you look at my skin biopsy, I don't have any ridges anymore.

NR: So if you're just looking at the skin, if you start with a baby at 100 in vascular density, at your age it would be what?

AC: I would say I'm at a two.

NR: Essentially, the homes for the MSCs—capillaries—disappear with age, so the MSCs also disappear with age because they die when the blood vessels diminish, is that correct?

AC: Yeah. With these skin biopsies, I can also tell whether a patient has diabetes or not because diabetics have half the blood vessel density of an age-matched control. That's why you see diabetic foot ulcers as such a difficult malady to treat, because their standard blood vessel density is so low.

NR: So they have fewer resources to repair.

AC: Right, so when they get a bleed, the number of MSCs that come in from the surrounding area is likewise diminished.

NR: Could you talk about the vascular density of liver tissue versus other tissues? And why the regenerative capacity of the liver is so good?

AC: The liver is organized like this: Arteries come in, then you have a bunch of liver cells, and then you have drain veins. Around every single arterial capillary in the liver, there are liver stem cells. Those stem cells divide, and their progeny begin differentiating into liver cells. The most differentiated liver cells, the hepatocytes, are sitting next to the vein. If you cut through a piece of liver in the just the right way, you can see the whole differentiation pattern from the stem cell to the most differentiated cell next to the vein. So blood comes in through the artery and gets detoxified as it goes to the vein. All of those cells, from the most primitive, newly differentiated hepatocyte all the way to the most highly differentiated hepatocyte has a certain capacity to detoxify the blood. What's interesting is that, when you cut off a hunk of liver, if you're going to survive, that liver needs lots of arteries and blood vessels. Sitting next to every one of those surviving arteries is a liver stem cell. They divide like wildfire, and they produce in rapid time the newly regenerated liver.

Sitting next to every single liver stem cell is an MSC pericyte, and that pericyte is obligatory for the expansion and differentiation of those liver stem cells. Those cells—the MSC pericytes that are sitting next to those stem cells—have a special name (hepatic stellate cells), have been studied extensively, and are highly unusual perivascular cells.

Every tissue in your body regenerates to some extent. You have a neural stem cell, a cardiac stem cell, a liver stem cell, etc. In all those stem cells there is a universal site that you could describe for every single stem cell, and the way to picture it in your mind is: that stem cell is sitting on top of a blood vessel's vascular endothelial cell. Sitting right next to it is an MSC pericyte. So both the stem cell and the pericyte are in contact with the endothelial cell. That's the universal stem cell niche, whether it's in your brain, your liver, or your heart, there is an MSC pericyte. Therefore, every time one of your tissues gets injured, the MSC pericyte is activated, which then activates the tissue-specific stem cell.

NR: I know there are not complete data on this, but if you look at the spinal cord—the vasculature of the spinal cord itself and the vascular density—there are data showing that the white matter, which is the majority of the cord, has one-fifth the vascular density of the gray matter. What would you think overall is the differential? The cord does have innate regenerative capacity but relative to the liver it is lacking. What would be the percentage?

to 30 years.[14] Those cells are 50 percent genetically distinct from the mother's cells, and yet her immune system allows them to remain. Again, this flies in face of what doctors learn in medical school—that foreign cells cannot remain in the body without the immune system mounting a strong, and sometimes fatal, response. And yet mothers house these foreign cells in their bodies for decades. In one report, a woman with hepatitis who had stopped taking medication despite her doctor's orders actually saw an improvement in her condition. An analysis of her liver cells found that her liver contained 400 male liver cells per square centimeter.[15] This woman was not a twin, had never received a blood transfusion and had therefore no reason to have male

AC: There's no way of doing that, but I would state the following: If you cut somebody's spinal cord and squirted in some MSCs from the outside, one of the things all MSCs do—all of them—is they inhibit scar formation. We know that, even in cut spinal cords, those nerves can regenerate, but they can't regenerate if scar tissue moves across the cut site. So therefore, in animals it's shown that if you cut the spinal cord in half and squirt in MSCs and no scars form, eventually the nerves will regenerate down the tracks that are already there.

It's the same with stroke. The important thing with strokes is you get this big blood clot, and that kills some of the axons, the nerves that are carrying information. If you make sure that no scar forms, those nerves can regenerate down the tracks that are there. That is how you can get coordinate function back—the tracks are still there. That has been shown in animal models and is one of the reasons why MSCs have a chance of being really useful for stroke patients. We normally teach stroke patients how to make new routings for their nerves. If you inhibit scar formation, the normal axons regenerate.

NR: One more question. What do you think of our facilities in Panama?

AC: As I tell people, I've gloved and gowned and gone into the GMP facility, which is as good as any GMP facility that I know in the United States. The fact that you have a way of selecting efficacious cells makes this an unusual facility. My mantra every time I talk to you is the same: publish, publish, publish. Because we need outcome data. That goes for every clinic in the United States and elsewhere.

NR: Our MS study data are complete, and I would love for you to look at it.

AC: Happy to do it.

cells in her liver. Follow-up studies revealed that a probable source for those male liver cells was likely a pregnancy between 17 and 19 years earlier. The male cells were morphologically indistinguishable from the surrounding liver tissue. It is possible that fetal cells that are transferred to the mother have the capacity to differentiate to various tissues and potentially home to a site of injury: once there, they may essentially "blend" with the mother's cells to aid recovery.[16]

It was once thought that mothers have a higher incidence of autoimmune disease, especially systemic sclerosis, but a prospective study in 2004 actually found a reduced risk for systemic sclerosis in women who had been pregnant compared with women who had not.[17] Additionally, a study of women with rheumatoid arthritis, another common autoimmune condition, found no correlation between the risk of developing the disease and whether or not the women had given birth, and how many times.[18] In women who had given birth, there was actually a lower risk of rheumatoid arthritis, such that the researchers concluded, "HLA-disparate fetal microchimerism can persist many years after birth and could confer temporary protection against rheumatoid arthritis." In fact, the life span of mothers increases linearly by about one-third of a year per each additional child up to 14 children,[19] further evidence that microchimerism—or the presence of non-self cells within the body—is not a danger and may even confer a health benefit.

For every stem cell type that we have used in the clinic, I was always patient number one. The first time we used bone marrow MSCs, menstrual blood MSCs, fat-derived MSCs, or umbilical cord MSCs, I was the first patient to undergo treatment. Since patient number one, we have successfully performed over 5,000 treatments for a range of chronic health conditions with no serious adverse events.

When considering the safety of stem cells, tumor growth is a top concern. Because embryonic stem cells, and in some cases fetal stem cells, are potentially tumorigenic, meaning they develop into tumors, regulators tend to be wary of the safety of any stem cells. In order to be approved by the FDA for investigational new drug (IND) use of stem cells for our Duchenne muscular dystrophy patient Ryan Benton, the FDA wanted to

Allogeneic Stem Cell Clinical Trials

Today, there are many clinical trials currently evaluating the use of allogeneic (donor) stem cells for a range of chronic diseases.

Condition	Number of Clinical Trials
Multiple sclerosis	5
Type I diabetes	10
Lupus	5
Rheumatoid arthritis	4
Sjögren's syndrome	1
Autoimmune hepatitis	1
Crohn's disease	5
Primary biliary cirrhosis	2

In addition to these, we are currently conducting seven National Bioethics Committee-approved clinical trials for multiple sclerosis, rheumatoid arthritis, autism, spinal cord injuries, asthma, and osteoarthritis. We do and have collaborated with doctors and scientists at major universities in the United States, Canada, and Costa Rica including the University of California San Diego, University of Utah, University of Western Ontario, Indiana University, and the University of Costa Rica.

see safety data that our stem cells do not enhance tumor growth. While some studies using MSCs from older donors have been found to enhance tumor growth, the vast majority of studies actually show the opposite—that they kill tumor cells.

We injected MSCs intravenously or intratumorally (into the tumor) into rats with glioma, a brain tumor. By both modes of administration, the tumors shrank by 50 percent, which satisfied the FDA's concerns.[20]

In a second study by researchers at Kansas State University, MSCs were injected either directly into tumors or intravenously. The tumors in both MSC-treated animal groups disappeared and did not reappear.[21]

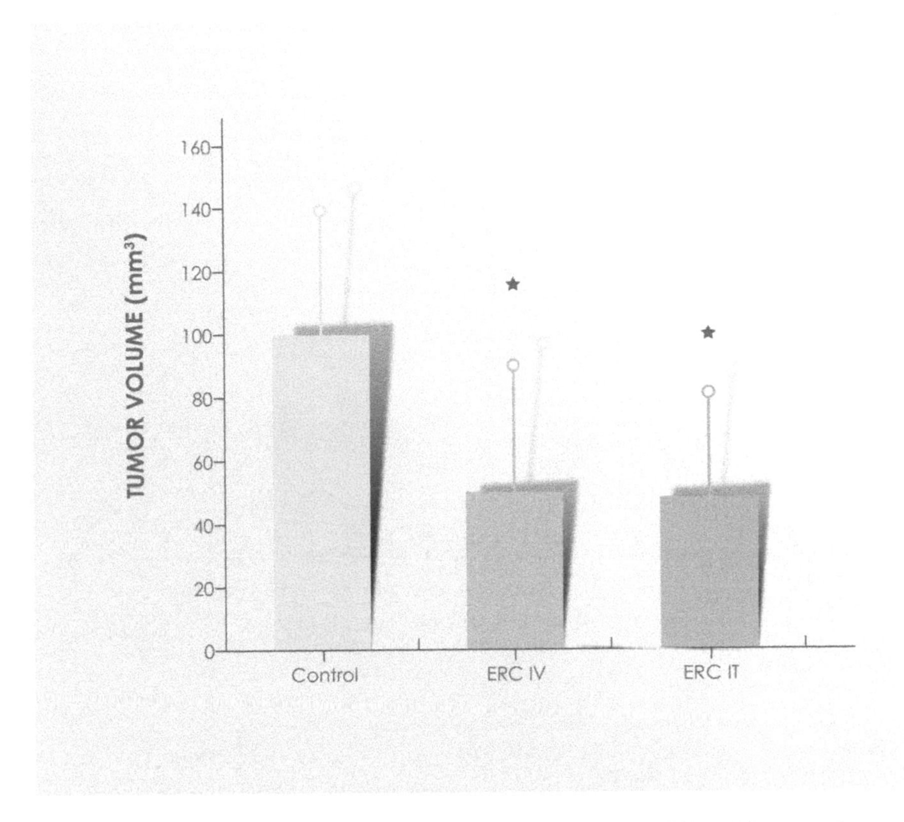

ERCs are mesenchymal-like cells derived from menstrual blood. Tumor cells were implanted into the brains of rats in three groups: 1) the control group (untreated), 2) a group receiving ERC into their veins, and 3) a group receiving ERC into the tumor. The size of the tumor was measured after 14 days.

Adapted from Han X, Riordan N., et al. Inhibition of intracranial glioma growth by endometrial regenerative cells. Cell Cycle. 2009;8(4):606-10.

As I mentioned in Chapter 2, my belief is that most solid tumors are caused by a dysfunction or lack of MSCs—cancer is a last-ditch effort to heal a non-healing wound. Replenishing the body's supply of MSCs has a healing effect and, as these studies show, has beneficial effects on suppression of tumor growth. In some studies complete eradication of all tumors in the body leads to the conclusion that MSCs can either kill directly or induce the death of the cancer stem cells themselves. See Chapter 3 for more about the anti-tumor effects of umbilical MSCs and their cell products.

Rat Umbilical Cord MSCs eliminate tumors with no recurrence.

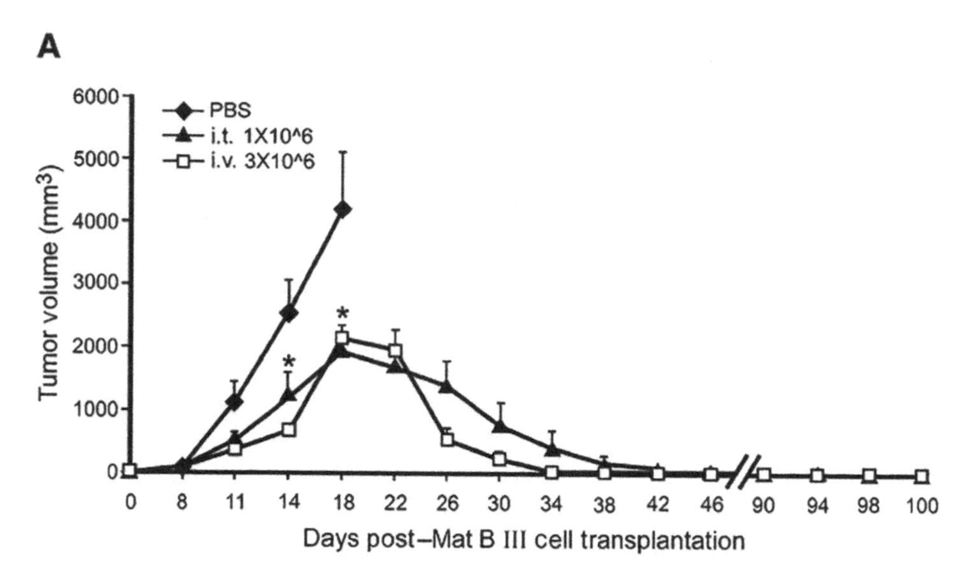

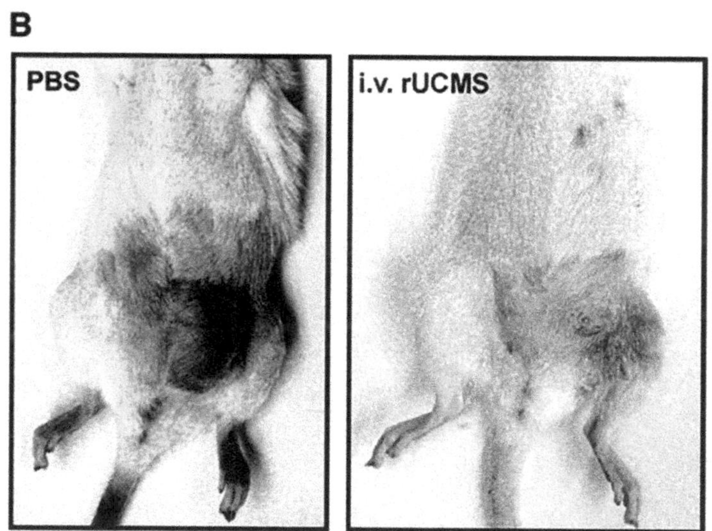

Cells from the Wharton jelly of rat umbilical cord (rUCMS) completely eliminate the tumors with no recurrence. The curve represents the growth of the tumor with time. Rats received either a placebo solution or rUCMS, representative examples after treatment are shown in the picture.

Reproduced with permission from Ganta C, et al. Rat umbilical cord stem cells completely abolish rat mammary carcinomas with no evidence of metastasis or recurrence 100 days post-tumor cell inoculation.Cancer Res. 2009;69(5):1815-20.

Interview with Robert Hariri, MD, PhD, Co-Founder and President, Human Longevity Cellular Therapeutics, and Founder, Chief Scientific Officer, Celgene Cellular Therapeutics

NEIL RIORDAN: Dr. Hariri, you are one of the true pioneers in cell therapy and a personal hero of mine. I've literally read every word of every patent you've written—and you've written many—in the field of regenerative medicine, in particular for isolating and making drugs out of mesenchymal-like cells from placenta. You founded a company called Anthrogenesis, which you later sold to Celgene and became the CEO of Celgene's Cellular Therapeutics division, correct?

ROBERT HARIRI: That's exactly right Neil. You and I are members of a mutual fan club.

NR: I am interested in your thoughts on the genesis of this research, where we are now, and where you think it's going to go.

RH: You and I have spent the last two decades believing that cellular medicine has the potential to transform how we deliver care for serious and life-threatening diseases. Much of our work has been based on trying to harness the regenerative power of these cells, and directing it to restore functionality in organs and tissues affected by either disease or injury. I think we both can admit that in the past 15 to 20 years, we've learned a tremendous amount. These cells are not simply replacement parts—they are master orchestrators of processes in the organs and tissues that restart functional renovation and regeneration of those tissues.

In 2012 a meta-analysis was conducted that included eight randomized controlled trials of patients receiving MSC treatment for a range of disease conditions.[22] The only adverse reaction the analysis detected was transient fever. They found no evidence of cancer, immune reaction, organ system complications, toxicity, infection, or death. Over 40 studies published on the use of MSCs in a wide range of chronic and acute health conditions have been found to have no serious adverse reactions. In particular, there have been no adverse events reported with the use of umbilical cord MSCs, which

> That's an important concept to keep in mind. As our friend and colleague, Arnie Caplan, who is credited with naming the mesenchymal stem cell, initially described these cells for their differentiation behavior, he is now very focused—as are we—on the synthetic and secretory behavior of these cells. That's how we all feel about how these cells exert much of their biological activity. That has been an important evolution in our thinking.
>
> I've personally spent quite a bit of time focused on what I've always felt to be the most reliable, abundant, economical, and scalable resource for deriving these types of cells—that is, the leftovers of birth. As you know, 20 years ago when the world was focused on stem cells derived from embryonic or fetal material, we went and explored the placenta as a source of these cells and found it was an incredibly rich harbor for pluripotent cells and more specialized stem and regenerative populations, which could be recovered in very, very high quantities with very, very high quality, and allowed us to procure under very rigorous control.
>
> As we've all been laboring to turn these living cells into medicines, we have faced the challenge of doing so in a way that meets the high quality standards necessary to satisfy the regulatory and clinical communities, as opinion leaders who are comfortable with delivering therapeutics in the form of discreet chemicals or biologic products.
>
> That said, I think we're on the threshold now of tremendous progress in using these products as therapeutics for two basic reasons: 1) because our understanding has grown

appear to have the highest safety profile among the four most commonly used MSC types: bone marrow, fat tissue, menstrual blood, or umbilical cord. For this reason, umbilical cord MSCs are the primary cells we use in our treatments.

Cell Selection Process

Our laboratory, Medistem Panama, Inc., is the only lab in the Western Hemisphere fully licensed by the government to isolate, manufacture, store, and use for treatment bone marrow, fat, and umbilical cord stem cells. We are licensed by the Panama Ministry of Health. Our 8,000 square foot laboratory utilizes state-of-the-art ISO-certified equipment and follows so much and we can begin to select clinical indications on the basis of that understanding; and 2) because cellular medicine has developed a fairly extensive clinical safety database. There are literally tens of thousands of recipients of cellular products, and that fundamental safety profile of living stem and progenerative cells administered as therapeutics is giving our colleagues in the regulatory community great comfort in knowing that these products can be deployed with a high level of confidence that they're not going to do any damage. We can begin to focus our lens on what they do beneficially, and begin to make decisions about how to use them, for what indications, at what dose and frequency, etc. I am very optimistic that we're entering into an era of a much more receptive community on the regulatory and clinical side, and we're going to see these products gain ever-increasing numbers of approvals and commercial authorizations so that we can begin to really build a much stronger clinical database to support their use in treating diseases.

NR: What indications has Celgene been pursuing with their cell products?

RH: We first focused on one specific attribute of cells from a placenta, which was linked to a unique biologic property of the organ that we found to be extremely intriguing and important—that's the unique immunobiology of the product. The placenta is very unique in that it's nature's professional allograph, meaning that it's designed to be transplanted across highly discordant HLA barriers without the need to change the immunology of the recipient. The placenta is an allograph that the mother accepts for nine months without

current Good Manufacturing Practices (GMPs), meeting the standards of the best laboratories in the United States.

Over the years of treating patients with chronic diseases, we noticed that certain patients experienced benefits above and beyond those of other patients. Miraculous recoveries were occurring on a regular basis. Other patients were improving after treatment, but the recovery of some patients astonished us. By this time, we had treated enough patients that we could take a good look at the activity of our cells to determine whether some cells were performing better than others.

We retrospectively analyzed cells used in highly successful cases, which we discovered were almost entirely limited to six particular cell lines. We then compared those cells to six cell lines of moderately successful cases rejecting. That particular unique relationship is even more evident in the case of surrogate pregnancy, whereby a woman carries a totally unrelated fetus and its placenta for nine months without rejecting it. That unique biological and immunological relationship is also conserved in the cells derived from the placenta.

We have treated hundreds of patients with placental cells without matching those cells between recipient and donor, and we've never seen a negative immunologic consequence from doing so.

We have treated hundreds of patients with placental cells without matching those cells between recipient and donor, and we've never seen a negative immunologic consequence from doing so. That, in its own right, is suggestive that the placenta has the ability to modulate the immune system of a recipient in a beneficial way. Our early work was to take these cells to treat autoimmune disease, in which an individual's aberrant immune response targets her own tissues. We observed, in clinical conditions, that the placental progenitor and stem cells could downregulate a host's immune system and suppress or control that autoimmune disease and, in some cases, put patients into full remission. That is obviously something we are very excited about and intend to pursue aggressively at Cellularity.

and six fibroblast cell lines, which have no activity at all. We then screened those cells, using high throughput screening, for the secretion of over 1,100 molecules.

What emerged was a molecular signature that was significantly different in the cells from the six lines given to highly successful cases compared with the other two groups. I call these highly effective cells Riordan Golden Cells.

This screening process took two and a half years because we first grew the cells in two dimensions, or on flat surfaces with the cells multiplying side by side. While this is the industry standard, it's a space- and medium-

NR: Can you talk about Cellularity? You and others are putting together a regenerative medicine company.

RH: For the last 15 years, I have been proud to lead an excellent group at Celgene, but I've always felt that this industry could benefit greatly from a broader, more diversified collaboration across businesses and academic centers whereby we operate from a position of strength—technological strength, intellectual property strength, and clinical development strength—and pool our resources in order to accomplish a great deal more that can be accomplished by an individual entrant into the field. The timing is right for leaders in the field to begin to align and consolidate our efforts in order to deliver these products to the clinical community—to the patients—at a much faster pace. That's been my dream for the last half a decade, and we're making a lot of progress in that direction.

NR: You and I were at a meeting a couple weeks ago and you were talking about the potential for modulating the life span of a mammal with these cells. Can you talk about that?

RH: Years ago our community was paying attention to stem cells in very specific clinical indications. While at Celgene, a leading biopharmaceutical company focused on oncology and hematology, I became interested in observations that the bone marrow, which is one of the body's most abundant reservoirs of stem cells, changes as a consequence of age. I learned, through data shared by Arnie Caplan, that bone marrow, as a source of blood and blood-forming cells, functions less efficiently over time and is less resistant to disease as the total number of stem cells in that tissue decline with age. There is a significant decline in the total number of available stem cells necessary to continually remodel and renovate tissue.

dependent process that we have been working to improve. The cells are anchorage dependent, so they require a huge surface area to grow. We have since grown the cells in bioreactors that allow the cells to multiply in three dimensions, a cutting-edge technology that allows us to grow more cells in less medium, with just the right density. We went through well over one year of screening to ensure that the Riordan Golden Cell molecular signature is preserved in cells grown in three dimensions. It is preserved. In fact, it's even pronounced.

At Human Longevity, the company I founded with Craig Venter and Peter Diamandis, over the last several years we did a comprehensive study in collaboration with Evan Snyder, looking at the change in stem cell compartments in tissues of animals as a function of age. Sure enough, we found these changes weren't limited to bone marrow, but occurred in other tissues. We then, based on the hypothesis that age-related degenerative changes are driven by a loss of the total number and quality of stem cells, attempted to modulate that loss with cells recovered from the placenta over the life span of the subjects; and looked at what that did to the stem cell compartments and, more importantly, to the quality and functionality of the tissues. We found that we could actually restore a more youthful functionality in tissues like muscles by giving back stem cells as these animals aged.

These studies are very supportive of the theory that one way to delay, reverse, or arrest degenerative disease associated with aging is to simply pay attention to the reservoir of stem cells in the tissues necessary to remodel and renovate them. We have at our fingertips a great tool—isolated, expanded cryopreserved stem cells that are coming from this newborn source. I believe this will be a very easy way to help maintain our tissues and organs as we age and potentially offset and reverse degenerative changes that I believe are a consequence of the loss of that regenerative engine. That technology is taking a center stage as we build a focus on placenta to address some of these degenerative diseases. I am very optimistic that we have a reasonable clinical rationale and a strong scientific rationale for using these products that way.

This is the first time in history that anyone has been able to retrospectively analyze which MSCs have more benefit. I like to say that an MSC is not an MSC. They are not all created equal. If you are picking a basketball team, would you want me on your team or LeBron James, possibly the best basketball player of all time? We are both humans, but our abilities on the court are not equal. It's the same with MSCs. Some perform better than others. That's why we've been working to select the best cells for use in patients with chronic disease. Now we can retrospectively analyze existing data of outcomes. We are the only stem cell company with the data to do that.

This new technology allows for us to continue to grow stem cells more efficiently, a crucial factor for the eventual large-scale use of MSCs for patients. With dosage costs of thousands of dollars, MSCs are not yet able

NR: One chapter in this book is about what we call "magic juice," or the secretions of these cells. Can you speak to the non-cellular products made from the expanded postnatal cells, that could be potentially useful?

RH: I've been a big proponent of what you've done. In fact, if you look at some talks I've given, including my TED talk on the role of stem cells and aging, I speak extensively about exactly what you're doing. My work has taught me that a stem cell is really a repository of the most intact, uncorrupted genomic information that we ever have in our lifetime. As our body is exposed to various environmental factors and other injurious stimuli, the DNA in our stem cell populations become, in many cases, subtly damaged and corrupted. The net result of that corruption in the software of our cells is that the synthetic repertoires of our cells are capable of generating a slow decline in quality or quantity.

> ***"The healthier and more intact the stem cell population you have, and the healthier and more normal the extracellular secreted product concentrations are, the more likely you are to maintain a healthy, youthful phenotype.***

I speak about the fact that aging echoes stem cell depreciation and accumulation of these subtle genomic problems that lead to an even more limited synthetic repertoire that I believe is essential to health and a youthful phenotype. It's clear to me that when you have cells from a youthful source—from newborn placental material—under cultivation conditions that produce and secrete factors into the supernate, as they would in the serum or the extracellular milieu, those factors are vitally important to cells that constitute the main structural and biological component of our organs and tissues.

to serve the large number of patients who need such treatment. We are the first stem cell manufacturer to grow these cells in three dimensions and are making major strides toward eventually reaching a wider population.

If we can replace those factors, which become deficient as we age, we can get many of the same biological benefits that we can by restoring the quality of those stem cell reservoirs. I believe the two clinical approaches are perfectly married: one is delivering very specific products in the form of soluble factors to patients; and the other is delivering specific living cells that take up residence either permanently or transiently, delivering factors that are lost or diminished in quantity in the aging individual.

The healthier and more intact the stem cell population you have, and the healthier and more normal the extracellular secreted product concentrations are, the more likely you are to maintain a healthy, youthful phenotype.

NR: Because of the embryonic world, and embryonic stem cells producing cancer, can you speak to the safety vis-à-vis the cancer perception with postnatal MSCs?

RH: Absolutely. Over the last twenty years we have recognized that the stem cells derived from healthy adult bone marrow or from healthy newborns can be delivered to recipients with essentially no significant risk of any adverse effects. These cells are incredibly stable, do not behave in an aberrant way, take up temporary residence in many cases, respond to local signaling, and secrete factors and products that have a selective advantage to the recipient.

I believe that some of the work done by our colleagues who are treating inherited metabolic disorders is, in essence, replacing a defective biological software system with one that can produce and secrete the appropriate factors, which can restore health or reverse or alter the natural history of a disease. That, to me, is very clear evidence that these products behave in an adaptive way to the environment they find themselves in, and they don't behave in an aberrant manner that puts the recipient at risk.

NR: Anything you want to close with?

RH: I am thrilled to be working with you in any way, shape, or form, and I believe our industry can really benefit from all of us finding pathways forward to meet the high standards that we want for these products, and from continually evaluating the combination of our clinical experience with the data so that it grows in size and quality. We are finally on the threshold of the decade of cellular medicine. I am happy to be working on it with you and our other colleagues.

Follistatin—Repair and Rebuild

One of the molecules secreted in higher amounts by the Riordan Golden Cells is the molecule follistatin. Follistatin is involved in tissue repair and rebuilding and is known to have anti-inflammatory effects. It is currently being investigated for its muscle growth ability. Follistatin is a natural inhibitor of myostatin, which inhibits muscle growth. The Blue Belgian Bull, bred to have decreased levels of myostatin, provides a visual for how the suppression of myostatin can increase muscle growth to impressive levels.

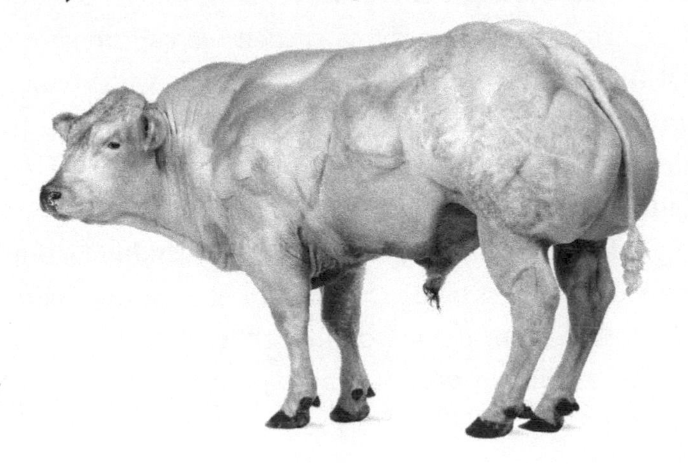

Licensed from Gettyimages by NH Riordan.

Now that our laboratory has established what makes an MSC a Riordan Golden Cell, we test the cells we receive to ensure that we only use those cells with the best molecular signature. Out of 100 umbilical cords that we receive, we now only use cells from fewer than ten.

Patient Selection Process

At the Stem Cell Institute we treat a handful of conditions for which we have developed institutional review board (IRB)-approved clinical protocols that are carefully followed. These conditions include rheumatoid arthritis, osteoarthritis, degenerative joint disease, multiple sclerosis, spinal cord injury, autism, cerebral palsy, and heart failure. We often receive requests to treat people with conditions that we are not currently taking patients for. These include amyotrophic lateral sclerosis (ALS), Alzheimer's, Duchenne muscular dystrophy, Parkinson's, and stroke. While we do believe that stem cells offer hope for a wide range of chronic diseases, offering stem cell treatment for any and all patients with simply the means to pay for it is not our practice. We are involved in cutting-edge medicine and are avidly collecting data so that we can continue to apply this treatment to the appropriate conditions and patients.

Our patient selection process involves a thorough review of medical history and a strict selection process so that we can be sure our patients get the most out of their treatment. For example, we generally treat only secondary progressive and relapsing remitting multiple sclerosis; spinal cord injury patients who were injured within the last ten years (the more recent, the better) and who are medically stable; autism and cerebral palsy patients under the age of 18; and heart failure patients with an ejection fraction of 10 or higher. Patients must be cancer free for at least five years and cannot have an active infection or open wounds. These criteria help us to identify the patients who will most benefit from treatment.

Chapter Six

SPINAL CORD INJURY—THE ULTIMATE REPAIR

Juan Carlos Murillo was a skillful pilot so deft in navigating a small plane that he was hired by a *National Geographic* photographer who wanted to take pictures of the mountainous Pacayas valley in Costa Rica back in May of 2008. The day was cloudy and the plane was buffeted by wind, but Juan Carlos and his passenger had been soaring smoothly over the valley floor and close to the highest peaks. Suddenly, two hours into the flight, Juan Carlos knew that something was wrong. The plane had endured turbulence off and on throughout, but it started to lose altitude. As he struggled to right the aircraft, he warned the photographer to get ready to make an emergency landing.

Juan Carlos wrestled with the aircraft, doing his best to make the impact as minimal as possible—what aviators call a controlled fall. The belly of the plane skipped twice over the valley floor before it came to a stop near a populated area. The plane was quickly surrounded by people. As Juan Carlos waited for the rescue vehicles to arrive, he thought he and his passenger were going to be just fine because their legs and feet, usually the first casualties of a crash, were intact. But when the helicopter arrived to transport them to the hospital and the emergency medical team maneuvered him out of the cockpit, Juan Carlos realized that something was very wrong with his back.

His doctor said that Juan Carlos would never walk again.

At the hospital, the MRI revealed that the spinal discs in his low back—at vertebrae L1 and L2—were completely crushed. There was nothing left of them. The doctors rushed him into surgery to stabilize his spine, but they had to stop the operation midway because of bleeding. The next day he had two more surgeries, one to stop the bleeding and another to stabilize his back. A week and a half later, his doctor transferred him to a long-term care hospital where he stayed another five weeks without making much progress in getting sensation below his waist. As he checked out of the hospital at the end of that discouraging stay, the looks on the faces of the staff told him what they believed his prognosis was. His doctor said that Juan Carlos would never walk again.

Immediately after the bleak prognosis at the second hospital, he checked in to another rehabilitation hospital that seemed as though it might offer some hope. There they kept him immobilized in a harness and strapped into a brace. Instead of soaring a mile above Earth in a plane as he was used to, the only thing he could see for the six weeks of his stay was the ceiling over his hospital bed. When he checked out of this hospital, the doctors again said they were sorry, Juan Carlos would never be able to walk again.

Undaunted, Juan Carlos signed up for a demanding course of physical therapy at the clinic run by a talented physical therapist, Eugenia Paris, who specializes in spinal cord injuries. What Juan Carlos didn't know when he committed to working with her is that Eugenia is a proponent of stem cell therapy. I have been sending my spinal cord injury patients to her physical therapy center since our clinic first started treating spinal cord injury patients with stem cells, but Eugenia had advocated for the treatment before that.

Eugenia had had a spinal cord patient who went to Germany for stem cell treatment and noticed some improvement in his condition. As she says, for a spinal cord injury, a little bit of improvement is a huge event for most patients. Patients who cannot move at all and then find they can manipulate a joystick, or stand in the kitchen with the help of crutches while their spouse makes dinner, are thrilled by these advances. Almost from the time Juan Carlos entered her clinic, Eugenia insisted that he try stem cell therapy for his injury. In fact, the first time Eugenia laid eyes on Juan Carlos she contradicted what every other medical professional predicted. "You are going to walk again," she said. "Don't worry."

At first Juan Carlos resisted. His family had sent him to several psychiatrists to help him handle the sad reality that he wouldn't be able to walk again. When he told his father, a respected obstetrician in Costa Rica, about the stem cell option, his father was very doubtful. He'd never heard of the treatments we were doing and suspected that they might harm his son. After all, Juan Carlos' father had paid for his son to travel to Miami and consult with some of the most respected spinal cord injury specialists in the world. Those doctors examined Juan Carlos' MRI and repeated the hopeless predictions of his Costa Rican physicians.

Eugenia was undaunted. She argued with Juan Carlos for two months, trying to persuade him that our treatment at the very least would do him no harm and, because he was so young and had been so active, had a good chance of making significant improvements. She knew he was a good candidate for stem cell treatment.

I had decided when we set up our clinic in Costa Rica that we would treat one local patient free for every twenty paying patients we took. I offered Juan Carlos one of the pro bono slots, and he persuaded his family this was the next best step, in fact the only step that offered some hope of recovery.

When a traumatic blow injures the spine, as happened to Juan Carlos, the impact pulls the nerve fibers apart and the pressure on the cord damages the blood vessels and the nerves. The pressure on the spinal canal rises and, as Juan Carlos experienced, there is a tremendous loss of blood. With the spinal cord depleted of blood and flooded with chemicals from the disrupted membranes, the body's immune response quickly forms scar tissue to protect the area. This is why spinal cord injury experts like to try to repair the area as quickly as possible—before the wounded spinal cord becomes scarred in.

Until recently, there was really nothing that could be done about spinal cord injury. A person with this injury would be disabled for the rest of his or her life. It makes sense, from an evolutionary standpoint, that the body puts great energy and resources into creating this wonderful cage, full of strong bones, around the spinal cord (the spinal column). It would have been a waste of resources to put a high concentration of MSCs in the spinal cord with all the protection already constructed. (This is similar to what has happened with vitamin C. At one point in our evolutionary history, humans lost the ability to produce their own vitamin C because we consumed enough of it from food. Mother Nature does not waste.) Capillary density of white matter is one fifth that of gray matter.[1] Capillary density of gray matter in the spinal cord is approximately three times less than that of liver tissue and ten times less than that of heart tissue.[2] Therefore we can assume that, since all MSCs live on capillaries, during a spinal cord injury many fewer MSCs are released, which is why the spine does not fully regenerate. This is in sharp contrast to the liver, which can nearly completely regenerate.[3,4,5]

Comparison of Vascularity

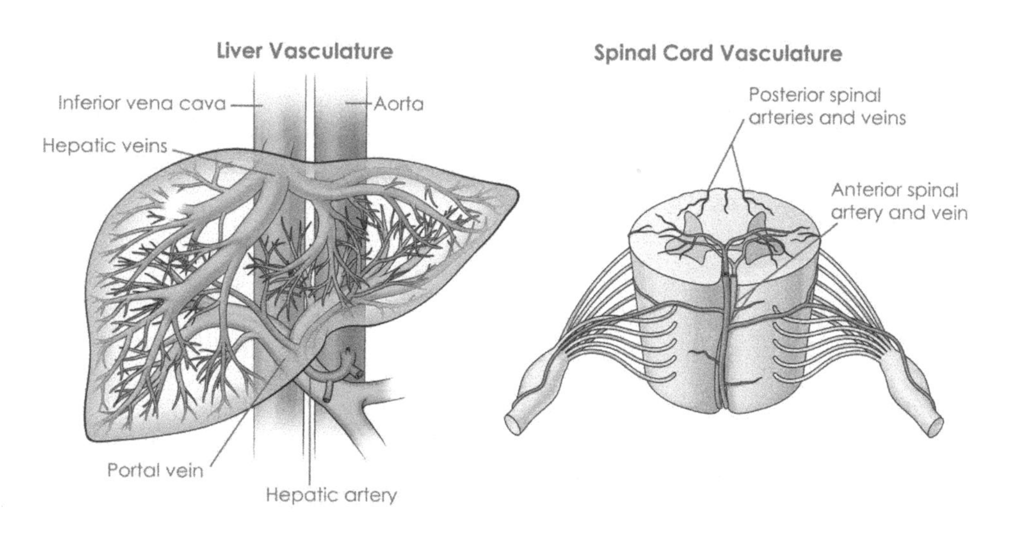

Comparison of the vasculature in the liver (very highly vascularized) and in the spine (sparsely vascularized).

Mesenchymal Stem Cells for Spinal Cord Injury

The spinal cord is a long, delicate bundle of nervous tissue encased and protected by the vertebrae and segmented into regions according to the position of the nerves: C1 to C8 (cervical), T1 to T12 (thoracic), L1 to L5 (lumbar), and S1 to S5 (sacral). A spinal cord injury (SCI) occurs when the tissue is torn, bruised, or crushed in an accident (traumatic) or by the progression of a disease or disorder (non-traumatic). The most common cause of SCI is physical trauma.

Magnetic resonance imaging (MRI) is used in SCI to pinpoint the level and extent of the lesion. The level of the injury depends on the vertebra (e.g., C3, T10). A complete SCI is one in which no function remains below the level of the injury whereas for an incomplete SCI some limited function does remain. Scales exist to measure motor and sensory limitations (ASIA scale, MEP/SSEP) and quality of life (ADL, SF-36, ODI) in SCI patients.

We'd had good results using umbilical cord cells to treat spinal injury, but Juan Carlos' dad still wouldn't agree to the procedure. He didn't want to subject his son to a treatment he considered to be unproven, partially because he'd never heard about it in medical school. Eventually Juan Carlos convinced his dad that it was his life and, in the shape he was in, he had nothing to lose. His dad respected his son's wishes and even provided umbilical cords from his own patients for the treatment. Once we received the cords, we harvested and expanded the stem cells to repair the damaged spinal cord, just as we continue to do in our clinic in Panama today. They are administered both intravenously and intrathecally (via the spinal fluid). We added the use of concentrated bone marrow to our protocol after Juan Carlos was treated. So, in addition to the umbilical cord cells, the bone marrow cells are given both in the vein and in the spinal fluid. Spinal cord injury is the only condition we treat using bone marrow. There are several studies now that show cells concentrated from the patient's own bone marrow as sole therapy can improve the functionality of spinal cord injury patients. The main reason we use the bone marrow is because in addition to containing MSCs, it is rich in CD34+ cells and endothelial precursor cells (EPCs). Both cell types potently stimulate new blood vessel growth. Most spinal cord

> Changes in motor and sensory functions are usually seen after a spinal cord injury, caused by a loss of neurons and axons as well as inflammation and damage to the protective nerve covering known as the myelin sheath (demyelination).[6] Since communication below the level of the injury is affected, significant loss of quality of life and many other complications may arise, such as hypersensitive sensations, pain with no sensation, extensive pain along the damaged fibers, involuntary spasms or reflex actions, respiratory infections, bone density loss, muscle tone damage, pressure ulcers, and problems with sexual function.[7]
>
> Researchers at Cambridge University in the United Kingdom, at Purdue University in Indiana, and at Washington University in St. Louis have had success treating spinal cord injuries in dogs and rats with stem cells. They tagged the cells with a radioactive marker so they could follow where the cells rested in the body as they migrated through the bloodstream. They tracked them to the site of the injury where some persisted and delivered growth factors that helped in the repair of the damaged spinal cord. Other researchers investigating how to regrow the spine looked into the immune system

injuries are traumatic and lead to a loss of blood flow to the spinal cord area, which has very few blood vessels in the first place, compared to other tissues and organs. Creation of new blood vessels with these cells is very important to stimulate healing.

Juan Carlos had his first treatment in October of 2008 and found great relief from his phantom neuropathic pain. It went from a ten to a three on a scale of one to ten and he was able to stop taking narcotic pain relievers. It wasn't until the second treatment at the end of February 2009 that he started to feel the stem cells working on restoring feeling. The next week, in the beginning of March, for the first time in almost a year Juan Carlos started to feel the muscles of his legs contracting, and he could move his toes. In physical therapy, Eugenia was working with him to move more, stimulating his legs electronically with probes—suddenly he started to feel his knee.

Eugenia began working with Juan Carlos to help him build up his strength. He'd lost nearly fifty pounds since the crash. Confined to bed and unable to control his bladder, he had been subsisting on liquids. He was embarrassed that he had to wear a diaper. His muscles were starting to atrophy. Eugenia and her staff put him on the parallel bars to help him stand response, which is complex. Spinal cord injuries trigger an autoimmune reaction to try to protect the other nerve cells from damage. It seemed clear that to help repair a human spine, MSCs would have to serve multiple functions: deliver growth factors to the spine that would help the cells regenerate, decrease scarring and inflammation, and shut down or modulate an inappropriate immune response.

Repair of the spinal cord is critical to recover mobility and function. The regenerative, anti-inflammatory, and angiogenic activities of mesenchymal stem cells (MSCs) have stimulated numerous preclinical studies in the area of SCI. The rationale for the treatment of our first SCI patient in 2007 came from a case report in Korea, in which a patient treated with umbilical cord blood stem cells was found to be able to move her hips and feel her hip skin 15 days after treatment.[8] After this, she began to elevate both lower legs about one centimeter, and muscle activity around her hips gradually improved. Tests taken 41 days after treatment showed regeneration of the spinal cord at the injured site and below it. This was supported by several studies of injured rats treated with cells from human

up while he practiced walking. They gradually coached him to put more and more of his body weight on his feet to help him regain control of his leg muscles and build up his strength. In a matter of just a few months, he went from walking with the help of a therapist and the parallel bars to a walker, then crutches, and finally to a cane. In May 2010, two years after the crash, Juan Carlos was able to walk without any assistance. That summer he was able to fly again, and requalified as a pilot. His recovery was amazing.

During the period when Juan Carlos was being treated, we had opened a new laboratory in Panama City, Panama, in the City of Knowledge, a converted military area located in the former Panama Canal Zone. The City of Knowledge is a government-sponsored cluster of academic organizations, research and technology companies, and non-governmental organizations. At the same time we opened the Stem Cell Institute, a research-based medical facility at the campus of Punta Pacifica Hospital.

In November 2010 when I was visiting the Stem Cell Institute, I was having a drink with some staff and a few friends in a bar near the clinic. Who walked in but Juan Carlos, holding hands with his lovely fiancée. With three treatments using carefully targeted injections of refined umbilical cord umbilical cord, showing improvements in function and some restoration of the spinal cord tissue.[9,10,11,12] In these cases, the cells survived without immune suppression, migrated to the site of injury, and enhanced recovery significantly. Treatment with bone marrow MSCs was also demonstrated to be safe and feasible for treatment of SCI.[13,14]

Perhaps the most compelling early animal trial for the treatment of SCI, published in 2008, contains both the rationale for their use in repairing the spinal cord and an elegantly designed study that demonstrated that the beneficial effects were from the secretions of the cells and not from the cell becoming spinal tissue.[15] The researchers completely severed the spinal cords of rats and then placed human umbilical cord mesenchymal stem cells over the fibrin glue that covered each severed end. The MSCs homed to the site of injury, secreting proteins that encouraged regeneration, calmed inflammation, and modulated the immune response in such a way that the spinal cord was able to regrow. The MSCs simply stimulate the natural repair process. As mentioned several times in this book, the beneficial effects of MSCs are due to their secretions and not from their "becoming" another

stem cells, Juan Carlos had regained 90 percent of what he'd lost because of the accident.

> ***I know this seems like a miracle, and it would be miraculous to the millions of people who suffer right now from paralyzing spinal cord injuries to think that with a combination of adult stem cells and extensive physical therapy they, too, could regain use of their spines, control of their bowels, and full sexual function. Yet it is not a miracle. It's basic, simple science that even some of the most prestigious specialists in spinal cord injuries have yet to attempt.***

I will never forget giving grand rounds at a prestigious U.S. university that is well known for its pioneering work on spinal cord injury. The researchers had never heard of umbilical cord cells or bone marrow from the patient

kind of tissue. An important contribution of this study is that the umbilical cord MSCs that had not been altered (had not been induced to become spinal tissue cells) worked better for repair than those that had. More importantly, because the cells were human, they could be identified in the tissue. After the spinal cords regrew, the human cells were found only between the regrown fibers and were not part of the spinal cord itself. It's not the cells themselves that are required for healing, you see, but rather, what they secrete.

Spinal Cord Repair

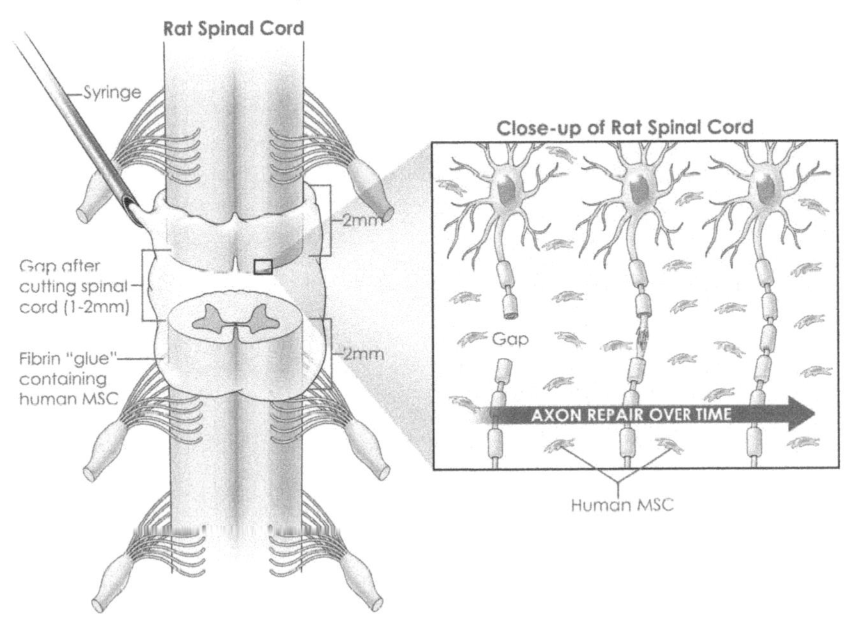

Adapted from data in Yang et al. Transplantation of human Umbilical Mesenchymal stem cells from Wharton's jelly after complete transection of the rat spinal cord. PLoS One. 2008;3(10):e3336.

as being useful for spinal cord injury. I presented six articles that were in the literature showing benefit in humans by treatment (i.e., restoration of neurologic function) with umbilical cord cells and bone marrow cells. They were unaware of the studies, having been focused only on their own cell type, for which they had a laundry list of patents. These included not just the cell type but the methods for isolating and growing them in culture. Oftentimes this is the biggest problem in clinical research for the treatment

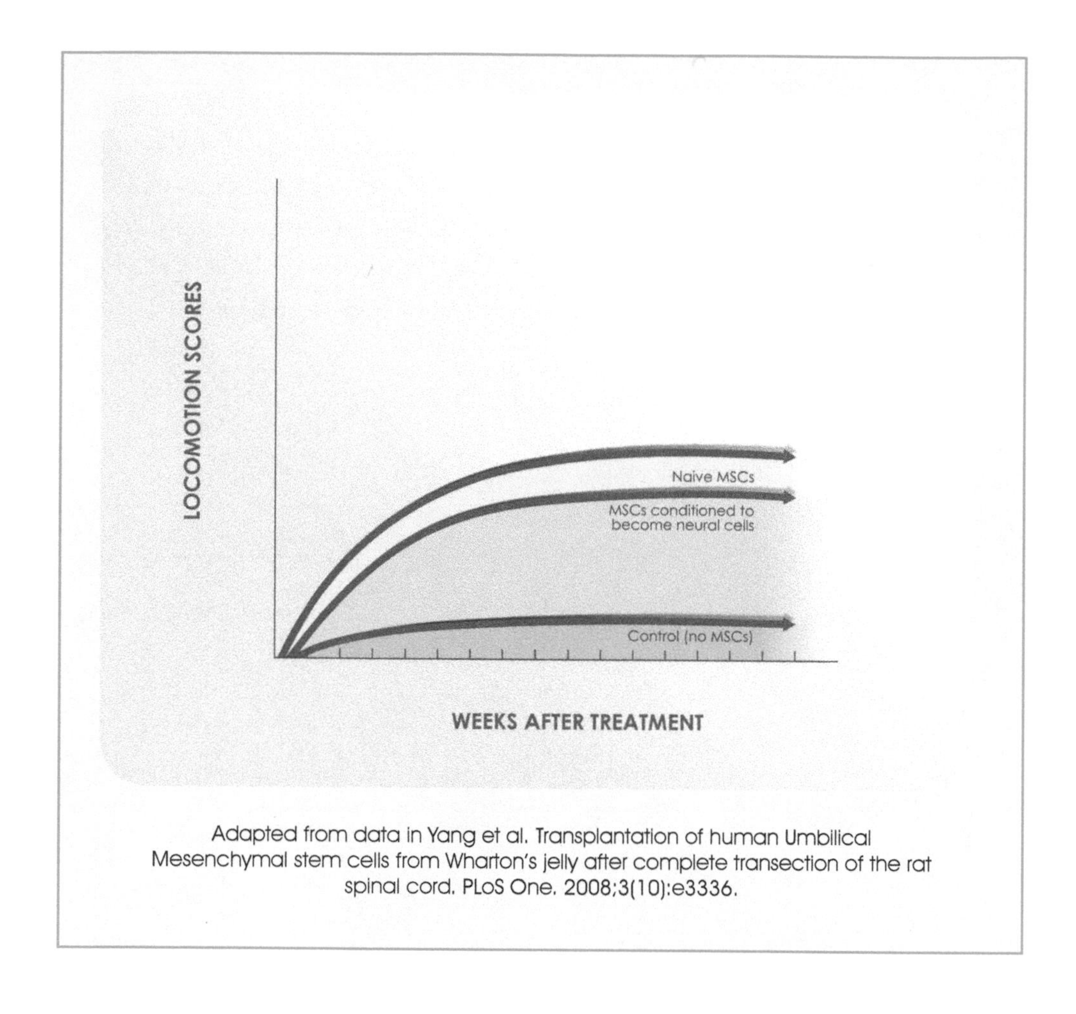

Adapted from data in Yang et al. Transplantation of human Umbilical Mesenchymal stem cells from Wharton's jelly after complete transection of the rat spinal cord. PLoS One. 2008;3(10):e3336.

of disease—conflict of interest. Rather than focusing on what works, industry and academia focus on what they own. I saw this with my own company, Medistem, Inc, a U.S.-based publically traded company. We had patents and patents pending out the wazoo on the menstrual mesenchymal cell (also known as the endometrial regenerative cell, or ERC). At the time, in 2007, we were doing some research on heart failure. We had a cohort of subjects that were treated with umbilical cord cells and the majority of them improve dramatically. The board of directors wanted to try using the menstrual cells, and we did. That cohort did not do nearly as well. We had to bring them back and treat them again with the umbilical cord cells. It was at that time that I knew we needed to part ways with the U.S.-based company, which was interested only in promoting what it owned. At the Stem Cell Institute we

Years after these initial studies, the effects of MSCs on SCI are still being demonstrated.[16,17,18] A recent review presents 21 animal studies with demonstrated therapeutic effects of MSCs in preclinical models, with significant improvements in mobility, sensory tests, and motor function.[19] Treatment with MSCs for SCI has entered clinical trials—a survey of ClinicalTrials.gov returns several ongoing and recruiting MSC trials.[20,21,22,23,24] A recently completed trial reported motor improvements in eight out of fourteen SCI patients safely treated with umbilical cord MSCs, with significant differences in ASIA scores as motor and sensory functions before and after treatment.[25] Other clinical trials with bone marrow MSCs also showed improvements for 50 to 75 percent of patients.[26,27] In our clinical experience, treating SCI with umbilical cord MSCs brought significant changes in pain scores and mobility, as well as recovery of bowel and sexual function, as we saw with Juan Carlos.[28]

We are conducting a phase I/II clinical trial in our Panama clinic to assess the safety and efficacy of intravenous and intrathecal allogeneic umbilical cord MSCs and autologous bone marrow MSCs for patients with spinal cord injury. Additionally, we are in the process of starting an umbilical cord MSC clinical trial in association with the University of Miami and Thomas Jefferson University, funded by the Marcus Foundation.[28]

were, as we always have been and are to this day, only interested doing what was best for the patients.

When I saw Juan Carlos in Panama he was visiting for a fourth treatment. He still had some stiffness in his right ankle and some spots on his right leg that were numb. He wanted to see if another treatment could eliminate the last traces of his injury.

Juan Carlos had made a remarkable improvement. He was so proud of what we had all worked so hard to achieve that he flew back to see the world-renowned back specialist in Miami who had glumly told him that he would never be able to walk. When he walked into the doctor's office for the appointment, the doctor didn't believe it was him. And his father, the conventionally trained obstetrician who was so skeptical of stem cell treatment at first, now educates other doctors and his own patients about the therapy.

Juan José Vallarino was 30 years old in 2009 when he tripped and fell down a river bank, landing on his neck. "It was like something snapped," Juan José said. He called his mom on the way to the hospital to say goodbye, unsure if he would survive. At the hospital, doctors determined that he had a complete C5, C6 spinal cord injury. He was completely paralyzed from the neck down. "I didn't know when I was being touched. It's a crazy feeling all over the body." After spinal surgery eleven days later, and hospital discharge seven days after that, he was wheelchair bound with difficulty breathing and without bladder or bowel control. He could move only his eyes and mouth.

After eight months of rigorous physical therapy, and with the help of two people lifting him into position, he was able to stand on his own while holding himself up. He had gained movement in his arms and could wiggle one of his toes. But he longed to do more. "The first two years were pretty bad," he said.

By the time he had heard about stem cell treatment four years later, he was still unable to wheel himself in his wheelchair, transfer himself from the chair to the toilet, or dress himself without great difficulty. He had no urinary control and was chronically constipated. He had very little independence. He would wake up in the morning screaming with neuropathic pain. "It was like 15 on a scale of one to ten," he said of his pain. "I feel as though I didn't sleep for four years. The pain was everywhere."

After his first stem cell treatment at our clinic in Panama, his pain subsided. He gained the ability to transfer himself to the toilet and into the car. He could pull himself up when needed and could put on his shirt. He started doing exercises on his own. "Putting the training together with the stem cells was great," he said. Perhaps best of all, he regained urinary and bowel control as well as erectile function.

> **"*When you can't move, it's like you're a plant, just waiting to be fed, given a shower, clothed, and put back in your chair where you stay. Now people can have a chance to get better.*"**

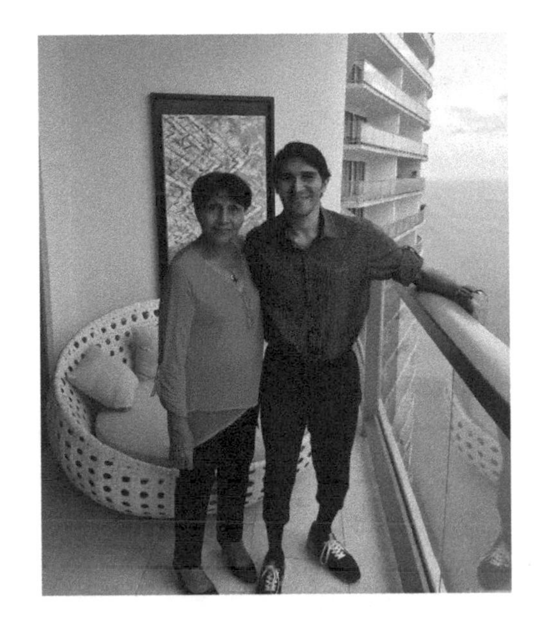

After his second treatment two years later, he has regained independence—he now lives on his own. He can completely dress himself and uses a gait training walker to move about the house and go outside. "When I stand up I can feel my glutes and my lower back muscles contracting. I can hold a fist now when before I couldn't." He continues to train twice daily, five days a week. "Every case is different, but what the stem cells have done to me is amazing. You have to put in a lot of effort." He's right. Our spinal cord injury patients undergo an intensive physical training regimen that we recommend they follow long term when they return home.

Juan José is enthusiastic about his progress with stem cells. "When you can't move, it's like you're a plant, just waiting to be fed, given a shower, clothed, and put back in your chair where you stay. Now people can have a chance to get better."

The first spinal cord injury patient we ever treated was in early 2007. He was a 23-year-old from Florida who had been in a motorcycle accident three months prior, which had paralyzed him from his T4 vertebra, at the level of his chest, down. He showed up with his doctor one day at our clinic asking to be treated, strapped to his wheelchair because he couldn't engage his abdominals or obliques to hold himself up.

He was treated for eleven days, and before he left he was able to bend from side to side and lean forward all on his own. He had gained feeling and movement down to his hips and was able to transfer himself out of bed and into his wheelchair for the first time. He came back a year later for another treatment and gained more function, including erectile function.

As of this writing, we've treated 116 patients for spinal cord injuries, including Iraq War veterans. Seventy percent of them have experienced restoration of some function. What we tell them at the first appointment is that they shouldn't hang all their hopes on walking again. The least we can work toward is for them to regain control of their bladder function. This is a great step forward from being hooked up to a catheter all day. We tell them to go slowly with their expectations. Just like relearning to walk, they have to take it one step at a time. But there is incredible hope here, particularly if we can get to the patients before significant scar tissue has had a chance to form, and if we can get them working with a physical therapist right away. We always tell patients that our spinal cord injury treatment protocol is 50 percent stem cell therapy and 50 percent physical therapy. You don't get the kind of results Juan Carlos did without a physical therapist who is always urging you to do more, to work harder, and to never give up hope.

Unfortunately, many people come to us after suffering for years with a spinal cord injury and we have to turn many of them away because too much time has passed since the original injury. But in patients with more recent injuries, our treatment, in combination with physical therapy, determination from the patient, and support from people around them, can lead to dramatic healing. As we continue to refine this protocol and learn from doctors around the world who are working on the same techniques from other angles, we hold out the hope that within the coming years we can end spinal paralysis.

Chapter Seven

MULTIPLE SCLEROSIS—CALMING THE IMMUNE SYSTEM

Of all the diseases and chronic conditions we treat with stem cells, the one that I have the best personal understanding of is multiple sclerosis (MS) because I had something very similar to it that time I got the bends.

They told me when I was being treated in the UK that the lesions that form in the brain after a severe case of the bends are the same as the lesions that form when someone suffers from multiple sclerosis. The thick, foggy feeling I experienced, the numbness in my extremities that made walking or any kind of movement a discouraging chore, and the way my days became dim and my mood sunk low were the same effects that MS patients struggle with every day. For me, though, there was hope that the treatments we undertook could reverse the worst of it. Not so with most of the people who suffer with MS.

Shortly before we set up our clinic in Costa Rica, articles started to appear in scientific journals that described experiments working with stem cells to alleviate MS symptoms in mice,[1] and one limited-success case study with a human patient who was treated by Iranian doctors.

The science behind using stem cells to treat MS made sense to me. Multiple sclerosis is an autoimmune system disorder in which the body's immune cells attack the central nervous system—the brain, the optic nerve, and the spinal cord—destroying the myelin sheath, the fatty substance that protects the nerve cells. Once that protective barrier is damaged, the nerve impulses that travel between the brain and the spinal cord are blocked or distorted, affecting walking, balance, coordination, and vision. As the disease progresses, those severely affected may lose control of their bowels and sexual function and can become confused and forgetful.

We'd had success working on other autoimmune disorders using stem cells to block the inappropriate immune response and to create the right conditions for tissue regeneration. I was eager to try our techniques on MS partially because I believed we could be very effective where conventional pharmaceutical treatments with steroids, immune modulators, and immune suppressants had not, and partially because I knew how these patients felt.

The goal of our umbilical cord MSC treatments for patients with multiple sclerosis really has nothing to do with repairing the damaged or destroyed myelin in the lesions found in the brain and spinal cord. Because multiple sclerosis is first and foremost an autoimmune disease, and not neurological, one goal is to address the immune dysfunction. At the root of the disease is a pool of immune cells called T cells, which actively proliferate, cross the blood-brain barrier (BBB), and attack myelin. These cells are not typically found in great numbers in the brain and spinal cord—they are found throughout the rest of the body. These T cells, for reasons unknown, clone themselves until they become an army of T cells. Our primary goal, then, is to interfere with myelin-specific T cell reproduction (also called *clonal expansion*). Mesenchymal stem cells have been shown in multiple studies to have the capacity to block this so-called clonal expansion of activated T cells. In a way, MSCs immunosuppress, but unlike some drugs that suppress the immune system, this specific blocking of activated T cells does not quash the entire immune system—the cells and their secretions only block the clonal expansion. Other drugs that suppress the immune system—for example, the steroid hydrocortisone—have an effect on the entire immune system, which can increase the risk to the recipient of infectious diseases and even some cancers. Steroids are catabolic, meaning they break down tissue. MSCs have the opposite effect—they are anabolic. They stimulate regeneration. They are the body's way of naturally keeping the immune system in check.

Multiple sclerosis is essentially the same condition as rheumatoid arthritis and type 1 diabetes. All three involve this proliferation of T cells—in multiple sclerosis they attack the myelin that protects nerves; in rheumatoid arthritis they attack the lining of the joints; and in type 1 diabetes they attack the beta cells in the pancreas. T-regulatory cells usually keep T cells under control but are unable to keep up with T cell proliferation in these autoimmune diseases. MSCs produce T-regulatory cells, which decreases activated T cells, addressing autoimmune dysfunction.

A new drug prescribed for relapsing-remitting MS called Tysabri® acts as a coating for T cells, preventing them from penetrating the blood-brain barrier or spinal cord. Preventing T cells from entering the brain may seem like a good idea, since activated T cells are responsible for destroying the myelin that leads to MS, but the drug also prevents inactive T cells from reaching

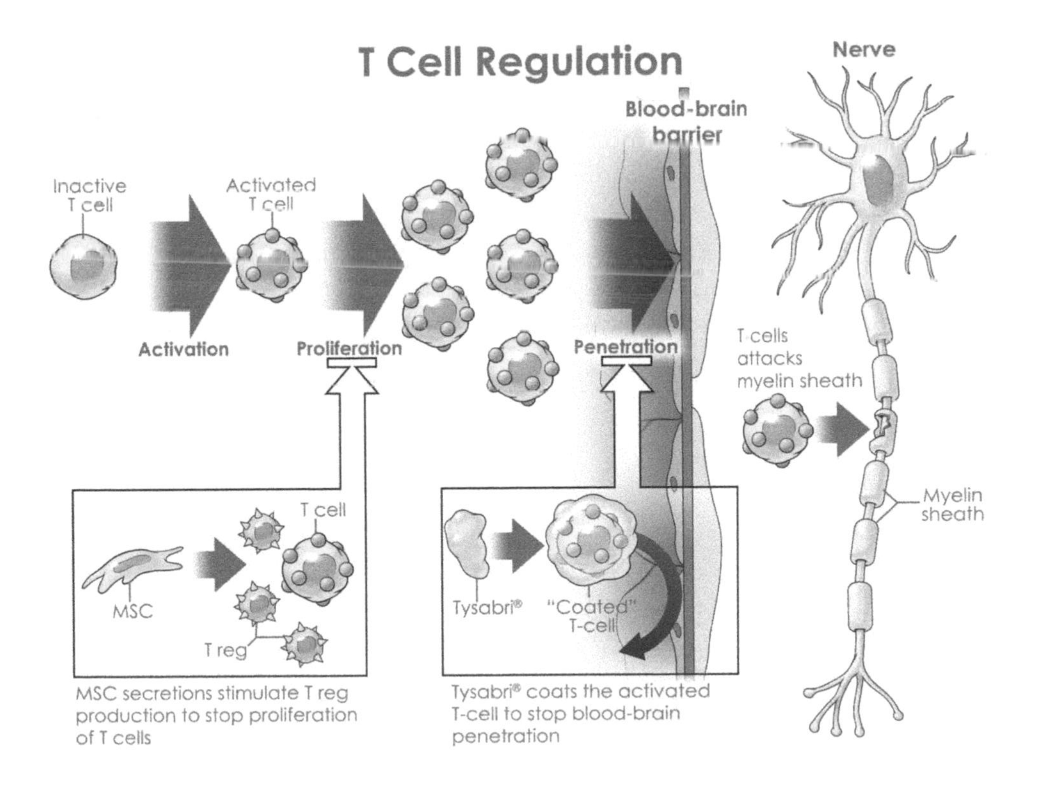

the brain to protect it from infection. Tysabri essentially compromises the brain's immune system. One of the worst side effects of this drug is a condition known as progressive multifocal leukoencephalopathy (PML), a potentially fatal viral disease that triggers inflammation throughout the brain. Because MSCs target the original clonal expansion of activated T cells, MSC treatment for MS obviates the need for a drug like Tysabri because it addresses the root cause of the problem.

If it were the goal of the treatment to induce remyelination, then certainly the route of delivery would be of greatest importance. You would want for the cells (or whatever proposed remyelination agent) to be as close as possible to the lesions requiring the repair. In my opinion, it will be difficult to successfully treat multiple sclerosis by remyelination alone because if you do not address the immune problem you will continue to lose myelin. Therefore, getting the cells to the lesions for myelin repair is not particularly important. Further support for this opinion is that there is very good evidence that the body has the innate ability to regenerate myelin without intervention. There are three good examples of this.

The first example comes from a condition called Guillain–Barré syndrome, an autoimmune disease that results from an immune attack on the myelin of peripheral nerves. It involves an ascending paralysis and can be life threatening if the paralysis gets high enough to affect breathing. Guillain–Barré syndrome is treatable and generally temporary. In 80 percent of patients the underlying nerves are not irreparably damaged, and there are no long-term neurologic symptoms, while 20 percent experience permanent nerve damage[2] because the axons of the nerves are damaged. The good news is that the disease is temporary. The better news is that in mild cases in which the axons were not destroyed, complete remyelination occurs—the body has the capacity to restore myelin.

The second example comes from a phenomenon seen with serial MRI images of the brains in people with MS. Fifty percent of these low-intensity lesions known as "black holes" revert within one month of appearance, indicating that remyelination has occurred spontaneously.[3]

Further evidence for supporting the immune system and not the central nervous system in MS comes from the work of several groups, including

Northwestern University, that are using chemotherapeutic conditioning whereby the immune system is wiped out (along with the bystanding hematopoietic stem cells), followed by bone marrow reconstitution using previously harvested bone marrow stem cells.[4]

Our turning point patient was Richard Humphries, a gregarious and affable Texan whose life spiraled downhill dramatically when he first suffered symptoms of MS in 2005 at age 50. At that time, Richard was a high-powered hospital executive, the administrator for a chain of nursing homes in Texas who supervised a staff of 140 people.

At first, Richard dismissed his symptoms as aberrations. At 6 feet, 5 inches tall, he's a big guy. He'd always been very active, playing a lot of golf, running three miles a day and biking six miles or more several times a week. One spring day he was cycling with his wife and noticed that his thighs were going numb, but he dismissed it. Then his wife started to notice that he was less coherent. One Saturday afternoon he came home from a golf tournament at his church and she told him he was acting like he was drunk, although there hadn't been any alcohol at the tournament. Still, he brushed this off as a one-time oddity. Until the seizures started.

Imagine this big guy, head of a big organization, dropping to the floor and curling up in a fetal position as his body rocked, his left arm contracting first, then his left ankle curling. Very quickly the number of seizures escalated from a few a day to so many that he lost count. Richard remembers one weekend when he had 132 seizures. Some hours he'd have one every six minutes.

He went to see a few neurosurgeons in his area, all of whom ran tests on him but couldn't diagnose his illness. One of the doctors prescribed anti-seizure medication, which slowed the number of seizures for a while, but they soon returned. When they came back, the seizures presented differently. After the seizure was over, Richard was out of it for quite some time. He wasn't conscious of what anyone was saying to him. He could repeat someone's words back to them, but he had no sense of what they meant. It was as if he were in a totally different world. Finally, in October 2005, he and his wife journeyed to the Mayo Clinic in Minnesota where the neurosurgeon quickly diagnosed his MS.

Richard was getting worse and so was his family's situation. He was fired from his job at the hospital because his bosses said he was unreliable and had become a workplace hazard. Richard entered a world of darkness. He had been the major breadwinner for his family of four children, two in college, and now no one would hire him. He had a tough time even being useful around the house. One day he went to the big box hardware store a few miles from home and couldn't figure out how to get back. "I didn't even have enough function in my brain to dial my wife," he said. "Everything kind of went gray, and I sat in the parking lot for a couple of hours until I figured out that if I got to that street right there, it would get me pretty close to my house. The street took me close to my house, but then I realized I missed the turn to my street. After a couple more mistakes, I finally find found my way home, but it took three and a half hours."

As he sat in his bed, struggling to make it to the bathroom on his own, he decided he was a terrible burden to his family. The most honorable thing to do, he thought, was to set them free of him. When his wife came home, he told her he knew she didn't sign up for this kind of life. If she wanted to divorce him, he was granting her permission. His wife, a surgical nurse, looked at him astounded. She had been at his side during the worst of seizures, massaging him and speaking softly to him until they subsided. She told him she took her vows to him seriously, and if he wanted a divorce he would have to be the one to initiate it. She wasn't going anywhere.

At first, Richard had responded well to the medicines that treat MS. His seizures decreased in 2006, but by 2007 they were back. The drugs he was prescribed had started to lose their effectiveness. The doctors changed his meds, with some improvement in his condition, but by the end of 2007 he was having 30 to 40 seizures a month.

In 2008, Richard's brother, a retired attorney, started looking into stem cell treatments for MS, and found our clinic in Costa Rica. He offered to finance Richard's treatment with us. Richard later told me he was pretty scared when he arrived, but it didn't affect his sense of humor. He was in a treatment room being assessed by one of our staff the first time he saw me. "Either you're the janitor, or you're the guy who owns this place," he said, not very impressed with my wardrobe.

After he got more comfortable with the clinic and saw with a professional's eye the quality of the service we provide and the high scientific standards for our treatments, he made a very unusual offer. He took me aside, placed his hand on my arm, and said, "If you've got anything you've wanted to try, something new you've been thinking of experimenting with, you can try it on me." Richard was willing to try something new because everything he had tried so far hadn't worked. He was hoping for a breakthrough treatment.

"I could see the wheels turning in your head," Richard later told me. "I could see the smoke coming out of your ears."

In fact, there was something we'd been talking about for a year, but we hadn't had a patient like Richard who was willing to be our subject.

We'd been having good luck with stem cells from umbilical cords, but we knew there was another repository of cells that remained untapped: fat. As we age and begin the middle-age spread, we have fewer and fewer stem cells, many of them stored in our fat. Some researchers had had success liposuctioning fat from mice and then culturing the stem cells for treatments, but no one had yet tried it on humans.

By that time I had had many conversations with Bob Harman, DVM, MPVM, the founder and CEO of VetStem Biopharma, the first company in the United States to provide fat-derived stem cells to veterinarians for use. He told me about a dog with the equivalent of rheumatoid arthritis they had treated successfully. Rheumatoid arthritis, as I discussed at the beginning of the chapter, is essentially the same disease as multiple sclerosis—the body mounts a Th1 immune response against the joints. In multiple sclerosis, the target is the myelin sheath that surrounds the nerves.

Richard said he was willing to let us try it with him. We were the first to use these stem cells from fat tissue in humans.

We were the first to use these stem cells from fat tissue in humans.

Interview with Bob Harman, DVM, MPVM, Founder and CEO of VetStem

I met veterinarian Bob Harman in the Bahamas back in 2003. He was checking out our clinic for a friend with liver cancer. He was familiar with stem cell therapies because the year before he had founded his own company, VetStem, the first United States-based commercial veterinary stem cell company. For 15 years prior to that, he was the CEO of HTI BioServices, a preclinical research company for veterinary and human pharmaceutical development. Bob and I catch up with each other on a regular basis.

NEIL RIORDAN: What is VetStem and how has it evolved over time?

BOB HARMAN: When we first looked at the technology, I thought that using these kinds of cells therapeutically would change everything about the dogma surrounding treatment of chronic and acute disease. Adipose-fresh cells could be something that was affordable

We consulted with a plastic surgeon who was willing to work with us on the experiment. Since plastic surgeons normally treat the fat from liposuction as a waste product, we had to sterilize his equipment and be extremely careful about the way the extracted tissue was handled after the liposuction was complete. A single bacterium in the mix would ruin the material. After a thorough sterilization of the plastic surgeon's room and his equipment, Richard went in for liposuction.

We took the fat into our laboratory and digested it with enzymes, isolating the stem cells so that we could culture them for Richard's treatment. I have to admit, I wasn't that familiar with the after effects of liposuction. I told him, "You will experience some bruising," because that was the way the plastic surgeon had phrased it. I was pretty shocked when Richard raised his shirt the next day and showed me a dark purple expanse of skin three quarters of the way around his midsection from just below his chest down to his hips.

For Richard's first treatment, it took nine days to administer the mesenchymal stem cells that we had isolated from his own fat. It took that long for two reasons. First, the gold standard for testing for sterility was culturing and doable in the short term in veterinary medicine. From day one, we determined that we eventually needed an off-the-shelf product in order for the treatment to be affordable. That meant that using autologous (self-derived) fat cells would be an interim solution that allowed us to get data, intellectual property, clinical experience, market exposure, and to build credibility. But eventually, the FDA's CVM (Center for Veterinary Medicine) would have to approve the allogeneic (donor-derived) treatments just like on the human side. That was the idea from the beginning, but it has taken longer than I originally thought. We're going on 14 years now. And we have only been working on development of allogeneic cells for three years.

NR: VetStem heretofore has been providing a service to veterinarians whereby they can do a biopsy of adipose tissue from their animals, right?

BH: In all these years, we have not sold one stem cell. All we do is provide a contract service for vets. It's a service. We operate under what's called "regulatory discretion," which means that the service is low regularity priority. We met with the FDA in 2003 before providing

the cells for 10 days to ensure there was no bacterial contamination. Second, MSCs like to migrate to inflamed areas, so we wanted the inflammation from the liposuction to dissipate. His own MSCs were augmented with umbilical cord stem cells. Richard reported no side effects but little improvement early on. In retrospect, I believe that the slow pace of improvement in that first session was due to some of the cells homing to the liposuction sites. The ideal treatment would be to harvest the stem cells from the fat, send the patient home to heal completely, and then have him or her return for treatment. That's one of the problems with operating outside the United States. Most patients don't want to make two trips for what is essentially one treatment.

The cells started to work a few months later, though. The pain Richard had been having in his neck and shoulders subsided, and two months after the treatment he had to lower the volume on his hearing aid because his hearing had improved. The big progress came three months after that first treatment when suddenly his brain started to work again. He wasn't confused anymore, and his seizures subsided. Plus, he was able to have sex again. I don't think we've ever had a patient who expressed such gratitude.

treatments for any veterinarians. We meet with the FDA regularly and they have continued to say this for over ten years because the service is provided legitimately, following FDA good tissue practices (GTP) guidelines and with no problems. They have inspected us and we talk with them every year.

NR: So the veterinarian does the biopsy, takes fat tissue from the animal, and ships the sample to you for processing. You then process the tissue into digested stromal vascular fraction (SVF), or the cellular part that includes stem cells, T-regulatory cells, and endothelial precursor cells (EPCs), and then you overnight the SVF back to the vet for injection into the animal.

BH: Yes. So we don't diagnose, prescribe, or treat. We are a processing lab. We provide data and continuing education to the veterinarians so that they have informed consent and knowledge about the possibilities for these SVF cells.

NR: How many animals have been treated?

In February 2009, Richard returned to Costa Rica for a second treatment. He thought if it worked as well as the first one, he might be able to ditch the hearing aid altogether. We treated him with essentially the same protocol, and his hearing did improve. The side benefit we didn't expect was that he also started to tolerate heat better. Richard lived in Texas, which is a very hot part of the world. And he loves golf. When the MS came on, he couldn't endure being out on the golf course. After the second treatment, Richard not only went out onto the course, he started teaching golf. For the first time in four years, he was bringing money home to his family.

Although we were the first to use autologous (self-donated) fat-derived MSCs, and we had a lot of success using these cells for many years, we discovered that the robustness of these cells varies, which we found correlates (inversely) with the benefits of the treatment. In those patients with less-than-robust cells, we augmented their cells with umbilical cord MSCs. Eventually, we replaced the use of fat cells altogether in favor of umbilical cord MSCs because we could better control the quality, select for cells with the best ability to control inflammation, and, maybe most importantly,

BH: Over 12,000. Mostly horses and dogs, split about evenly, plus a couple hundred cats. We also got the opportunity to be funded by the Office of Naval Research to study adipose stem cells in therapy of wound healing primarily in the dolphin, but also have done work in the sea lion. We have published one study and are preparing a manuscript for a second paper in which we took adipose cells by liposuction from the dolphin, did a full characterization[1]—flow cytometry, all the things you do to characterize the cells—and did a blinded controlled study of those stem cells in treating skin wounds.[2] After that we became known as the "exotic animal guys." So we have now done work for multiple zoos and private collections. We're probably at 30-plus species now, including giraffes, rhinos, elands, antelopes, pilot whales, beluga whales, orcas, and penguins. There will be a segment on an education channel on the treatment of an eye problem in an injured wild caught seal. So it really is helping this wild population, in particular endangered species like the northern white rhino, when they don't respond to typical pharmaceutical therapy. This isn't something we do for profit.

reduce the time of treatment and eliminate the waiting period between harvest and treatment.

Richard and I became friends partially because we share a strong spirit of adventure, and also because we have a very similar sense of humor. He and I communicated by phone or by email several times a week. At his last treatment in May 2010, he made another unusual request.

By then, I'd decided to concentrate our research and our clinic facilities in Panama. Richard said that when he came for his fourth treatment, he wanted to swim in both the Atlantic and the Pacific Oceans in the same day. I realized that despite all my years as a competitive swimmer and a professional diver, I'd never thought of doing something like this. I told Richard yes. It was a great way to celebrate his return to health.

We started at a resort next to the Pacific that had a beautiful golf course. Richard, the guy who couldn't even find his way home from the hardware store a few years back, shot a 68, four under par. I did less well. But I made up for it that night at blackjack.

NR: You have a registry of the stem cell treatments. Have there been any serious adverse events?

BH: I think there have been none that are "likely or probably" related to the therapy [this is an FDA classification]. As you know, from the beginning we decided to be data driven, trying to get peer reviewed trials before we make recommendations. We've created our own internal library here, always trying to comply with FDA guidelines on tissue processing and handling. We operate as a tissue bank and processing bank, fully under good tissue practices. I don't think anyone else in the vet industry does that.

NR: You're about to issue a press release about your new GMP facility right? And you are in the process of being approved by the FDA for a product that would be off-the-shelf (donor-derived) and not autologous (self-derived).

BH: That's correct. We have three FDA veterinary investigational animal new drug applications. It's very similar to your investigational new drug (IND) approval on the human side. We filed for use in horses, dogs, and cats. When approved, the use will be under review

The next morning, we jumped in the Pacific for a pretty good swim, nothing too athletic for two middle-aged warriors. We changed our clothes and got on the road for the three-hour drive to the Atlantic.

When we got to the Atlantic, I think both of us were a bit underwhelmed. There was no easy way to get into the ocean from the place where we parked. We had to clamber over rocks trying to figure out the best way to enter the Atlantic. We were standing on the edge of a dock with Richard trying to estimate the depth of the water, hemming and hawing, and I thought we should just go for it. I jumped in and told him the water was beautiful, even though it was not exactly crystal clear like the water we'd splashed in a few hours before.

"Come on, coach!" I yelled.

He hesitated for a few moments more and took the plunge.

We only stayed in the Atlantic a few minutes, but we were grinning the whole time. This was a victory for both of us—for me and my research, and for Richard, his family, and the rest of his life. The next time he visited his of the FDA. We created what we believe is the only veterinary-specific, GMP-compliant cell production facility in the world. After approval, we will have cells available "out of a bottle" in the freezer at the clinic. The advantage to allogeneic (donor-derived), is that the animals will not have to undergo anesthesia and fat biopsy, and then wait a day or so for treatment. The cells will be available at lower cost, with no surgery, and available for same day injection.

NR: What conditions are vets using the cells for now, and for what indications will the allogeneic cells be used?

BH: In both the dog and horse, by far the primary use is in orthopedics—osteoarthritis; tendon, ligament injury, and joint therapy; sometimes bone repair—for acute and chronic orthopedic diseases. The first allogeneic dog product will be for osteoarthritis in the dog—intraarticular (into the joint spaces) injections for the treatment of chronic degenerative joint disease.[3] We are expecting approval in 2018 for that. Our commercial marketing partner, Aratana Therapeutics, will deliver the product to market for us.

neurologist, the doctor was amazed. Although the MRI showed Richard still had the lesions on his brain, he'd moved from primary progressive MS to relapsing-remitting MS, the version of the disease that has the fewest episodes of pain, seizures, and confusion.

Speaking of coaches, Sam Harrell was a Texas High School Football Hall of Fame coach who was diagnosed with multiple sclerosis in 2005 at age 50. He first noticed something was wrong when his vision changed. About two years later his lower legs were affected and walking became difficult. He soon needed to use a golf cart to get out on the field and became extremely sensitive to the heat. By age 55 he had to retire from the career he loved due to his loss of mobility and coordination.

At that time Sam was only able to take small steps, shuffling his feet—even turning around was a big effort. He would focus his attention on the movement of each leg as he walked and had to concentrate on how he was going to get from point A to point B. His days were filled with routine. He'd

NR: You have had some cases of dogs with a rheumatoid arthritis-like disease that recovered with SVF treatment.

BH: Most dogs that are treated have osteoarthritis, but dogs can also get immune-mediated polyarthritis. They don't have RA factors like humans, but the disease is very similar. It's systemic. There is an attack of the inside of the joint by the immune system. And we treat it systemically as well (by IV injection). We have seen multiple dogs with this condition. We get reports back from the owner or the veterinarian. They see improvements clinically. When we see something like that, it has real potential to cross over into the human field. You have treated RA cases with a substantial degree of success since our early discussions about our applications in dogs.

NR: Yes, our first RA patient had a fantastic response to SVF injections of her own fat. That was the beginning of our use of SVF in patients with autoimmune disease. You and I have coauthored papers on this.[4,5,6,7]

wake up, eat breakfast, read his bible, watch television, and answer email. Then he'd look up at the clock and it would read 10:30 a.m. "Well, in another hour and a half I can make myself a sandwich. That will take about 30 minutes. Then in five more hours Cindy will be home and at least there will be someone else in the house," he told himself. They would go to bed around nine or ten o'clock and wake up the next day and do it all over again. The monotony of his routine wore on him. He felt an immense lack of purpose in life and became depressed.

Around that time, a friend of Sam's told him about Richard Humphries' recovery after stem cell treatment. Sam knew he had to meet Richard, so he tracked him down and invited him to lunch. After hearing his story and seeing Richard's results in person, he decided to contact our clinic.

Sam came down for two treatments but did not gain impressive benefits. And yet, he knew something was happening inside and was drawn back for another treatment. After his third treatment, everything changed. His transformation didn't happen overnight, but he slowly gained movement, balance, and coordination. He could lift his leg again, then walk, and

BH: Yes. Interesting aside, we started out by injecting the therapeutic cells into the injured tendon or joint. But in our CE course, we educate about how cells work. Based on Arnold Caplan's work, we taught about the migratory nature of these cells. So I was telling small animal vets to inject the cells into the joint, but they began asking about intravenous injections. The literature supported the safety of such injections. Those veterinarians—every one of them—would tell us that the dogs did better, faster, and it appeared to have more longevity of effect when given both intravenously and intra-articularly. Nearly 100 percent of treating veterinarians do both now. I think we help the dogs feel better right away by reducing global inflammation by the IV therapy.

NR: What do you think are the potential applications for MSCs, from what you've seen, in the animal world as well as human?

BH: Clearly from the observation that an autoimmune disease—the polyarthritis—can be transferred to use for multiple sclerosis, lupus, rheumatoid arthritis, and other autoimmune diseases. We have seen immune-mediated skin diseases in dogs as well as

eventually even ride his bike. Before long, he was back to coaching. "I'm the luckiest guy in the world," Sam said. "It's given me my life back. I'm coaching again, standing out in 100 degree heat every day and not riding the golf cart." He no longer needs to wear a brace to walk or use a walker—he can run, jump, and turn on a dime. He doesn't have to think about moving from one place to another—he just moves. He went from taking a maximum of 200 steps a day to clocking 10,000 steps a day on his Fitbit®. "I tell people I'm 60, but I feel 40."

> ***I'm the luckiest guy in the world," Sam said. "It's given me my life back."***

Sam's experience with stem cells is a sharp contrast to his experience with conventional medical treatment of multiple sclerosis. "I had never heard about the possibility of improving when I went to doctors in the United States," he said. Doctors told him, "Let's keep taking this medication so that you might get worse at a slower rate." The difference stem cells have made in Sam's life is remarkable. He has since been back for two more treatments, lupus and conjunctivitis. UC Davis recently published a study on the use of lacrimal-gland injection of stem cells for conjunctivitis in dogs[8]. I personally think they could have given the cells IV, and it probably would have done the same thing.

UC Davis also treats gingivostomatitis, a horrible dental disease in cats marked by severe and chronic inflammation of the gingiva (gums) and mucosa. Standard treatment is to remove all of the teeth. A few IV stem cell treatments have been shown[9] to turn off the autoimmune disease.[10]

IV therapy can turn off gut inflammation in dogs with inflammatory bowel disease , which is very similar to inflammatory bowel disease in humans. Atopic dermatitis in dogs is another area of stem cell therapy.

In cats, kidney disease is a big one. I don't suspect that this disease is too different across species. We have treated close to 200 cats with this disease and are working on a manuscript.

which have continued to improve his condition. "I think it's the next huge wave of medicine, myself," Sam says.

Holly Huber had big dreams and aspirations. She was well, active, and didn't have health concerns because she was living a health-conscious life in San Diego. But when she was diagnosed with multiple sclerosis in 2004, an explanation for the years of clumsiness, forgetfulness, dizziness, and weight loss that had gone unnoticed or had been explained away by doctors finally came to light. Prior to her diagnosis, Holly had noticed a loss of sensation when urinating, along with difficulty viewing her computer screen, and she knew something was wrong. She had told herself that she'd get it checked out "when this big work project is finished." And so, more time passed. She had seen a few doctors but was never quite sure what to ask. She was misdiagnosed for quite some time.

When Holly finally had an MRI done with contrast in 2004, a neurologist was able to diagnose her with progressive MS. "He rattled off a list of drug

You know, if I speculate too much it sounds like snake oil. It's not easy to figure out which of these diseases are worth putting the effort on. There is a lot of discussion about ocular diseases, corneal injuries, retinal disease. I know a vet group in Israel that is treating retinal degeneration—similar to macular degeneration—with sub-retinal stem cell injections in the dog. There is clearly evidence for treating or preventing sepsis. I think the emergency room is a place you can envision using a migratory repair cell in patients with multiple organ and tissue trauma, just like they do today by hanging a bag of fluids with steroids as the standard of care.

NR: Drowning in opportunity, right? You've got to pick your battles and run down one track or another.

BH: True, and you've done the same, Neil, with clinical trials. We have tried to do the same. We just published a blinded, placebo-controlled, 93-dog, nine-site randomized clinical trial.[11] It's the first and largest one done in veterinary regenerative medicine. And we just initiated a 240-dog, 17-site trial. So that kind of data, and trials you are doing in Panama,

names during a very short appointment, saying, 'Go read about them. There's one medication I can give a patient on Friday, and she has flu-like symptoms over the weekend, but she's okay to take care of her kids on Monday.'" That was the extent of the visit. Holly was so distraught that she cancelled her upcoming vacation to Australia.

From there her MS progressed rapidly, and within a few months Holly collapsed on her floor, unable to walk. She went through all the standard MS medications, none of which worked to halt her disease progression and most of which left her with side effects. She spent $400,000 on medications over the course of four years.

When she came to our clinic in 2008, she was in constant pain from the numbness in her limbs. She could no longer have intelligent conversations and was often at a loss for words. She fell more times than she could count and stayed barricaded in her home. She felt as though she had wax paper over her eyes due to the optic neuritis caused by one of her brain lesions.

After her first stem cell treatment Holly began to feel her arms and legs again. Her balance improved. She could gargle again—a benefit only is the only way to escape the stigma of being snake oil. Papers are so hugely important because the industry gets accused of treating patients unnecessarily and without data. It's the way it is with new technology. But as we get better data, pharmaceutical companies gain interest, and vet schools add programs in regenerative medicine. Ten years ago they said I was crazy, inappropriate, and didn't have data.

NR: In Panama we just finished our multiple sclerosis trial, with 1800 data points per patient. It's a safety trial with efficacy signal. The next one is a 33-patient autism trial with one-year follow-up. After that is our rheumatoid arthritis trial.

BH: Obviously, you are from the United States and you have a perception of quality standards. I have visited about a dozen offshore clinics in the past decade, but there is no place I would go to or send family to except your facility. As you know, I brought my own daughter down to be treated because I had the comfort level in your SOPs (standards operating procedures), clean rooms, hoods, and staff. I have a problem with many kit manufacturers and in-clinic systems. Literally hundreds of doctors' offices that do SVF

MS patients would appreciate. Since her first visit, she has been back thirteen times. She now walks, thinks clearly, and is able to maintain a normal lifestyle driving, cooking, climbing stairs, and flying on her own. "You changed my life and gave me a future," she told me. "Everything was so fogged when I was diagnosed and on all those medications. There was a moment when everything became clear again—all of my hopes and dreams."

"You changed my life and gave me a future," she told me. "Everything was so fogged when I was diagnosed and on all those medications. There was a moment when everything became clear again—all of my hopes and dreams."

therapies do not even have an SOP written down. People are trained over the phone or in a few hours. As you know, it takes months to years to train qualified people to handle tissue. You took that standard with you to the Bahamas, Costa Rica, and Panama. We do the same thing here. There are dozens of vet clinics across the country that do in-clinic without a hood, no sterility tracks, no cell counts. You followed that same pattern of having really good release criteria, data, cell counts, and sterility checks. It's not that I'm worried about the cell therapies, it's that the clinicians are dangerous if they do not follow high quality standards.

NR: There are about five cases that keep getting rehashed. I could say that all of them are due to bad medical practice.

BH: We have 400+ SOPs here. It's cumbersome, but it's the right way to do medicine. We don't even let a small animal clinician use our products in the field unless they take our continuing education course and pass the exam.

NR: What is your overall take on the stem cell world?

BH: When I started in 2002 and I saw a beating heart in a dish at a stem cell meeting in San Diego, I thought, "Oh, this is really easy. All you have to do is make this tissue and put it anywhere." Back then that's how we thought these cells worked. But over the next five years, the Arnold Caplans of the world went from talking about creating tissue to talking about the trophic effects. I just followed what the animals were telling us. When you see that the cells aren't working like you think, but they are giving you a really positive outcome, you follow the clinical evidence, collect data, and do good studies. All of that tells you how it appears to be working, and shows you how to change your approach to use those mechanisms better. Follow the patients, go look at the science, and then come back to the patients. To reverse the old cliché, I think it goes from bedside to bench.

Jason Upshaw was diagnosed with MS over twenty years ago. He first came to our clinic in Costa Rica in 2008 with relapsing-remitting MS. He boarded the plane to Costa Rica on a wheelchair, unable to walk even a few feet without exhaustion. "I still had a lot of numbness and tingling," he said. After his first stem cell treatment he was able to walk off the plane, collect his luggage, and walk out to the parking lot. "It improved my life in one treatment," he recalled. His numbness and tingling gradually faded, his fatigue improved.

Two years later his fatigue began to increase. "I wanted to get a head start on it, so I came back," he said. "Before I got to rock bottom, where I was before I went to Costa Rica, I wanted to get back down to try to stay ahead of the curve." By then our clinic had moved to Panama, so he flew down to our new clinic there. "I have been coming back ever since," he said. For Jason, periodic treatments and not pushing his known limits of exertion keep his symptoms at bay. "If I'm smart and listen to my body, I really don't have any problems," he said.

Mesenchymal Stem Cell Treatment for Multiple Sclerosis

Multiple sclerosis (MS) is a chronic and progressively debilitating disease in which the immune system wears down the protective myelin sheath that insulates the nerves. Nerve damage may be observed by magnetic resonance imaging (MRI) as plaques in the nerves of the brain, spinal cord, or the optical system. Symptoms include visual, motor, sensory, balance, and cognitive problems.

Certain medications that have some efficacy in modulating the immune system have been incorporated as the standard of care for MS.[5] However, the benefits are lost as the disease progresses, and they do not help with regeneration of the nervous tissues that have already been damaged.[6]

Mesenchymal stem cells (MSCs) secrete anti-inflammatory, antifibrotic, immunomodulatory, and regenerative molecules that stimulate the repair and regeneration of inflamed or damaged tissues, and as such are being tested as an option for the treatment of various conditions.[7,8] In the case of multiple sclerosis, MSC secretions stimulate the body to produce more T-regulatory cells (key for keeping the immune system in check), further modulate the immune system by decreasing the activity of dendritic cells (immune system activators), and exert a direct protective effect on the central nervous system.[9]

Treating MS patients with MSCs has been shown to be a feasible alternative in animal and human studies. MS mouse models have reported improvements in neurological functions and on repair rates, which illustrates the potential for MSCs to modulate an overactive immune system[10] and to reduce inflammation.[11] An early study that caught my eye was published in 2003 by researchers from Northwestern University's Feinberg School of Medicine.[12] The 21 patients in the trial, ages 20 to 53, had relapsing-remitting MS that

Jason's wife Michelle has been with Jason through every step. She is impressed by our facilities.

When it comes to MS, people often ask, "How many treatments does it take to get me over my disease?" We are trying to push a rock up a hill. People have different sized rocks and different sized hills. When the activated T cells are diminished, they can no longer attack the myelin in the brain. When the myelin is not being attacked, the body has an amazing ability to remyelinate nerves that have not been denuded. The smaller the rock and the smaller the hill, the fewer treatments are necessary to remyelinate the nerves.

had not responded to at least six months of standard treatment. The study showed reversal of neurological dysfunction in early-stage MS patients by killing off their own immune stem cells with chemotherapy (while also killing off the bone marrow), and reinfusing previously harvested bone marrow stem cells to restore the bone marrow. This treatment in effect "reset" the subject's immune system—depleting it of the activated T cell population that could penetrate the blood-brain barrier. The disease stabilized in all patients, and 81 percent of patients improved by at least one point on a disability scale. This validated the fact that immune modulation can shut down MS, without affecting CNS myelin/neuronal damage directly—most importantly it demonstrated that remyelination occurs naturally and that remyelination should *not* be the focus of MS therapy. In 2011, researchers from the University of Cambridge completed a phase I/II clinical trial with 10 patients and showed that treatment with autologous MSCs was safe.[13]

A recent systematic review of 83 studies reported 24 applications of MSC treatment for MS.[14] The progression of MS has been shown to slow or stabilize for most patients in the first year after MSC treatment, with no serious adverse events.[15] Improvements in vision[16] and in disability scores[17] have also been reported. Several MS clinical trials are currently approved and recruiting for MSC treatment in many countries, including the United States,[18,19,20] France,[21] Spain,[22] as well as at the Karolinska Institute in Sweden.[23]

Patients with MS have been safely treated at the Stem Cell Institute since 2010 with no adverse effects, and the group has consistently published case studies and proposed the use of MSCs to treat MS.[24] Preliminary results of our completed clinical trials, to be published shortly, as of this writing suggest significant differences between pre- and post-treatment responses to the Multiple Sclerosis Impact Scale questionnaire.[25]

Chapter Eight

HEART FAILURE TURNAROUNDS — A NEW APPROACH

Daniel Wills, like most people, didn't think much about his heart. There was no history of heart disease in his family. At the age of 45, Daniel was still an athlete, running daily as he had when he was a cross country star in high school. He had no trouble keeping up with the younger jet mechanics at the hangar where he worked at O'Hare International Airport outside Chicago.

One crisp fall day in 2005 Daniel went on a short jog, but when he got home it seemed as though he couldn't recover. He felt nauseous and "kind of blah" instead of experiencing the usual endorphin high. "I didn't suspect anything," Daniel remembered. "I thought, 'Oh, it's one of those days when it's just not there.' I didn't tell anyone." That night he went to bed sweating and feeling queasy, but the next morning when he woke up refreshed, Daniel brushed the whole episode aside.

Three weeks later when the same symptoms recurred, Daniel could not deny that his body was sending him some powerful signals. He called his doctor who told him to get checked out by a cardiologist. He was diagnosed with congestive heart failure, a fatal condition in which the heart pumps less blood than the body needs to survive. The failing heart still pumps, but as the heart's blood flow slows down, the blood returning through the veins backs up, causing congestion in the tissues. People with congestive heart failure get short of breath and tire rapidly when they exert themselves.

"If you don't get this valve repaired, you could die within six months," Daniel's cardiologist said.

He sat there for a few minutes trying to absorb this new reality. A diagnosis of congestive heart failure would be a shock to anyone, but it's a rare diagnosis for someone so young and healthy. The long-term prognosis for him was shocking too—his doctor told him that people diagnosed with this form of heart failure have a life expectancy of only seven to eight years. "I could feel my face flushing. I was overwhelmed like I'd never felt before."

When he left the cardiologist's office to start back to work, Daniel had to pull over and rest a minute in the Walmart parking lot. "It was likely that I wouldn't die tomorrow, but I knew I wouldn't live to see eighty," Daniel said. "I had a thirteen-year-old daughter and an eighteen-year-old son." His new reality weighed heavy on him.

Daniel scheduled the surgery for three weeks from the date of his diagnosis. The heart valve repair was successful, but his recovery was very slow. A neighbor friend came over every day to take Daniel out for a walk, but the walks were labored. "This thing changed my life." He altered his diet to mostly vegetables and very lean meats and stopped drinking beer, but despite all these changes he couldn't build his abilities back up to where he was before.

"I couldn't sustain exercise at first," Daniel said. "But some months after the operation I found I could bike, although not as far as I wanted to go."

Despite his rigorous discipline, the repair of his heart valve hadn't made much of a change in Daniel's condition. Doctors gauge the health of the heart by watching the readings of the heart's left ventricle ejection fraction, a measurement of the volume of blood pumped out of the left ventricles, or heart chamber, during a heartbeat. In a normal, healthy heart, the ejection fraction ranges between 50 and 70. At the time of Daniel's diagnosis, his ejection fraction was 30, half the healthy amount. Three years after the operation, his ejection fraction numbers continued to decline. He dropped from 28 to 26. Sleep was increasingly difficult for him, as it is for many congestive heart failure patients, because when they lie down fluid collects in the lungs and causes shortness of breath.

The fact that he'd been so healthy all his life before the heart condition actually worked against him getting a heart transplant, the next step in his treatment. Heart patients qualify for a heart transplant when their ejection fraction hits 30, but Daniel was still active when his fell to 20, so the doctors hadn't yet put him on the transplant list.

"I asked my doctor where we were at. How could we change this? He said, 'All we can do is manage your condition until you qualify for a heart transplant,'" Daniel recalled. Many people die waiting for a heart transplant.

Daniel's marriage collapsed, and he became depressed and started seeing a psychiatrist. In fact, the whole Wills family was in despair about Daniel, who they thought might die at any time. In 2008, Daniel's mom went online searching for something—anything—that might offer Daniel another chance. What she found was that prestigious medical institutions such as the MD Anderson Center in Texas and Cedars-Sinai in Los Angeles were having success treating congestive heart failure—a disease that stubbornly defied all pharmaceutical and surgical attempts at a cure— with stem cells.

My staff and I started treating congestive heart failure shortly after I opened my clinic in Costa Rica in 2006. Our first patient was a physician from Texas whom I'll call Dr. Bill. He was a man like Daniel—in his early 50s and slowly dying of congestive heart failure—one for whom doctors held little hope of long-term survival. Congestive heart failure has many causes, but in Dr. Bill's case, his genes were the root of his trouble. His mother had died of heart failure at the age of 24, and other family members had also succumbed.

When he first contacted our clinic, Dr. Bill hadn't been able to practice medicine for some time. His ejection fraction was 30, and he was on the heart transplant list, but it was a procedure he wanted to avoid because he knew it was no guarantee of a cure. A heart transplant is extremely painful, invasive, and dangerous, and would have cost him at minimum a quarter of a million dollars—that is, if a suitable heart could be found. Hearts are transplanted from people who are brain dead but still on life support, and they have to match the tissue type of the recipient to reduce the potential of the body rejecting the new heart. It's a highly selective process. After the transplant, he would endure a lifetime of immunosuppressant medications to prevent him from rejecting the foreign heart. Taking drugs to suppress the immune system increases the risk of opportunistic infections that, because of the medication, the body would be too weak to fight off.

He called our clinic a number of times asking to be treated with stem cells. We hadn't treated a heart failure patient up until that time, so we declined his request a few times. He believed, however, that stem cells could heal his heart. He was persistent. When he finally got through to me, he told me, "I am going to die waiting for a heart. I will never get a new heart due to my age. Please treat me. I don't care if I die trying—I am going to die anyway."

At first we were skeptical about using stem cells to repair the heart. There was some research on this. In 2003, scientists published papers that described how adult stem cells circulating in blood can be used to repair hearts, and that it is not necessary to take the stem cells from bone marrow.[1] In 2004, they found that stem cells use different methods to morph into the two kinds of cells needed to restore heart function. In animal studies, research showed that to make new heart muscle cells, the human stem cells fuse onto cardiac cells to produce new muscle cells called myocytes.[2] But to form new blood vessel cells the stem cells differentiate, or mature, by themselves to provide new endothelial cells that patch vessel damage. There was a study in Germany that showed that, when injected into mice that had had heart attacks, umbilical cord blood stem cells were drawn to the damaged areas where they stimulated the growth of new blood vessels.[3] Other studies conducted in Germany and the Netherlands showed how stem cells could transform into cardiomyocytes (heart muscle cells), but there hadn't been a reported case of a human patient being treated for heart failure with stem cells. Still, Dr. Bill's situation was desperate and, based on our experience treating other diseases with stem cells, we knew with a high degree of certainty that our treatment would do him no harm.

We decided to use umbilical cord blood CD34+ and mesenchymal stem cells from the umbilical cord matrix. We knew, from experience and research, that CD34+ cells would home to damaged tissue and to hypoxic (low-oxygen) tissue. We had seen the way these cells arrived at the tissue damaged by low oxygen and then released factors that stimulated new blood vessel growth (angiogenesis).

Many studies have shown that new blood vessels, called collateral vessels, can help out a failing heart. To encourage the cells to do this work, we also added intravenous vitamin C after the umbilical cord MSC injections. This was based on the results of another study that had been conducted at Harvard Medical School that showed vitamin C could promote differentiation of stem cells into heart muscle cells.[4]

Mesenchymal Stem Cells for Congestive Heart Failure

Congestive heart failure (CHF) is a disabling and potentially deadly condition in which the heart weakens and cannot pump blood at a fast enough rate to meet the needs of the body. As a consequence, the flow of oxygen and nutrients to organs and tissue is reduced. Common symptoms of CHF are fatigue, shortness of breath, chest pain, and a limited capacity for physical exercise. CHF usually develops following an injury to cardiac tissue, for example after an infarction, or heart attack. The resulting acute inflammation may become chronic—elevated levels of inflammation markers[5,6] and cytokines[7] have been reported in CHF patients. For many heart failure patients, heart transplantation becomes the only treatment option after medications fail to increase ejection fraction.

Mesenchymal stem cells (MSCs) have properties that make them a viable option for CHF treatment. MSCs exert potent anti-inflammatory activities, regardless of tissue of origin.[8,9] Mechanistically, MSCs suppress inflammation and modulate immune reaction through the secretion of cytokines.[10,11,12] MSCs can also differentiate into cardiac-like cells[13] and promote angiogenesis, delivering nutrients to the affected area and allowing regeneration.[14] MSCs have been shown to stimulate myocardial regeneration, to inhibit pathological remodeling, and to stimulate angiogenesis in cases of ischemic heart failure.[15,16] The administration of

MSCs post infarct (after heart attack) has been demonstrated to decrease the production of the inflammatory molecule tumor necrosis factor alpha (TNF-α) and to regulate inflammatory and anti-inflammatory cytokines, correlating with therapeutic benefits.[17]

Over 73 CHF animal studies have used MSC treatment,[18] showing that they are effective in models of CHF.[19,20,21] Treatment with MSCs for heart failure has also been shown to be safe in clinical settings,[22,23] with significant reduction in reversible defects and improvement in ventricular function.[24] The results of several randomized clinical trials have been published in the last decade; a recent review of 23 trials (1,255 participants) concludes that there is evidence that bone marrow MSCs have a beneficial clinical effect in the long term.[25] Another review of 31 clinical trials (1,521 participants) reports a significant reduction in mortality and hospitalization, as well as an improvement in quality of life.[26] In 2010, our group reported positive results in quality of life questionnaires as well as chemical and physical improvements in a three-year follow-up of a patient treated for heart failure.[27] In a very recent study led by my colleague Amit Patel, MD at the University of Utah, 18 patients receiving umbilical cord MSC infusion showed improvements in heart failure, as demonstrated by an increase in the ejection fraction of the left ventricle.[28] Studies are still ongoing to establish the therapeutic effects of MSC treatment for CHF, to understand the mechanisms at the molecular level, and to find which type of stem cell is ideal for cardiac diseases.[29,30,31,32]

Before he finished the series of injections, Dr. Bill reported that he had more energy and less shortness of breath. When the treatment was complete, he said that he felt so good he wanted to visit a doctor friend in Panama before going home. I had heard great things about Panama and asked him if he minded if I tagged along. He agreed.

We flew to Panama and met his old friend Jorge Paz-Rodriguez, MD. We also met Lic. Rodolfo Fernandez, owner of the largest clinical laboratory company in Panama. The three of us hit it off instantly. Dr Paz, called Georgie by his friends, and Rodolfo were very interested in what we were doing in Costa Rica. They said they wanted to come up and see our operation. Sure enough, six weeks later they jumped on a plane and came to visit me in Costa Rica. I recall them saying in unison, "We need to get this in Panama." They went back to Panama and hired an attorney to look into the legal situation regarding stem cells in Panama. What they found was a law that had been passed in Panama a few years earlier. The law, which was passed in 2004, simply banned the use of embryonic stem cells, and allowed physicians to treat patients with adult stem cells, including umbilical cord stem cells, as long as the patient gave informed consent. Shortly thereafter, I took another trip to Panama and we started planning to set up operations there. We met with the Director of the City of Knowledge. Ultimately, we set up a small lab there and began operations in 2007. Georgie and Rodolfo are partners in our operation there. Georgie is the medical director of the clinic and Rodolfo is the laboratory director.

While visiting Panama, Dr. Bill and I made the obligatory visit to the Panama Canal, just a short drive from downtown Panama City. The Miraflores Visitor Center and museum stands at the side of one of the locks on the Pacific side of the canal and is a good place to observe the ships as they make the passage between two oceans. The observation deck is on the top of the building on the third floor. Excited to see the ships, we climbed the flights of stairs to the observation deck. As soon as we got to the top, Dr. Bill paused and put his hand on my shoulder as we gazed at the huge containership in the lock.

"This is incredible," he said.

"Yes, this canal is an amazing feat of engineering, and this is a great view of the ships," I replied.

"No, not that—I'm not short of breath!"

That was twelve days after his first treatment.

Dr. Bill went back to Texas and had an echocardiogram four months after his treatment. His ejection fraction had gone from 30 to 52. His cardiologist didn't quite believe it. An improvement like that never happens in heart failure patients. A month later, his doctor repeated the test and found his ejection fraction had gone up to 55. Dr. Bill has since returned to work and enjoys a relatively normal life as of this writing.

As far as we can tell, when we treated Dr. Bill it was the first time congestive heart failure had been dramatically improved using umbilical cord cells in a human. By the time Daniel's mother was searching the Internet for a solution three years later, she found information on the clinical trials and experiments on animals. At MD Anderson, Dr. Edward Yeh's experiments on heart attack-induced mice showed again that the CD34+ cells survived in the left chamber of the heart for twelve months.[33] While they lingered there promoting new blood vessel formation, ejection fraction increased from 37 to 50 after the treatment. In another MD Anderson research project led by Dr. Yeh, he and his team discovered a "sticky" protein that helped adult stem cells fuse with heart muscle cells to grow new cells that would repair the damaged organ.[34]

But while these researchers are still conducting their investigations, we have since treated 26 more people with congestive heart failure. All but two of them have had positive responses. One of those successes is Daniel.

Daniel's mom had found many clinical trials underway researching the efficacy of this exciting new treatment, but Daniel wasn't interested in participating in a clinical trial, even if he qualified. In a clinical trial, half the patients are treated and half get a placebo, or false treatment, so that scientists can compare the difference between treated patients and those who are not treated. Without any kind of treatment, Daniel was sure he wouldn't last many more years. He didn't want to risk being in the placebo group. Instead, he and his mom found our clinic.

After we accepted Daniel as a patient, he took money out of his retirement fund to finance his trip to the clinic. Then he called his family to tell them what he was going to do. Although his brother was skeptical, ten days after Daniel's announcement, Bryan and his wife decided that they would accompany Daniel when he came to get his treatment. His parents decided to come along too.

At the clinic, our understanding of stem cells and how they help the heart repair had grown dramatically since our first case with Dr. Bill. Research performed on hamsters in the United States by Dr. Te-Chung Lee changed the way we looked at treating heart disease. Dr. Lee did an interesting study on hamsters that had heart failure.[35] He had noticed that although a very small percentage (one to two percent) of cells injected into the vein of animals were actually found in the heart, CHF symptoms improved. He designed what I consider a groundbreaking experiment to discover what was happening. For the experiment he used a hamster model of heart failure, which is considered by many to be clinically identical to human heart failure. His team injected one set of animals with MSCs into the hamstring muscle; they had previously demonstrated that cells injected there would stay there and not travel to other parts of the body, including the heart.

Additionally, they collected the growth medium that the cells were grown in (typically called the supernatant) and injected it into the hamsters' hamstrings. The liquid in which they were culturing the cells was rich in trophic factors—the chemicals in the bloodstream that encourage healthy cell growth. When either the cells or the culture medium was injected into the hamstrings, the hearts of the hamsters got better. So it wasn't that the cells necessarily needed to become heart cells, or that they even had to be injected intravenously—the cell-secreted trophic factors, whether from implanted cells or from the injections of only the trophic factors, would migrate to where they were needed and stimulate repair of the heart. The treated animals had improved heart function, decreased heart cell death, decreased damaged tissue, and an increased number of repairs in the heart.

Daniel received stem cell treatment over the course of five days. His treatment was the same, morning and afternoon. "And between times, we got to tour Costa Rica!" Daniel said, noting that it was one of the best vacations his family ever had.

As he headed home we told him, as we tell all our heart patients, don't expect big changes right away. Sometimes it takes up to six months to feel a difference. Yet we were very optimistic about Daniel because he was relatively young and, besides his heart, very healthy. We told him he might begin to experience some positive changes in as little as eight weeks.

Sure enough, eight weeks later Daniel started to notice he had more energy during the day and that he wasn't having breathing issues anymore. The big test, however, was the day that Daniel went to see his cardiologist for his regularly scheduled check-up.

Daniel had been apprehensive about telling his doctor about being treated with stem cells. A month before he was scheduled to fly down for treatment at our clinic, he had an appointment with his doctor. He was going to tell him what he was about to do, but he feared that the doctor might be so alarmed that he'd fire Daniel as a patient. Would the doctor forbid him from doing it? Just as Daniel was girding up for the battle, he got a call from the doctor's office informing him that his doctor had slipped in the bathtub and had to cancel his appointments for some time to come. When Daniel next saw his doctor, he'd already received his stem cell treatment.

Daniel's previous echocardiogram in January had been pretty grim—it was the one that showed his ejection fraction to be 26. Daniel looked on with concern, trying to read his doctor's face as he listened to Daniel's heart. He feared that the doctor sensed Daniel's condition was worsening. He ordered an echocardiogram and told Daniel he wanted him to take it right away, that day.

"Now I'm really nervous," Daniel recalled thinking. "What did he hear?"

Normally it took the doctor a few weeks to get back to him after he received the results of an echocardiogram. Daniel was so nervous about the outcome that he didn't pick up when he saw his doctor's number on his cell phone.

"Dan, we got your echo results," his cardiologist said. "I think you're going to be really pleased. Your echo came back with a 40 percent ejection fraction."

"Holy crap!" Daniel said out loud. "That's really good!"

He was scheduled for a follow-up call with our clinic, and shortly before the appointment he faxed a copy of his echocardiogram, which showed him having some ejection fraction numbers as high as 45. When I saw it, I knew I wanted to speak with him. His first question was a bit of a surprise.

"How do you know that the stem cells are causing this improvement?" Daniel asked.

"There are some cases of spontaneous remission in people with your condition, but the vast majority of those are chronic alcoholics who quit drinking. Most people do not get better in a six-month time frame for no reason," I told him. "You could ask any cardiologist in the world. You typically do not go from an ejection fraction of 26 to 45 on your own."

As Dr. Lee's work had helped to clarify, the heart was repairing itself by being "kickstarted" by the secreted trophic factors that encouraged the growth of new, healthy tissue in an ailing heart.

Morris Gray was diagnosed with heart failure over twenty years ago. He had 11 stents put in his heart, of which the last three blocked an artery and triggered a heart attack. Four years later he had an EKG and a nuclear scan, and his doctor told him there was nothing more he could do for Morris. A friend of his from Corpus Christi, Texas told him about our stem cell facilities in Panama. He looked into it and decided to come down for treatment in October 2011. "I didn't feel anything for 30 days," Morris said. "Then I started feeling better. I really felt good."

> ***Morris's doctor asked him, "What have you done? You have a normal EKG. You've never had one of those before."***

Morris went back for another EKG in January 2012, and his doctor asked him, "What have you done? You have a normal EKG. You've never had one of those before."

Morris hadn't told his doctor about the stem cell treatment. "Do you think I ought to tell him?" he asked his wife. She said yes. When Morris told his doctor about the treatment, the doctor looked shocked. "How did they do it?" he asked. Morris explained the procedure to him.

Morris's next three EKGs were normal. He received another stem cell treatment that repaired his kidneys, unexpectedly. "My kidneys have been bad my whole life, but now they're fine," Morris said.

The turnarounds these heart patients like Daniel, Dr. Bill, and Morris experienced seem nothing short of miraculous. Rigorous studies like those being performed by my friend and colleague Dr. Amit Patel at the University of Miami hopefully one day will lead to effective cell/trophic factor therapy being broadly available in the United States and around the world.

Chapter Nine

FRAILTY OF AGING—REVERSING THE INEVITABLE

Getting old sucks!

As we age our bodies undergo, at varying rates, a series of changes that move us away from homeostasis—or perfect biological balance—and toward a decreased ability to adapt to both internal and external stress, which leaves us more vulnerable to disease. In some people the effects of aging are pronounced, characterizing them as frail—with decreased strength, endurance, physiologic function, and activity, all associated with poor health outcomes. Perhaps you have known people who were dependent on others for their everyday needs—shopping, cooking, and caring for themselves. These are the hallmarks of frailty of aging.

Frailty as a consequence of aging is a major health concern. Rather than an inevitable outcome in the elderly, frailty has recently been considered a medical condition. Frailty is defined as a clinical syndrome with three or more of the following criteria: unintentional weight loss, self-reported exhaustion, weakness, slow walking speed, and low physical activity.[1] There is no specific treatment for frailty,[2] though exercise, nutrition changes, and hormonal therapy have been proposed to delay further deterioration.[3] Loss of skeletal muscle mass (sarcopenia)[4] is driven by inflammation and contributes to weakness and weight loss associated with frailty. In particular, changes in inflammatory cytokines (chemical "messengers" such as interleukins, tumor necrosis factors, and insulin-like growth factors) are linked with sarcopenia.[5]

One cause for frailty of aging may be the decreased capacity of the body's organ systems to perform under stress, a function known as organ reserve. The body's pool of mesenchymal stem cells (MSCs), as discussed in chapter 5, is depleted in number and robustness with age. Each person is born with a certain number of adult stem cells. This number can be thought of as the amount of money in a bank account. A person "withdraws" money as needed throughout life. As in real life, not all stem cell bank accounts are created equal. Some people are born rich while others are born poor. Most people, however, can be thought of as middle class when it comes to the amount of stem cells they have.

This fact helps to explain why some people are able to enjoy health and longevity despite very unhealthy lifestyles while other people may enjoy neither robust health nor longevity despite healthy lifestyles. In other words, some people are able to "spend" their stem cells more extravagantly than others simply because they have more to spend. Most people fall somewhere in the middle—both the length and the quality of our lives may be influenced to some degree by our choice of lifestyle. Environmental factors also play a key role in determining how rapidly one's bank account of stem cells is depleted.

As an example, you probably know someone who's 80 and looks 60 and someone else who is 40 and looks 60. Think of Dick Clark for the former. I'll let you choose the latter.

Even under ideal circumstances, stem cells continually diminish with age. Our stem cells exist in every part of the body to repair damage such as broken bones, cuts and bruises, inflammation, radiological and chemical exposure, etc., all of which require stem cells for healing. You may draw on your bank account, like going to an ATM machine, whenever you need to do so until you run out of stem cells. Depending upon how you live your life, and whether you were born with a large or small bank account, after a certain point you may or may not be able to withdraw from your account.

The ATM works quickly and efficiently when someone has a large number of stem cells in the bank. But when the account is almost empty, which ordinarily happens later in life, the ATM does not distribute the stem cells as readily. In biological terms, this happens for two reasons: 1) the density of capillaries (the home of MSCs) throughout the body diminishes, and 2) the division rate of the stem cells slows considerably. Simply going from a stem cell doubling time of 24 hours to 72 hours can make a 90-day difference in the amount of time required to reach the critical mass of cells required to heal a wound.

As an example, MSCs from a newborn will divide approximately every 24 hours; from a 35-year-old every 48 hours; and from a 65-year-old every 60 hours. If one of those cells were placed in an incubator in growth medium, the yield from that one cell at 30 days would be 1 billion, 32,000, and 200, respectively. If your body needed 10,000 cells to heal, you would be in trouble if you could only produce 200. Not only time and lifestyle affect the overall number of stem cells in your body—if you were to have a massive heart attack or were hit by a truck and broke many bones in your body, there would be a substantial withdrawal from your stem cell ATM as your body tries to repair all of the damage. Below are two graphs—one showing a normal decline in stem cell number over time, the other showing what happens if you have a major heart attack or accident.

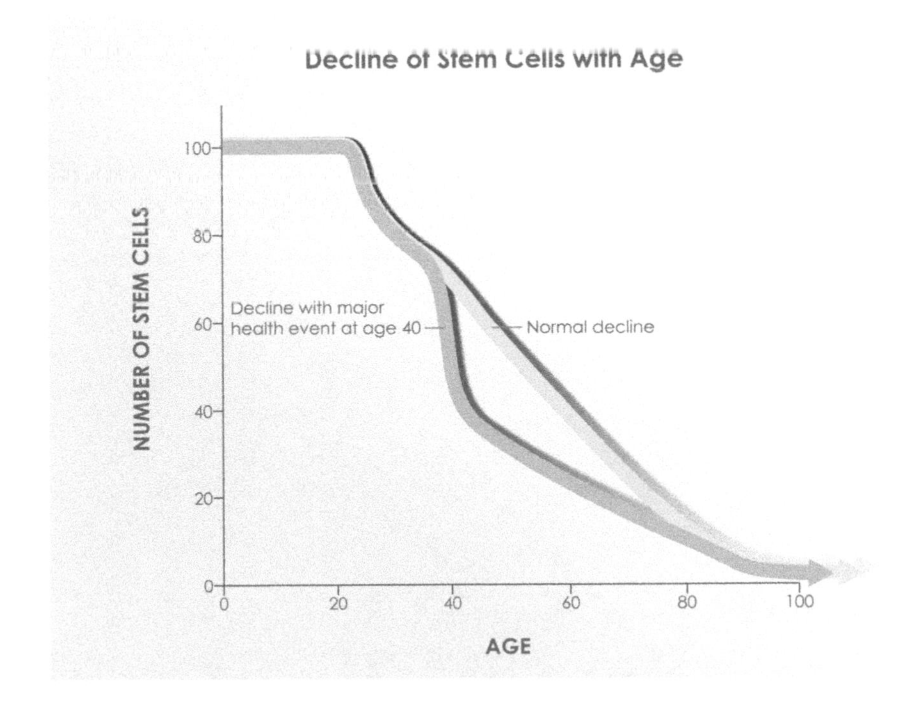

If you were fortunate enough to be born with a large amount of stem cells—stem cell rich—then you might be able to smoke, drink, eat unhealthy food, and not exercise, but still live to a ripe old age because you run out of stem cells later than if you had been born stem cell poor. But if you were born on the other end of the spectrum, with a small amount of stem cells, an unhealthy lifestyle will have a more immediate and detrimental impact upon the quality and length of your life. As your bank account approaches zero, physiological healing will become increasingly difficult, until it finally ceases altogether. It's like your own bank account. When you have plenty of money, it's easier to spend. When you are broke, it becomes more difficult to part with each dollar. Likewise, the fewer stem cells that exist in your "account," the stingier the ATM becomes in distributing the contents of that account. Most people are somewhere in the middle. If we think of maintaining health, or homeostasis, as a balance between degeneration and regeneration, we can look at it as a balancing act, much like a teeter-totter with degeneration on one side and regeneration on the other.

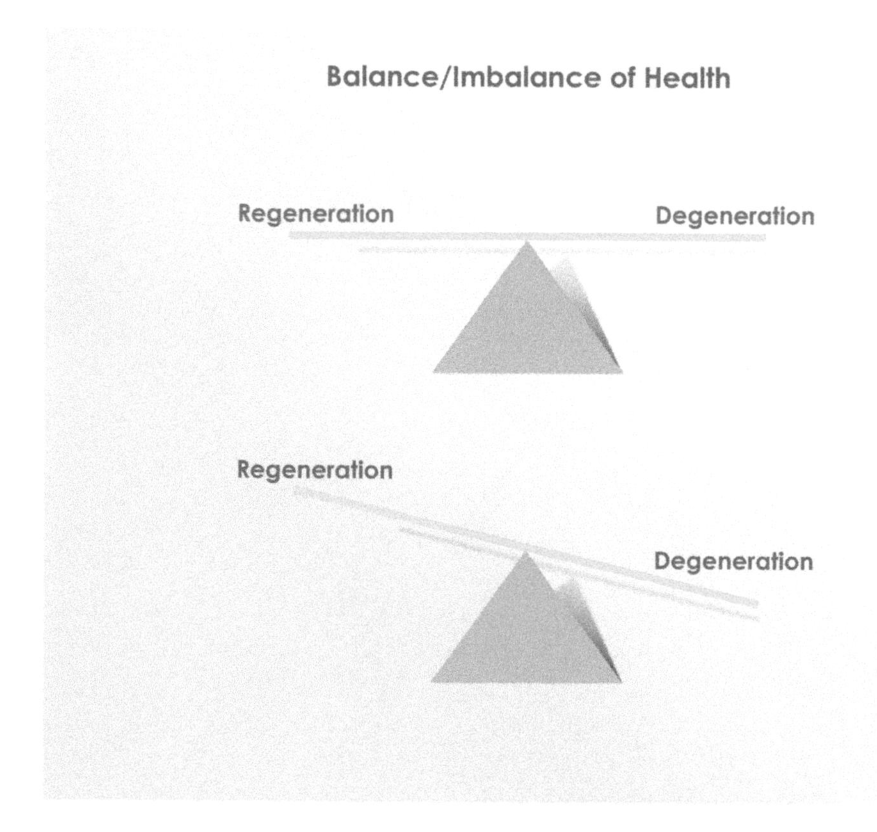

At a certain point in life, which may vary by individual, a disequilibrium between the body's capacity to regenerate and its tendency to degenerate will occur. This imbalance can happen naturally, or it may be accelerated by a health condition or event. When stem cells run low—both those in bone marrow and the MSCs throughout the body—frailty sets in.

When someone has mostly or fully depleted his or her stem cell reserve, the only possible way to get more stem cells is from an alternate source. This is where stem cell therapy comes into play. A fresh supply of regenerative MSCs in someone with a highly depleted reserve may go a long way toward renewing health in that person. MSCs secrete trophic factors and cytokines with a demonstrated anti-inflammatory effect for many conditions. As such, MSCs are positioned as an interesting potential treatment for those affected by frailty or those on the fraily spectrum. I believe the majority of people over the age of 50 are well on their way toward frailty.

Mesenchymal Stem Cells and Aging

Mesenchymal stem cells (MSCs) derived from older individuals lose some of their beneficial characteristics. Cellular environment changes with age,[6] and the amount of circulating cytokines and growth factors is altered, which may affect MSC function and growth.[7,8,9] Younger MSCs are distinctively spindle-shaped, whereas MSCs from older individuals are larger and flatter.[10] The number of MSCs that may be obtained from bone marrow declines with age,[11] and colonies from older MSCs produce a lesser number of viable, newer MSCs.[12] The growth rate of older MSCs as well as the capacity and time to divide are slowed down,[13] and the life span to proliferate is shorter[14,15] than in MSCs derived from younger individuals.

This decline in functionality, or robustness, of older MSCs has critical implications for their participation in the healing process and may be associated with diseases that develop with age.[16] MSCs from an older individual would take much longer to obtain the same regenerative results compared to MSCs derived from younger sources,[17] such as the umbilical cord from healthy, live births. Aside from having faster replication times and a longer life span for proliferation, umbilical cord MSCs secrete abundant cytokines and growth factors necessary for repair and regeneration of the inflamed or injured site and are therefore an attractive source for MSC treatment.

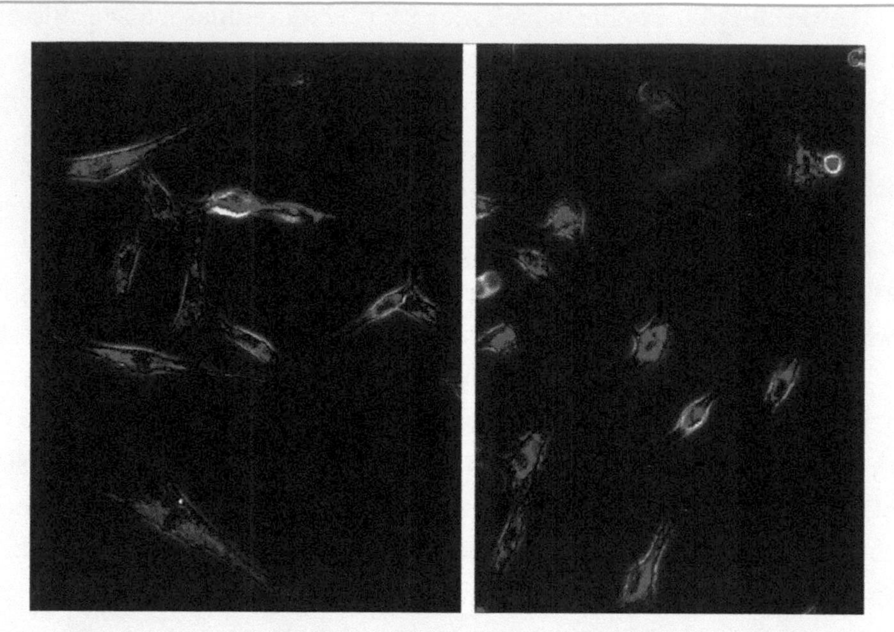

The MSCs in the images above were cultured from the bone marrow of a 65-year-old. The cells on the left were treated with secretions of amnion, a tissue rich in MSCs derived from the amniotic sac of healthy newborns; the cells on the right were cultured with a standard growth medium. Notice the red mitochondria in the cells on the left are evenly distributed throughout the cell body, indicating healthy cells. On the right, the mitochondria are limited mostly to the area surrounding the nucleus, and the morphology of the cells is flattened and more fibroblastic, indicating the cells are near exhaustion, or terminal differentiation. If we measure the trophic factors from the cells on the right, the number and concentration will be much lower than from the cells on the left. This phenomenon highlights the ability of MSCs derived from younger tissue to retrain the MSCs from an older individual to behave like younger MSCs.

The Interdisciplinary Stem Cell Institute at the University of Miami is currently investigating the use of donor MSCs for people aged 60 to 95 with aging frailty in a phase I/II clinical trial.[18] The study aims to demonstrate the safety and effectiveness of donor bone marrow MSCs administered in this population of frail adults. "Allogeneic human MSCs not only help replenish exhausted and/or senescent native stem cells but also have demonstrated systemic anti-inflammatory properties," note the researchers. They are hoping to ameliorate, or even reverse, some of the changes associated with aging. Noting that stem cells can reduce chronic inflammation that erodes the body's repair mechanisms, Goldschmidt, one of the researchers, said,

"In many cases, these seniors can resume walking, cooking, and other daily activities, so they can enjoy a more independent lifestyle."

We have had success at the Stem Cell Institute treating frailty of aging. Mel Gibson's dad Hutton ("Hutt") is a great example. When he was 92, Hutt's health was rapidly deteriorating. His kidneys were backed up and he was in chronic kidney failure due to prostate trouble, his lungs were congested, his heart was failing, and his heartbeat was irregular due to a prolapsed heart valve—Mayo Clinic doctors gave him a grave prognosis. His hips were also in bad shape—one had been replaced and the other had deteriorated badly with severe arthritis, but his current state of health was so fragile that surgery was not an option. On top of all this, his memory was not as sharp as it once was, and he rarely spoke.

The Mayo Clinic was able to stabilize Hutt over the course of ten days, but Mel worried that his father's lack of mobility had been the cause of his declining health. "If only he could get that hip working," Mel wondered. Surgery was out of the question at his age, so when Mel's brother contacted him to tell him about stem cell treatment in Panama City, which he had learned about by searching the Internet, Mel was interested. Mel's good friend Brad Hillstrom, MD, a Mayo trained doctor, was not for it in the beginning, but Mel convinced him to get on the phone with Dr. Paz-Rodriquez, our medical director, and me.

After two lengthy phone calls, a review of studies and papers I had sent him, and consultations with other stem cell researchers who discreetly gave our clinic in Panama—over any other clinic—the green light, Dr. Hillstrom said, "Maybe I'm wrong, but what's your dad got to lose?" They brought him down for treatment. He received IV injections as well as a single injection into his hip. On the plane ride home, Hutt was able to walk without pain. "I have personally taken care of hundreds of patients acutely with hip replacements, and I've never seen anything like it in my life," Dr. Hillstrom told me. "When he went down there he could not sit, walk, stand, or even lay down without pain." Within six weeks, he put on 20 pounds, gained strength, improved mentally, and began walking again with no pain. His kidney and lung function improved, and his prolapsed heart valve even resolved. His eyesight improved and the pigment of his hair darkened. When another set of Mayo Clinic doctors later followed up with him, they were astounded. He was even taken off several medications.

Hutt has been to Panama three more times and continues to benefit from the stem cell infusions. He has experienced a progressive improvement of health rather than the expected decline people undergo at his age. Hutt is now 98 years old and still going strong. "It was almost like it wound the clock back a few years," Mel said. "He's had six more years of life, and I believe it's a direct result of the stem cells."

About six months after Hutt's treatment, Mel invited me and Dr. Paz out to Beverly Hills to give a lecture to many of his friends who wanted to learn more about stem cells after seeing Hutt's results. After the lecture, which was held at the Beverly Hills Hotel, we went to see Hutt at his house in Agora Hills. When Hutt first came to Panama, he was accompanied by one of his nurses, named Nelly. Nelly's body language the entire time she was in Panama said, "I don't believe in any of this crap." When I walked into the house, she came up to me with open arms, gave me a big hug and said, "Oh, Dr. Riordan! Come over here and look at Mr. Gibson." She showed me his hair and described how it was thicker and some of the white was now black. Then she said to Hutt, "Get out of that chair, old man, and show him what you can do." Hutt proceeded get out of the chair, walked across the room, and then moonwalked back—something I have never been able to do. He was making all sorts jokes the entire time. I was astounded at the turnaround he had achieved. And I was most happy about Nelly thinking differently of me.

It was almost like it wound the clock back a few years," Mel said. "He's had six more years of life, and I believe it's a direct result of the stem cells."

Because of the amazing recovery Mel and his doctor friend saw in Hutt, Mel, Dr. Hillstrom, and Dr. Hillstrom's wife Tina came down for stem cell treatments themselves. Mel experienced improvement in his shoulders from bone spurs, the doctor experienced relief from knee pain as well as more stamina and reduced depression, and the doctor's wife experienced improvements in stamina as well as skin and hair health after having suffered through a previous bout of pneumonia. "From an anti-aging standpoint, there is nothing like it," Dr. Hillstrom said.

At the age of 86, Ricardo's health wasn't what it once was. He could no longer drive and opted to stay at home most of the time. He became lost in conversations, and his memory failed him on a regular basis. His energy declined, and he could no longer visit his farm, where he loved to work. Ricardo happens to be the father of Rodolfo Fernandez, laboratory director of Medistem, our clinic's parent company. So when Rodolfo noticed the decline in his father's health, he knew stem cells might help. Ricardo agreed to treatment and received umbilical cord MSCs intravenously. A week later the results were evident. His memory improved, and he regained so much energy that he felt confident to drive again. He even went back to work on his farm. He is now going on 90 and continues to feel well. He is looking forward to another treatment to maintain the benefits he has gained.

Rodolfo's mother, Teresita, has an even better story. Asthmatic since the age of five and later diagnosed with emphysema, Teresita became quite sick when she contracted flu at the age of 80. She was hospitalized, given many medications, and put on oxygen. The pulmonologist told her she would need to stay on oxygen and could no longer travel to her farm, which was at an elevation of 5,000 feet. When Rodolfo saw how successful his father's stem cell treatment had been, he wondered if his mother might qualify to enroll in a clinical trial for asthma that we were undertaking at the clinic. She did qualify, and received her treatment using intravenous MSCs along with intranasal (inhaled) trophic factors. Two months after her first treatment, she called Rodolfo. "I'm feeling different," she said. Her breathing had improved. At that time, her oxygen tank had run out, but she felt so good that she didn't need to use it anymore. That was over two years ago, and she hasn't needed oxygen since. She has traveled to Europe, Costa Rica, the United States, and yes, back to her farm.

The Body's Energy Powerhouses

Within most cells of the body are small yet powerful organelles called mitochondria, responsible for 90 percent of the body's energy production. Remember learning about adenosine triphosphate (ATP) back in science class? ATP is the body's energy currency. Without it, we could not function. Mitochondria produce ATP out of molecules derived from food. The function of our mitochondria is very important to our overall health.

Mitochondria degrade by a process known as oxidation, which essentially means the mitochondria do not get the maintenance they require, so they wear out. Mitochondrial oxidation is inversely related to life span—the more your mitochondria are oxidized, or worn out, the shorter your life span.[19] Oxidation is the biggest predictor of death of an organism.

One risk of frailty in older age is dementia. The brain experiences aging just as the rest of the body does. In some people, this process begins earlier than in others. At the Stem Cell Institute, we generally don't treat Alzheimer's, the most widely recognized form of dementia, largely because it requires frequent treatments that become too costly for most patients. There is one exception, however. A patient whom I will call Wilma has a strong family history of Alzheimer's disease—both her parents and her grandmother had had it. Wilma was tested and discovered that she carried both alleles that strongly predisposed to her the disease. By 2008, when she was 61, they began to notice symptoms, and she was diagnosed with early-onset Alzheimer's disease. While she is not yet considered frail, her condition would put her down an early path to frailty if left to conventional treatment, which does little to help this devastating disease.

Wilma is married to a highly successful businessman—a man with the means to seek out cutting-edge treatments that may be expensive. They learned about stem cell treatment at our clinic from my close friend Dr. Bob Harman, founder and CEO of Vet-Stem, and began visiting regularly, first

Very interesting research in the past few years has discovered that MSCs are the only cells we know of that donate their mitochondria.[20,21] MSCs actually triage cells, just like in the hospital when a nurse triages patients to determine who needs immediate treatment and who can wait a while. When an MSC encounters another cell, if it detects a need for help, it will actually donate its mitochondria via small vesicles (containers) or tubules (tubes), to the cell in an effort to replace the oxidized mitochondria with healthy mitochondria.

This scientific discovery deserves a Nobel Prize in my opinion. In the future, I believe we will be able to bioreact MSCs, optimizing them to produce these microvesicles and microtubules of mitochondria that will perhaps allow people to live a healthy life span of 200 years. MSCs as mitochondrial factories may one day be one of the most important science breakthroughs of our time.

to our clinic in Costa Rica and then to Panama. As a matter of fact, Wilma has been down for 10 treatments in Panama and has received a total of 52 injections—796 million cells since August 2010. "She never feels any type of side effect with intravenous stem cell treatment," her husband said. She has received more intravenous stem cells than any other patient we have treated. The only other treatment she receives for Alzheimer's disease is gamma globulin infusions biweekly, which was added in 2014.

While her disease has progressed some, Wilma and her husband believe that it is progressing at a much slower rate than it would without stem cell treatment. She is still fully functional. She can drive and is independent. She still goes to the grocery store and shopping with her friends. Only her short-term memory is somewhat challenged. I had dinner with Wilma and her husband a few months ago with several other patients—no one could tell she had that diagnosis. Given that the average time to death is seven years for people with her diagnosis, I find it incredible that she is doing so well eight years later. "The stem cells,

> ***"The stem cells, I think, are the key," said her husband. "She can tell after receiving the cells that her memory improves for a period of time."***

I think, are the key," said her husband. "She can tell after receiving the cells that her memory improves for a period of time. Sometimes her memory starts getting "iffy" and she says, 'When are we going to Panama?'"

Hendrikje van Andel-Schipper was once the oldest woman in the world. She died in 2005 at the age of 115, at which point her body was donated to science at her request. Interestingly, scientists studying her body found that all the white blood cells in her blood were derived from just two stem cells, suggesting that her stem cells had all but run out by the time she died.[22] The telomeres, or DNA tips, of her white blood cells were greatly worn down, a sign of cell aging and deterioration. This research begs the questions, as the scientists put it, "Is there a limit to the number of stem cell divisions, and does that imply that there's a limit to human life? Or can you get around that replenishment with cells saved from earlier in your life?" Did this woman live to such an old age because her stem cell supply was abundant? Could she—or anyone for that matter—extend life by increasing her supply of stem cells? These are the questions that we will be faced with as this field moves forward.

A colleague recently sent me the test results of a 79-year-old man with pulmonary fibrosis who had undergone three treatments with IV umbilical cord MSCs. The telomeres in five of six different cells—lymphocytes, granulocytes, naïve T cells, memory T cells, B cells, and NK cells—increased in length over the course of a year. His cells now have a much "younger" telomere length than prior to treatment. Idiopathic pulmonary fibrosis patients have shorter than normal telomeres, which is thought to be, at least in part, the etiology of the disease. Once telomeres become too short, the cell cannot divide and therefore senesces, or deteriorates. Senescent cells are the root of all evil in aging and lack of repair. In fact, they not only do not contribute to repair and remodeling, but they also actively inhibit those activities in neighboring cells. There is active research on how to selectively remove senescent cells to increase health, decrease disease, and increase lifespan.

This is the first time I've seen a human's telomeres increase in length. They increased after stem cell therapy, a completely nontoxic treatment that is also improving his health. Scientists have been searching for a way to increase telomere length for many years, believing it to be the key to the "Fountain of Youth."

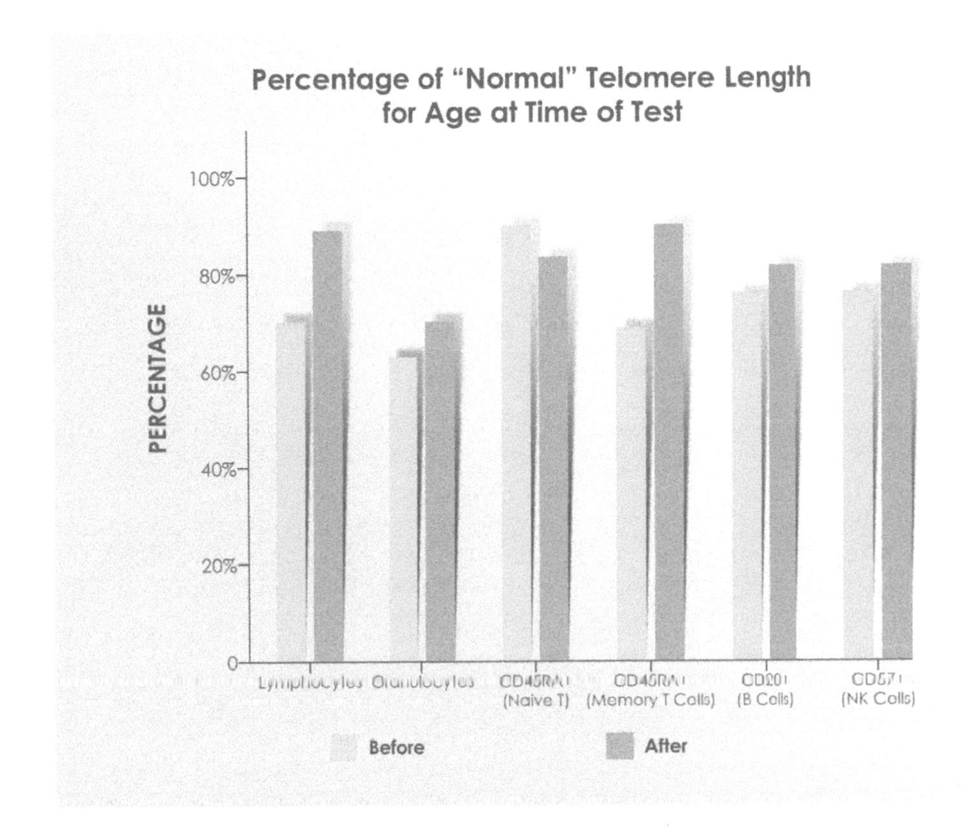

Telomere Length in Various Immune Cells Before Stem Cell Treatment

Sample Dates (mm/dd/yy) **Draw:** 12/02/15 **Received:**12/03/15 **Resulted:** 12/16/15

Lymphocytes			Granulocytes			CD45RA+ (Naïve T)			CD45RA+ (Memory T)			CD20+ (B Cells)			CD57+(NK Cells)		
MTL	MTLN	INT	MTL	MTLN	INT	MTL	MTLN	INT	MTL	MTLN	INT	MTL	MTLN	INT	MTL	MTLN	INT
(kb)	(kb)		(kb)	(kb)		(kb)	(kb)		(kb)	(kb)		(kb)	(kb)		(kb)	(kb)	
3.8	5.4	L	4.7	7.4	VL	5.1	5.7	N	3.5	5.1	L	5.7	7.2	L	4.0	5.2	N

MTL = Patient Median Telomere Length

MTLN = Normal MTL at age (50th percentile)

INT = Telomere length interpretation

VH = Very High (≥ 99 percentile)

H = High (≥ 90 and < 99 percentile)

N = Normal (≥ 10 and < 90 percentile)

L = Low (≥ 1 and < 10 percentile)

VL = Very Low (1 percentile)

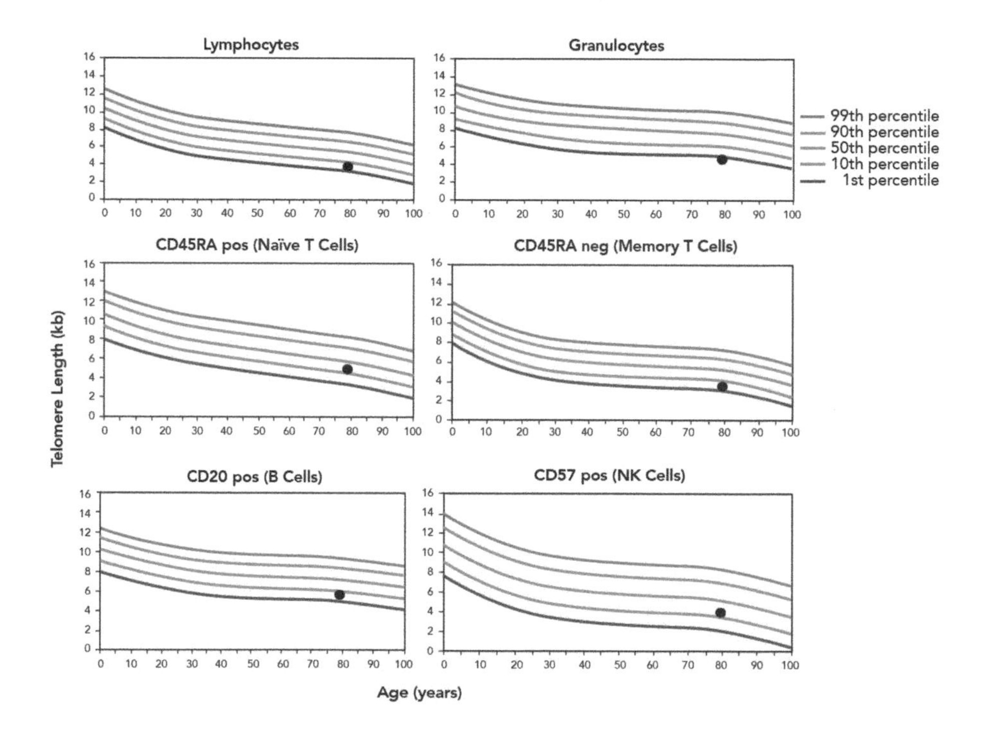

Telomere Length in Various Immune Cells After Stem Cell Treatment

Sample Dates (mm/dd/yy) **Draw:** 11/16/16 **Received:**11/18/16 **Resulted:** 11/30/16

Lymphocytes			Granulocytes			CD45RA+ (Naïve T)			CD45RA+ (Memory T)			CD20+ (B Cells)			CD57+(NK Cells)		
MTL	MTLN	INT	MTL	MTLN	INT	MTL	MTLN	INT	MTL	MTLN	INT	MTL	MTLN	INT	MTL	MTLN	INT
(kb)	(kb)		(kb)	(kb)		(kb)	(kb)		(kb)	(kb)		(kb)	(kb)		(kb)	(kb)	
4.8	5.4	N	5.2	7.4	L	4.8	5.6	N	4.6	5.1	N	6.4	7.2	N	4.3	5.1	N

MTL = Patient Median Telomere Length

MTLN = Normal MTL at age (50th percentile)

INT = Telomere length interpretation

VH = Very High (≥ 99 percentile)

H= High (≥ 90 and < 99 percentile)

N= Normal (≥ 10 and < 90 percentile)

L= Low (> 1 and < 10 percentile)

VL= Very Low (1 percentile)

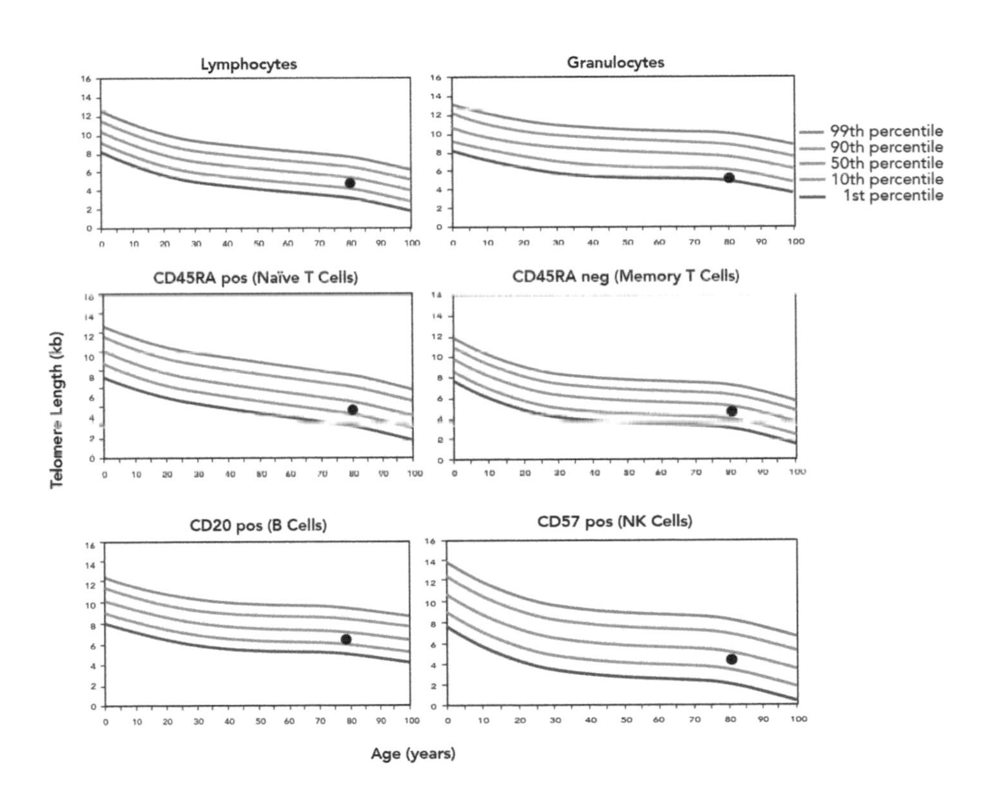

Chapter Ten

RESPIRATORY DISORDERS— A FRESH BREATH

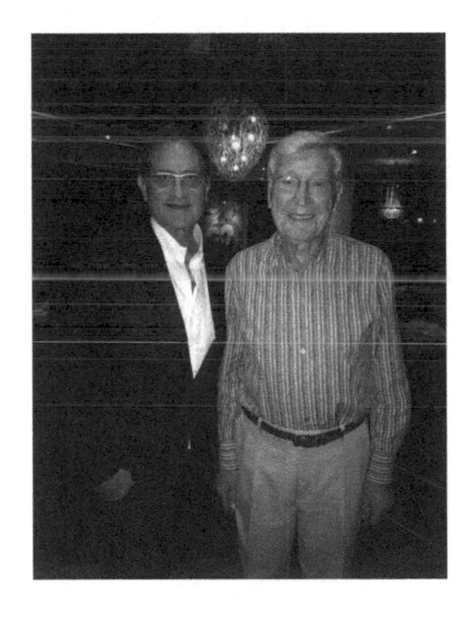

Bernie Marcus, cofounder of Home Depot and the company's first CEO, suffered from bronchiectasis, a chronic lung condition that caused him to have difficulty, especially when public speaking. As a prominent businessman and active philanthropist, Bernie is a sought-after speaker. When his condition worsened and interfered with his speaking ability, he knew something had to be done. "I would get hoarse and cough ten to fifteen times every hour," he said. "It was difficult to handle and progressively getting worse." He went to the nation's top respiratory hospital—National Jewish Health—where the doctors told him he would have to take antibiotics for two years to address the bacterial infection in his lungs. This treatment would do a number on his digestion, however, so he sought an alternative.

His physician recommended that he try stem cell treatment in Panama. Another good friend of Bernie's had already been down to Panama to treat a stomach disorder that completely cleared up, so he felt comfortable with the recommendation.

Bernie was treated with stem cells and shortly thereafter stopped coughing and was able to return to his work. "I was able to go back to public speaking without embarrassing myself," he said. The next time he came down for treatment he brought his wife, who had two osteoarthritic knees that her orthopedic doctor recommended be replaced. "As you know, total knee replacement means being out of action for six months per knee, which would mean a year of not being able to do the things she likes to do," Bernie said. "She's a very active woman."

So he brought her to Panama for stem cell treatment. "We had to carry her onto the plane because she couldn't take any steps at all without tremendous pain." Just three weeks after her treatment she was back to playing golf four times a week with no pain. Fourteen months later she is still doing well. "When I go down again I'm going to take her with me to double up so it doesn't happen again," Bernie said.

When two more of Bernie's friends came down to treat back pain after undergoing back surgery and experienced amazing recoveries, Bernie knew that stem cell treatment was a worthwhile investment. "Both were crippled, in pain 24 hours a day, couldn't sleep, couldn't lie down—and both had orthopedic doctors who said stem cell treatment wouldn't help," said Bernie. "They were reluctant to come to Panama, but they didn't want surgery. Today, both of them are functioning very, very well. They are both without pain, able to function normally, and are playing golf again without the painful aftermath they experienced before."

When Bernie later returned to National Jewish Health, the doctors were amazed to discover that his bacterial infection, which never really goes away in patients with bronchiectasis, was almost undetectable. And he felt much better. "My symptomatology has improved 90 percent," he says.

I believe that Bernie's bacterial infection was impacted by a particular protein known as LL-37, originally discovered by Stanford University scientists. LL-37 is secreted by mesenchymal stem cells and has been found to be one of the most powerful antimicrobials around. Younger MSCs produce more LL-37. The stem cells Bernie received may have produced enough LL-37 to kill off the bacteria in his lungs.

We actually tested the antimicrobial effect of our MSCs in the lab. We inoculated our MSCs with *Staphylococcus* bacteria in a petri dish. What we found was a zone of inhibition around each of the cells where the bacteria could not grow. The cells were protected from the bacteria, which I believe is due to the LL-37 they secrete.

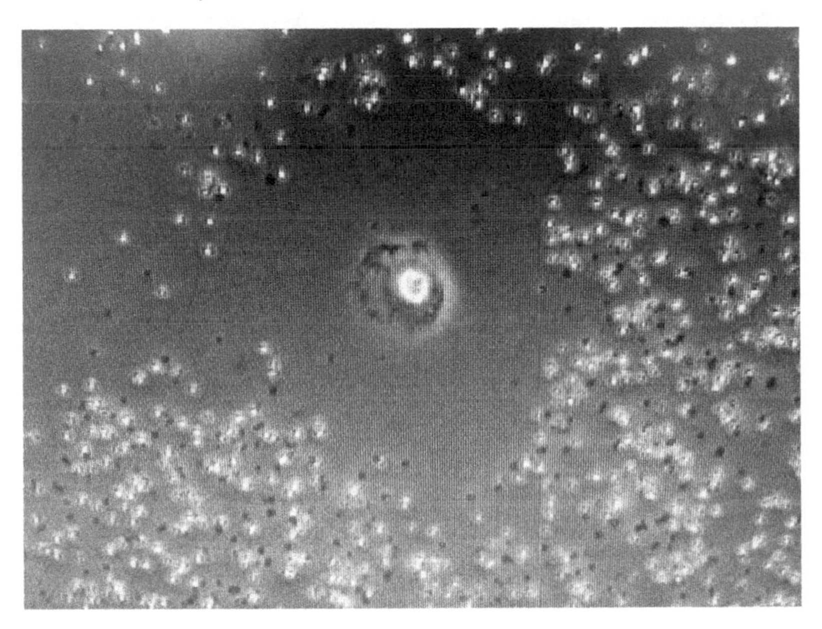

MSC with zone of inhibition, protected against *Staphylococcus* bacteria.

A group from Russia published a study of a group of 27 patients with untreatable, drug-resistant *Mycobacterium tuberculosis* infection who were treated with their own bone marrow-derived mesenchymal stem cells.[1] Every patient experienced a positive clinical effect. In 20 patients, bacterial discharge stopped after three to four months—these patients were no longer drug resistant. In nine of the 16 patients who were followed for a full one and a half to two years, remission of the tuberculosis process occurred. When I asked the Russian doctor who led this study about his rationale

Mesenchymal Stem Cells for Treatment of Asthma

Allergies are caused by an overreaction of the immune system to an external substance that is normally harmless (an allergen), triggering an inflammatory response. Common symptoms (watery eyes, runny nose, sneezing, skin rash, swelling, etc.) depend on the type of allergen and on the manner in which it enters the body. Asthma, a closely related condition, is a chronic inflammation of the airways with frequent spasms in the muscles near the airways of the lungs known as the bronchi. As the airways narrow and too much mucus is produced by the inflammatory response, breathing becomes difficult. Asthma

for using MSCs in these patients, he replied, "When I have nothing else, I give them MSCs."

Bernie Marcus founded and chairs The Marcus Foundation, whose focus on children's health, medical research, free enterprise, and Jewish causes has converged with his support for stem cell research. "It's done such amazing things for me that I've become an advocate for stem cells," he says. "My experiences in Panama have really moved me to try and get stem cells into the United States. I don't know where it's not going to be useful. The work in Panama is proving to be a blessing in disguise for a lot of people. It's the opening of a new era, and especially umbilical cord stem cells."

"*My experiences in Panama have really moved me to try and get stem cells into the United States. I don't know where it's not going to be useful. The work in Panama is proving to be a blessing in disguise for a lot of people. It's the opening of a new era, and especially umbilical cord stem cells.*"

Bernie is a strong proponent of stem cell treatment and research. In fact, as of this writing, he and Newt Gingrich are may be triggered by an allergic reaction in the presence of an allergen (allergic asthma), but non-allergic factors may also come into play, for example stress, weather, or a respiratory infection such as a cold or the flu. Chronic asthma may cause an eventual change in the structure of the airway, known as airway remodeling, or the presence of excess scarring (fibrosis).[2,3]

Via their secretions, mesenchymal stem cells (MSCs) have been shown to have anti-inflammatory and regenerative properties as well the capacity to influence immune response. MSCs have been used safely to treat a multitude of conditions, in particular autoimmune conditions, which involve a strong inflammatory response. The potential of MSCs for the treatment of lung conditions has been well documented,[4,5,6] leading to clinical trials with improvement in the clinical condition and quality of life.[7,8]

trying to convince Gingrich's daughter, who has suffered from rheumatoid arthritis since she was in her twenties, to try stem cell treatment. "She has a very severe case," Bernie says. "Her father and I are trying to convince her to come down to Panama."

Another patient, we'll call her Sylvia, came down to Panama with an antibiotic-resistant lung infection that was suspected to come from her work with animals, horses in particular. She was a strong woman who had always been well, with no previous health problems. Over a period of about 18 months, her condition worsened so much so that her family didn't think she would make it. She couldn't finish a sentence without coughing and wheezing and couldn't walk without losing her breath. Her lung function was at 41 percent. A friend of hers was aware of successful treatments with stem cells and offered to send her to our clinic in Panama for treatment.

She was skeptical about the treatment at first, as some patients are, but about two months after receiving the stem cells, Sylvia's lung function returned to 100 percent. Her voice was strong again, and she felt great and continues to be well as of this writing.

Recent studies with animal models of asthma have investigated the molecular mechanisms of MSCs and their interactions with immune system cells as they lessen airway reactivity and lung inflammation.[9,10] Most experiments have been on mouse models of asthma; such studies have demonstrated a decrease in airway inflammation and a reduction in airway remodeling.[11,12,13] MSCs have also been found to significantly reduce allergic symptoms, improve lung function, and significantly inhibit proteins that coordinate the response to allergens.[14] A growth factor derived from MSCs known as TGF-β was shown to be a key component for signaling a stop to the excessive immune response found in asthma.[15] In an allergic rhinitis mouse model, MSCs were found to significantly reduce allergic symptoms and to lessen inflammation by inhibiting inflammatory cytokines.[16]

Some concerns have existed that the capacity of MSCs to regenerate new tissues could contribute to airway remodeling in a harmful way, but the opposite has been shown—MSCs helped *improve* faulty airway structure.[17] This study also concluded that repeated doses of MSCs might be necessary to keep up the beneficial anti-inflammatory effects. Similarly, a cat model of asthma showed a short-term improvement in stopping airway remodeling, but the effect was lessened after a year, prompting the authors to propose repeated doses of treatment with MSCs for further studies.[18]

Mesenchymal stem cells, once injected into the veins, will travel first to the lungs. If a lung condition exists, the cells will go to work in the lungs before they head to other parts of the body. For this reason, MSCs have a lot of potential for treating lung disease. In fact, a seven-year-old autism patient of ours who had terrible asthma that put him in the hospital a couple times each year experienced a resolution of his asthma after one stem cell treatment. He was able to come off of his asthma medications and no longer had asthma attacks. His parents were able to use the money they would have spent on hospital bills to bring him down for a second stem cell treatment.

We are currently doing a clinical trial in Panama on patients with asthma. The patients in this trial receive inhalations of the MSC secretome—the trophic factors secreted by the MSCs. Without disclosing too much information about the results, the first four patients have been able to get off all their asthma medications after six weeks. We hope to have the results of this trial published within the next couple of years.

While there are many experiments on animal models of asthma and allergy and a great interest in MSC treatment for these conditions,[19,20] there are still not yet many results of studies with human patients. In a laboratory setting, MSCs have been shown to have a direct effect on human cells that coordinate the response to harmless allergens and suppress excessive immune response (regulatory T cells CD4+, CD25+ and CD127-).[21] A clinical trial is ongoing to treat autoimmune urticaria (allergic skin disease) with fat-derived MSCs.[22] Our group is conducting a clinical trial to investigate the safety and feasibility of treating asthma with trophic factors derived from umbilical cord MSCs administered via inhalation.[23] A preparation of cytokines and growth factors are collected from the secretions of these MSCs grown in a laboratory setting. These mesenchymal trophic factors (MTF) allow for patients to receive the benefits of MSC therapy without the need to administer cells. This allows for more widespread accessibility of treatment, as well as potential lower costs of treatment. MTF has been demonstrated to possess anti-inflammatory,[24,25] antioxidant,[26] antifibrotic,[27] and regenerative properties[28] in vitro (out of the body) and in vivo (in the body).

Chapter Eleven

ARTHRITIS— A NEW SOLUTION

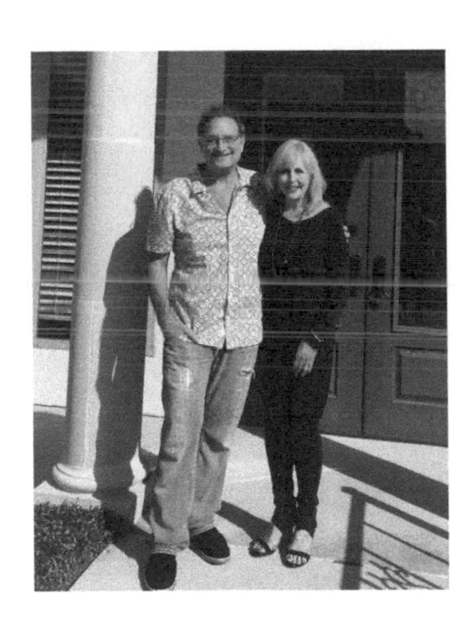

Marian D'Unger lives in a menagerie. The house she and her husband own near a creek in a suburb of Dallas sits on one and a half acres. There she tends to four cats, two love birds, two dogs, a rose-breasted cockatoo and two geese. Every night she feeds the fifty raccoons that gather on the property, including one named George, who she lets come into the house. When her fingers swelled up in November 2008 and she had trouble writing, at first she wondered if she'd gotten an insect bite or something else from one of the animals.

Marian is a real estate agent who loves her work. She sells seven days a week and shows an average of fifty to seventy-five houses a week. She always wears boots with her glitzy jeans and tailored blazers because she never knows when she's going to have to make her way around a construction site. The night that her hand started to give her trouble, she was writing a marketing report for one of her properties. She looked down at her right hand when it started to stiffen up and saw that it had turned beet red. "I took all the pain killers in the house, the stuff we had left over from the dentist," she said.

One of her friends thought she might have gout, a chronic form of arthritis that occurs when uric acid builds up in the joints. The pain and swelling returned the next night. When Marian saw a friend of hers who is a doctor, he took a look at her hands and said he thought she had rheumatoid arthritis. He was able to diagnose that at a glance by examining Marian's fingers. From the middle joint up, her fingers were slanted toward her little finger, a characteristic of rheumatoid arthritis. The arthritis in her joints appeared to have mangled her hands.

"I had never noticed it before," she said, amazed. "Before that night I didn't have any hand pain. I'm 65 and I have aches and pains, but I thought what was going on in my hands came from something I did that day."

Arthritis is a common condition that affects nearly 30 million people in the United States, or 10 percent of the population. There are more than a hundred different kinds of arthritis, a condition of the joints that causes pain, swelling, and stiffness and limits range of motion. The cause of these difficulties is the breakdown of cartilage, the sinewy and flexible connective tissue that is not as stiff as bone and not as flexible as muscle. The cartilage helps hold your body together, keeping the bones in alignment and allowing the joints to flex and the whole body to move.

Cartilage is unique in that it is a kind of tissue that doesn't contain blood vessels. As a result, it grows and repairs more slowly. In osteoarthritis, the most widespread form of the disease, affecting 27 million people in the United States, the pain in the joints is due to the wearing away of cartilage, which leaves no protection for the joints as they move. When a sufferer bends a knee or an elbow, bone rubs on bone, causing great pain. Often with osteoarthritis, the joints wear out where the cartilage has been thinned out by overuse.

Marian's type of arthritis was rheumatoid, an autoimmune disease. The body's immune system is designed to seek and destroy invaders, particularly infections. Autoimmune diseases are those in which the body mistakenly identifies healthy tissue as a foreign substance and begins to attack its own cells. As the attack on the cartilage advances, those who suffer from rheumatoid arthritis can notice the shape of their body changing, as Marian did with her fingers. The disease can attack other joints too, resulting in swollen knees, cramped up toes, and bumpy fingers with raised nodules on the knuckles.

There is no cure for arthritis, only an array of drugs that may or may not help calm the inflammation. As Marian was about to find out, these drugs may have horrible side effects. The doctor first gave Marian methotrexate, which helped with her symptoms for a few months even though it made her feel nauseated for most of the day. When its effectiveness started to ebb, the doctor switched her to Enbrel®, which he told her to inject into her legs. That treatment only lasted two weeks because she broke out into huge rashes at the spots where she injected the drugs. "It looked like I had big red pancakes plastered on my legs," Marian said.

The next drug was Arava®, which helped with some of the pain and swelling but gave Marian terrible diarrhea two or three times a day. She was also taking Celebrex® and ten to twelve aspirin a day. Celebrex, too, stopped being effective after a while. Again she was having trouble holding a fork or a pen. When she and her husband went out to dinner, she'd just push the food around on her plate. She couldn't hold a fork well enough to maneuver food to her mouth, and she certainly wasn't going to eat with her hands. "It was impossible for me to work," Marian said. "The quality of my life was going downhill fast." She got to the point where she couldn't drive because she couldn't shift gears.

In the beginning of 2010, the doctor suggested Marian return to methotrexate, only this time to take it in an injectable form. The side effects were horrible. "It was like I was injecting myself with food poisoning every Monday evening. My hand would be shaking so badly when I tried to inject it. I was so frightened by what I knew was going to happen. The next day after the injection, I'd be lying on the floor, gagging and throwing up constantly.

I couldn't work Tuesday and Wednesday. Thursday I could go back and by Friday I'd be feeling pretty good but by Saturday I was a wreck thinking about what was coming on Monday."

How was this helping Marion battle her disease? She thought the drugs were only making things worse. She was still stiff when she got up in the morning, and the days of lying at home too sick to move contradicted the advice to stay physically active to maintain some mobility and flexibility in her joints. Worst of all, she was losing hope. No one knows the cause of rheumatoid arthritis, and all of the treatments focus on easing the symptoms, not eliminating them. In Marian's experience, none of the available drugs worked for her.

A friend of Marian's who lives in Corpus Christi said she had heard of something that might help. She knew a man there, Dusty Durrill, who had been to Panama for stem cell treatments for his osteoarthritis. He had gone down to Central America shuffling, stooped over, using a cane to support

Biologic Response Modifiers for Rheumatoid Arthritis

In recent years, a new group of drugs called biologic response modifiers, or biologics, has been approved for the treatment of rheumatoid arthritis in patients with moderate to severe forms of the disease who do not respond well to the standard drugs. These drugs are genetically-engineered proteins derived from human genes that inhibit certain components of the immune system. They can be prohibitively expensive, to the tune of $20,000 every two months, and come with a host of side effects. For example, the disclaimer for one of these biological medications reads, "Humira® can lower your ability to fight infections including tuberculosis. Serious and sometimes fatal infections, and cancers including lymphoma, have happened, including blood, liver, and nervous system problems, serious allergic reactions, and new and worsening heart failure. Before treatment get tested for TB, tell your doctor if you've been to areas where certain fungal infections are common, and if you've had TB, hepatitis B, are prone to infections, or have flu-like symptoms or sores. Don't start Humira if you have an infection."

his weight, and unable to shake anyone's hand. He returned from treatment able to walk into the room without any assistance. He was telling everyone he knew about this miracle.

Researchers have found that the cartilage-forming cells of those who suffer with osteoarthritis don't divide as quickly as the cells of healthy individuals, so they can't replenish the cartilage tissue in a robust fashion. In experiments with animals, injections of the animals' own stem cells boosted the cartilage-forming capacity in the area of the animals' greatest suffering and pain.[1] In fact, there are veterinary services throughout the country that routinely use stem cells derived from dogs to treat animals with arthritic hips.

Dusty Durrill had a gradually worsening case of osteoarthritis that had started when he was in his fifties. He'd had perfect health for the decades when he was a Navy pilot, but by the time he reached his fifties he had trouble walking more than a block or climbing half a flight of stairs. When he reached his sixties the doctors told him he would need to have both knees replaced as well as at least one of his hips. A friend who had been married to a veterinarian told him that dog owners would bring in their pets that couldn't walk. Once they were treated with stem cells, the dogs were running and barking just as they had been when they were puppies.

"What the hell?" Dusty asked. "We can fix dogs but we can't fix humans? They've been fixing dogs for eight or ten years. There's got to be someone who can fix humans."

That's when he found our Stem Cell Institute in Panama on the Internet. He applied, described his case, and was accepted for treatment. "I went down there and got treatment, and ten days later—ten frigging days—I had no symptoms," Dusty said. "I had been suffering from this for twenty years, and they cured me with stem cells in only ten days."

> ***"I had been suffering from this for twenty years, and they cured me with stem cells in only ten days."***

Dusty has a great way of explaining how the stem cells work. I like to explain it scientifically so that people understand that it makes sense medically. But because of Dusty's background in the military, he likes to use the language of war. "The best I can describe it to you, when you have something wrong with your body it's like a battlefield. When you get stem cells it's like you get a combat battalion of U.S. Marines, and they start fixing all the broken bridges and roads, and killing the enemy, attacking all the bad stuff. They don't need a road map. They just go in there and go to work," Dusty said.

A few weeks after Dusty's visit to Panama, he sent Dr. Paz an email that detailed all of the changes in his body since he'd received the stem cells. The good news was that his arthritis was in remission, but there was other

Mesenchymal Stem Cell Treatment for Osteoarthritis

Osteoarthritis (OA) is an inflammation of the joints, caused by wear and tear, which can be severe enough to impair movement and cause pain. OA is a leading cause of disability in patients over age 65[2] and commonly affects the hands, knees, hips, and spine. Wearing down of cartilage in the joint area may lead to the eventual need for a major replacement surgery with prosthesis. Existing treatments for OA are aimed to reduce pain, but the progression of the condition is not stopped.[3]

OA occurs when inflammatory and oxidative stresses progressively wear down cartilage.[4] Mesenchymal stem cells (MSCs) have been shown to produce factors that are anti-inflammatory[5] and that are key for tissue repair and regeneration.[6] MSCs can also directly become new cartilage tissue.[7] In particular, umbilical cord MSCs have been shown to have a superior potential for cartilage regeneration over other MSC sources.[8]

Animal models have shown that treatment with MSCs is effective for OA. Goats that received MSCs for knee OA had evidence of regeneration in the meniscus and less wearing down of the cartilage in the joint.[9] Similar regenerative effects have been reported in rat,[10] rabbit,[11] sheep,[12] and dog[13] models, and a single dose of bone marrow MSCs has been shown to be enough to slow the progression of OA in sheep.[14]

good news as well. The cells had gone to work on other issues that had been troubling Dusty. The clicking and soreness in his right knee disappeared, his hair turned from white to grey, his skin cleared up and smoothed out, the folds on his lower neck disappeared, his erectile dysfunction was no longer an issue, his bladder incontinence came under control, and his office staff and son claimed that he was more alert and involved in his business than before.

The dramatic nature of his recovery turned Dusty into a stem cell evangelist. He wanted to help alleviate other people's suffering because he knew how hard their lives were and how much they hurt. He was a successful businessman and very generous. That's why he flew Dr. Paz up to Corpus Christi's Del Mar College in June of 2010 to spread the word about

Treatment with MSCs for OA has been shown also to be effective and safe in clinical settings.[15,16,17] Recent clinical trials reported pain relief and improvements in cartilage quality in OA patients treated with bone marrow MSCs,[18,19] as well as cartilage regeneration with MSCs derived from fat.[20] Another study reported improvements in walking distance and stiffness for 30 months after treatment.[21]

One very exciting breakthrough for osteoarthritis is the development of Cartistem®, a drug manufactured from umbilical cord MSCs by Medipost, a Korean regenerative medicine company.[22] Cartistem was approved for the treatment of OA in January 2012 by the South Korean equivalent of the FDA (the Ministry of Food and Drug Safety). In other words, a tier-one country's regulatory body approved an allogeneic, or off-the-shelf, stem cell product made from donor tissue. They would not have gotten approval had the product not been shown first to be safe and then secondly to be effective. As of February 2015, more than 2,000 doses had been given safely, with excellent results in a third phase (follow-up) clinical trial seven years after treatment,[23] and with a clinical trial well underway in the United States at the Cartilage Restoration Center in Chicago, IL and the Cartilage Repair Center in Chestnut Hill, MA.[24]

There are currently several clinical trials listed on ClinicalTrials.gov to treat OA with MSCs from bone marrow, including one trial in the United States at the Regenerative Pain Center in Illinois.[25] Other countries also have ongoing MSC clinical trials.[26,27,28] Our group is currently conducting a phase I/II trial to assess the safety and efficacy of intraarticular knee injection of umbilical cord MSCs.[29]

the potential of this treatment. And Marian D'Unger was in the audience that day.

Marian was very impressed by Dusty's improvement. Even though they had different kinds of arthritis, Marian thought the stem cells might be as useful for her as they had been for Dusty. Excited by what she had heard at the seminar, she asked her doctor what he felt about adult stem cell therapy for arthritis. Her doctor was very discouraging and told her not to go to Panama for treatment. He said that she wasn't that bad yet.

"What does that mean?" Marian thought. "I have to be in a wheelchair before I should consider alternative treatments?"

The medicines she had been prescribed for her condition were taking a toll. While she was at the doctor's office, they asked her to check the lot number of the methotrexate she had injected into her system a few months earlier. The FDA had recalled some batches of the drug because they found that some of them had inadvertently contained ground glass. Marian was stunned. "This is the medicine that's supposed to be helping me, and it's approved by the FDA, yet in reality it's destroying my life," Marian thought. "I think I'm going to try the stem cells."

Marian, her husband, and her daughter all flew to Panama for the two weeks she needed to be there for treatment. They rented an apartment overlooking the Pacific Ocean and viewed the whole journey to help Marian's arthritis as a family vacation. "We cooked most of our meals in the condo because the fish in the marketplace was so fresh," she said. She even hooked up with a local real estate agent and is thinking of starting a business selling condos to retirees who want to move to Panama—all because she is feeling so much better.

Marian was injected with her own stem cells and some cells cultured from umbilical cord blood. Most mornings before treatment, she had to hold on to the furniture to move around her room. By the time she got home, she was no longer limping and sore when she got out of bed in the morning. "Within two months I was 95 percent better, virtually pain free and with no swelling," Marian said. Before the visit to our clinic, she couldn't hold a pencil in her hand. Now she can write with a pencil and use a fork when she

Mesenchymal Stem Cell Treatment for Rheumatoid Arthritis

Rheumatoid arthritis (RA) is an autoimmune condition in which otherwise healthy cells in the body are mistakenly recognized as a threat and are attacked by the immune system. In the case of RA, the lining of the joints is attacked by the immune system and becomes inflamed, leading to an eventual loss of physical function and disability. RA affects approximately 0.5 to 1 percent of the population worldwide,[30] with rates between 20 and 50 cases per 100,000 people in North American and Northern European countries.[31] Persons affected by RA frequently suffer from other diseases (cardiovascular, pulmonary, and renal, for example) and show higher rates of infection.[32]

RA is usually treated with anti-inflammatories to relieve pain, and with disease-modifying antirheumatic drugs (DMARDs) to stop the progression of the disease. Some of the newer DMARDs include both biologic and non-biologic medications. They work by targeting immune system cells and cytokines involved in inflammation, such as tumor necrosis factor (TNF). However, 30 to 40 percent of RA patients do not respond to DMARD treatment.[33] Additionally, DMARDs affect the performance of the rest of the immune system, leaving the body at risk for opportunistic infections and certain cancers such as lymphomas. No current treatment reverses or corrects the joint damage that has already occurred in RA.

goes out to eat. Also, she's cut the use of painkillers by 75 percent. She's gone from taking twelve aspirin a day to two. Plus, she's cut her use of Celebrex from 400 to 100 milligrams, and she doesn't take it every day. She returned to real estate and continues to work full time at age 74.

Marian's rheumatologist, after reviewing her records, told her that he couldn't believe she had experienced such dramatic results. She should have been in a wheelchair at the rate of rapid deterioration she had experienced before stem cells. In June 2016 she returned to Panama for a second treatment. "I've been very fortunate to get to go to Panama. It took four minutes to get across the room before stem cells. I had to hold on to something to be able to walk. People don't know that I have arthritis now. I am pretty active for my age. I outrun people who are 15 years younger than I am. It was the cells in Panama that did that, even my rheumatologist attests to that," Marian said.

Mesenchymal stem cells (MSCs) can modulate the immune system[34,35,36,37] and have been used safely to treat certain inflammatory conditions[38,39,40,41] in clinical settings. Additionally, MSCs have the ability to regenerate worn-out cartilage,[42] with umbilical cord-derived MSCs showing greater capacity than other MSC sources.[43] Treatment with MSCs has been shown to be effective in animal models[44,45,46,47] of RA, and MSCs have been effective at inhibiting production of inflammatory cytokines from cells derived from RA patients.[48,49] MSC infusions are almost always followed by an increase in T-regulatory cells, which calm down the inflammatory T cell inflammation response common in rheumatoid arthritis. In 2010 we published a case report showing improvement in a 67-year-old RA patient, along with our proposed rationale for treatment with MSCs.[50] Additionally, we reported no major side effects in 13 RA patients given a total of 35 injections of cells from their fat in 2012.[51]

Angela was diagnosed with rheumatoid arthritis in 2008 after doctors misdiagnosed her with flu symptoms and joint pain. She was on the usual concoction of pharmaceuticals in addition to monthly infusions of a biologic that cost $6,500 each month and yet only partially controlled her condition. She still had a difficult time getting up in the morning and had to take a nap each afternoon. When her brother, who was treated with umbilical cord MSCs and is a proponent of stem cell therapy, suggested she try the treatment, she was skeptical because her doctors told her it was an unproven treatment.

> ***"People don't know that I have arthritis now. I am pretty active for my age. I outrun people who are 15 years younger than I am. It was the cells in Panama that did that, even my rheumatologist attests to that," Marian said.***

Angela came to our clinic in 2014 and received four stem cell infusions over the course of one week. By the second day she felt so good that she wanted to take a

One particularly remarkable trial of umbilical cord MSC treatment for RA was published in 2013: 172 patients were divided into two groups; 36 received treatment with DMARDs alone (the control group) and 136 received DMARDs plus MSCs.[52] The treatment was shown to be safe with no adverse events. Compared to the control group, those treated with DMARDs plus MSCs showed statistically significant improvements in the HAQ and DAS28—two scales used to measure the extent of RA impact on the patient. The DMARD plus MSC group also had a decrease in levels of the inflammatory markers corticotropin-releasing factor (CRF) and rheumatoid factor (RF), and an increase in T-regulatory cells (associated with clinical benefits). Patients were assessed after three-, six-, and eight-month intervals, with improvements for all three time points, but at eight months the effect was not as significant. The most exciting part of this study was the finding that a single treatment of 40 million MSCs reduced the amount of TNF-α and interleukin-6 (IL-6) in the treated patients by approximately 50 percent. TNF-α and IL-6, sentinel molecules in autoimmune disease, are the primary targets of the newer, and costly, biologic DMARDs (such as Humira® and Enbrel®). Additionally, a subset of patients who were treated a second time with the same dose of cells experienced a 25 percent further decrease of TNF-α and IL-6, for a total 75 percent reduction of TNF-α and IL-6.

walk in the mall. At the airport on her way home, she opted to walk instead of take the escalators. She followed up with her doctor the next month and found that her inflammatory markers, usually quite high, had gone down considerably. Another month later her rheumatoid arthritis was no longer detectable and she was off all of her medications. She lost the thirty pounds she had gained due to all the medications she was previously on. Her doctor was amazed.

Angela's husband had been putting off retirement because he needed his insurance to help pay for the high cost of her previous medical treatments, but after she received the stem cells, she no longer needed treatment and he could finally retire. Two years later at the time of this writing, she is still doing well after one stem cell treatment.

MSCs are therefore a potential therapy for RA that would promote the regeneration of damaged tissue and would address the underlying immunological abnormality. There are currently several clinical trials registered on ClinicalTrials.gov using MSCs to treat RA, including a nationwide trial using allogeneic (donor) cells with the participation of The University of California at Los Angeles and clinics in states including Arizona, Florida, and Maryland, among many others.[53] The trials are proposing umbilical cord MSCs.[54,55] Our group in particular is conducting a phase I/II trial to assess the safety and efficacy of allogeneic umbilical cord MSCs with DMARDs to treat RA patients.[56]

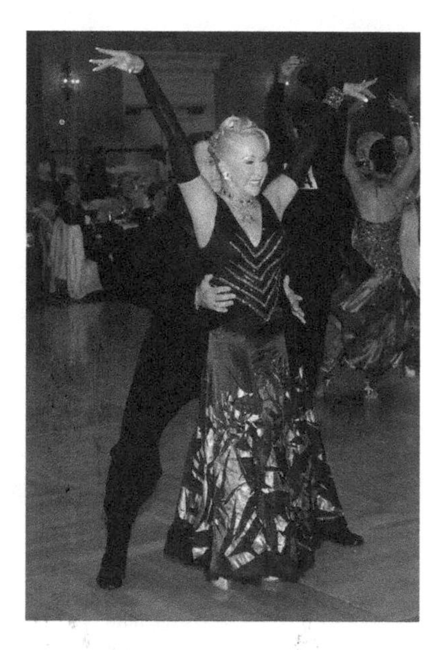

Janet Vaughan is a competitive ballroom dancer and orthodontist. She regularly participated in 10 to 12 American Rhythm or American Smooth style dance competitions every year, and loved every minute of it. During the final round in the 2000 U.S. National Championships American Rhythm Division, while dancing the swing, Janet heard a loud pop and felt excruciating pain in her right foot. But she refused to leave the dance floor and finished strong, winning third place with a dislocated joint. The injury left her later unable to walk, however, and she was diagnosed with osteoarthritis and a dislocated toe that required surgery. Her doctors told her that she would never dance again. She was devastated.

She found a specialist in Houston who performed the surgery and even proved her doctors wrong—she did dance again. But not for long. She suffered a knee injury while practicing one day. Numerous injections and eventually an arthroscopic surgery failed her miserably, gave her a swollen knee, and put her on crutches. Her condition became worse with every new treatment.

Undeterred, Janet communicated with clinics all over the United States in search of the right treatment. Some clinics said her injury was too severe to treat. Others didn't give her the confidence she needed to know the treatment would be helpful. Then she met Dusty Durrill. When she heard his story about the Stem Cell Institute, she knew stem cells were the treatment for her. She applied immediately and came down for treatment.

> ***"Stem cell treatments, for me, were life changing. I am back to the dance floor with no pain and regaining the confidence to dance full out, not tentatively."***

Janet began feeling the effects of her first stem cell treatment about six months afterward. The change was dramatic, and she felt it in all of her joints, not only her knee. She felt relief from a neck injury that had occurred twenty years earlier and from the arthritic joint pain in her hands. Since her first treatment Janet has been down a few more times for maintenance treatment, "for fighting the degenerative disease that osteoarthritis presents," she says.

Best of all, Janet is dancing again. In fact, she won the U.S. American Rhythm title with world champion Tony Dovolani, "a dream come true," she said. "Stem cell treatments, for me, were life changing. I am back to the dance floor with no pain and regaining the confidence to dance full out, not tentatively."

Chapter Twelve

BIOLOGICS IN ORTHOPEDICS—THE RIORDAN MEDICAL INSTITUTE

Over the years, I've followed the adoption of biologics in orthopedic surgery practice among my colleagues. Biologics are medical products derived from living sources; stem cells are a type of biologic. Many physicians started out by using the only biologic available to orthopedic doctors in the United States at the time: platelet-rich plasma (PRP). PRP is essentially made up of the growth factors from whole blood - in orthopedics, PRP is actually a mixture of white blood cells and platelet-rich plasma. PRP is used to augment the healing response in soft tissue injuries such as tendon and muscle tears. Before biologics came into use, patients were usually given steroid injections to ease pain from soft tissue injuries.

Steroids make the injury feel better short term, but in the long run, they actually tear up the tissue, breaking down proteins and sometimes worsening the injury rather than healing it. They do nothing to address the underlying problem, which is how to regenerate damaged or degenerated tissue. Eventually, the patient may need surgery due to the damage.

Do Steroid Injections Help or Harm?

Inflammation of the joints can be treated with a combination of a local anesthetic and corticosteroids to reduce pain. However, this treatment can induce death in cartilage cells,[1,2] especially at higher doses,[3] raising questions about the benefit when used for osteoarthritis. Animal models, particularly in horses, show a detrimental effect of corticosteroids on cartilage:[4] treatment with corticosteroids alters cartilage and collagen production not just in the treated joint(s) but also in untreated joints, an effect that may spread to the rest of the body.[5] Similar negative effects to cartilage tissue have also been observed in dog models in vivo, and in vitro.[6,7]

MSCs Action in the Body

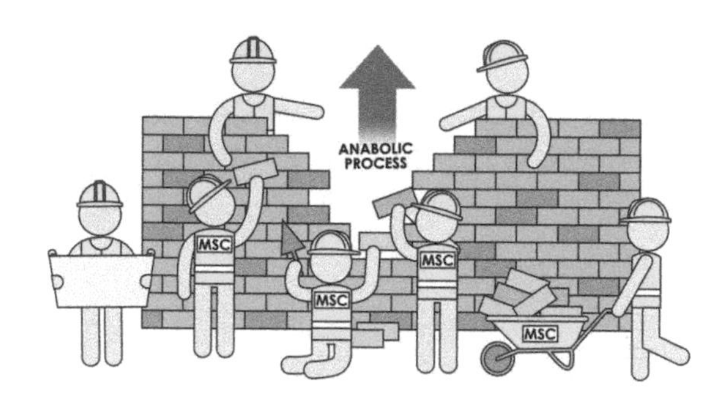

Steroids Action in the Body

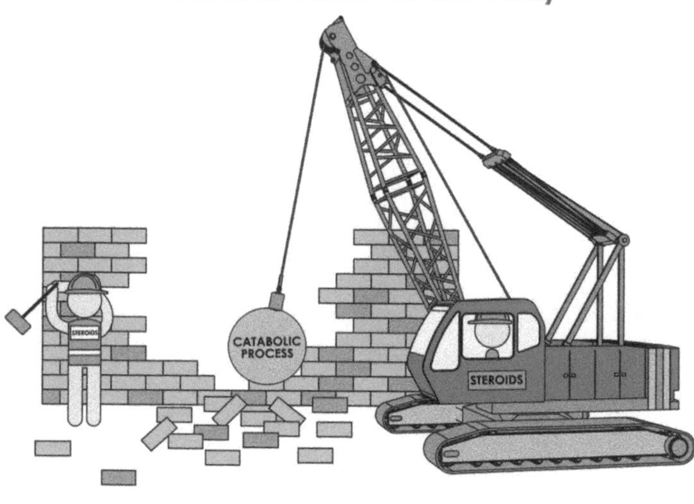

Steroids are associated with damage to cartilage cells and with avascular necrosis of the joints, along with other negative effects on the body:

- Decrease overall immunity
- Toxic to stem cells
- Destroy body's capacity to repair tendons

The progression of osteoarthritis was shown to continue regardless of corticosteroid treatment as early as 1993: the knees of steroid-treated patients showed more degeneration (78.6 percent) than the knees of those who did not receive treatment (52.4 percent).[8] More recently, the use of corticosteroids has been shown to have fewer long-term benefits for lateral epicondylitis, more commonly known as tennis elbow—an inflammation in the elbow region with damage to the tendons and muscles in the joint area. Despite positive short-term effects, injections with corticosteroids have been found to be no better in the long term than injections with a placebo,[9,10,11,12] with higher recurrence rates after a year.[13]

Interestingly, steroids are naturally secreted in the body by the adrenal cortices in response to stress only in the absence of sufficient vitamin C. The adrenal cortices have the highest concentration of vitamin C of any tissue in the body. When the body is under stress, vitamin C is secreted from the adrenals first, having a potent anti-inflammatory effect in the body. We routinely put our orthopedic patients on oral vitamin C, and we give a vitamin C IV after every surgery to replenish the body's and the adrenals' supply.

It makes sense evolutionarily that if the building blocks of repair are not available to heal a wound, the wound will remain in a chronically inflamed state. Vitamin C is crucial for collagen production and therefore wound healing. If the adrenals are out of vitamin C, the secreted corticosteroids may have an anti-inflammatory effect, but their catabolic action is inferior to the vitamin C they are replacing.

Early on, orthopedic specialists used PRP to treat a variety of inflammatory conditions like infrapatellar tendonitis, also known as jumper's knee. They knew that surgery would likely make this condition worse in many patients, especially in athletes. Reports were coming in of patients being treated with PRP for a variety of tendon conditions, without needing surgery. Very few doctors were using PRP treatments, but then

Arthroscopy for Orthopedic Injuries

Arthroscopy is a surgical procedure performed with the aid of an arthroscope, a small camera-like optical instrument that allows the surgeon to see the interior of an affected joint. This procedure usually requires two small incisions, one for the arthroscope and the other for the surgical instrument, making it a minimally invasive intervention under local, regional, or general anesthesia. Arthroscopy may be used in cases of ankle, wrist, shoulder, or elbow damage, but is most commonly used for the knee in meniscal tears or anterior cruciate ligament (ACL) reconstructions.

While recovery time is not as long as it would be with arthrotomy (fully opening the joint), arthroscopy patients still experience swelling and pain, and necessitate physical rehabilitation to be able to bear weight in the joint. There is great interest in augmentation in arthroscopic surgery—in particular, the use of biologics to speed recovery time and to promote healing in the affected area. Therapy with platelet-rich plasma (PRP) containing high levels of growth factors has shown promising results; studies summarizing multiple clinical trials report pain reduction and a decreased risk of reinjury after PRP treatment for certain conditions.[14,15,16]

again, their options were limited. PRP turned out to be a good choice for infrapatellar tendonitis. Patients did much better with PRP than they would have with arthroscopy, the most common surgical procedure for that condition.

Without the growth factors from PRP, a tendon has little chance to heal due to the low blood supply—much like cartilage in people with arthritis. Platelets are designed to heal a wound and stop bleeding as well as recruit cells from the bloodstream and bone marrow to induce healing. When PRP is injected, it sends the message, “this tissue is injured” to the body so that the body responds accordingly. With a minimally invasive procedure taking fewer than 30 minutes, athletes could now be back on the field in six weeks, playing with no pain.

As PRP technology matured, physicians moved from pulling growth factors out of blood to pulling growth factors out of bone marrow, as well as stem cell concentrate. Whole blood contains very few stem cells, but bone marrow is a rich source of these cells. It is particularly rich in stem cells that promote angiogenesis, or the development of new blood vessels, which helps to bring needed nutrients to the site of injury. When working with tissues that naturally have less blood supply, growth of new blood vessels to the area can make a big difference.

Also during this time, orthopedic surgeons performed microfracture surgeries, the standard of care for patients with damaged knee cartilage. The procedure involves drilling holes into the knee that go just deep enough to let bone marrow leak out. In microfracture, the bone marrow is key to prompting healing of the cartilage. Stem cells and other growth factors from bone marrow home to the area of damage and promote healing of the cartilage. Whether or not the procedure is successful is largely dependent on how robust the stem cells are. The problem is, many patients who undergo this procedure do not recover from the injury, or they only recover for a couple years because they were not able to heal the cartilage well enough. Unfortunately, this procedure has poorer outcomes than other cartilage repair techniques,[18] and a paper that reviews 20 years of data in 28 studies has found that there is insufficient data available on its long-term effects.[19] As it turns out, the protective covering that grows back to heal the cartilage after a microfracture procedure is not hyaline, the type of cartilage we are born with, but fibrocartilage, which is inherently less stable than hyaline within joints. Fibrocartilage breaks down more easily than hyaline, which is why so many microfracture procedures fail.

The relatively poor success rate of microfracture surgery spurred doctors to look for a better alternative and some began adding a concentrated bone marrow aspirate to help heal the knee better than the few drops that are extracted during microfracture. The problem was, at the time, the procedure involved extracting bone marrow with a tool called a Jamshidi™, a long nail-like needle that is driven into the hip bone using a mallet. The old Jamshidi procedure was painful, required the patient to be put under anesthesia, and involved multiple bone marrow draws to get a good sample. Jamshidi design improved over the years and nowadays, an experienced doctor can use a

Platelet-Rich Plasma (PRP)

Treatment with platelet rich plasma (PRP) is a technique to enhance the healing process after injury. Blood is drawn, generally from the patient's arm vein, and is then centrifuged to obtain platelets and cytokines in higher concentrations than in circulating blood. This process separates the PRP product into three distinct layers: 1) red blood cells at the bottom; 2) white blood cells and inflammatory cytokines (the buffy coat) in the middle; and 3) plasma (the liquid part of the blood), containing platelets and growth factors at the top.

There are actually two products that are commonly referred to as PRP. One of them is pure PRP. This classical, or true, PRP is made by centrifuging the tube gently so that the platelets remain suspended in the plasma. The plasma is then transferred to another tube, which is centrifuged harder so that the platelets separate to the bottom.

In the field of orthopedics, PRP is not only PRP—it also includes the white blood cells (from the buffy coat). Most machines that automate this process will also include the white blood cells (commonly known as the PBMCs, or peripheral blood mononuclear cells). So, in the literature there are many articles that refer to PRP when in fact they are describing PRP with PBMCs. Preferably, you would want the white blood cells in the PRP mixture if the goal is to heal the wound, because it includes cellular components that aid in healing.

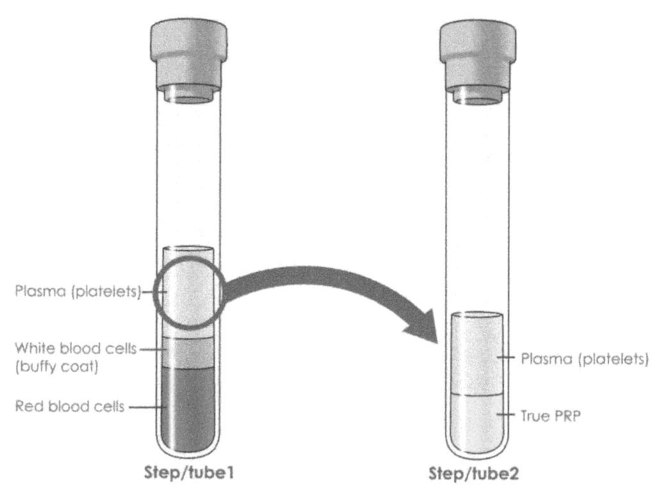

Once the platelets are activated inside the body, they release more growth factors, which promotes blood vessel formation. This newly formed blood vessel network allows nutrients and other cells to be delivered to the area, resulting in a faster recovery with less pain and reduced scarring of the injured tissue. Treatment with PRP is especially useful in orthopedics and in sports medicine, with notable successes in arthroscopy (anterior cruciate ligament and meniscal repairs), muscle tears, Achilles tendon injury, and tennis elbow, among many other injuries.[17]

PRP plus PBMCs can be described as "bone marrow lite." The bone marrow is a very rich environment of stem cells, including CD34+ cells, which are the precursors to all blood cells, and endothelial progenitor cells (EPCs), which are very important for inducing new blood vessel growth. EPCs and CD34+ cells both contribute to new blood vessel formation. The bone marrow also contains MSCs, which also can enhance new blood vessel growth as well as secrete many trophic factors that stimulate regeneration and decrease inflammation.

specially designed Jamshidi to quickly harvest bone marrow with minimal discomfort for the patient. Processing the bone marrow aspirate in a vertical axis centrifuge enables doctors at RMI to maximize the concentration of extracted mononuclear cells, which includes stem cells, compared to older machines like the Magellan.

Given the current regulatory environment in the United States, one of the very few stem cell options available to us is bone marrow aspirate concentrate (BMAC). Even though it is available in the United States, it is rarely paid for by insurance. I believe that soon, that is all going to change.

Stem cells from bone marrow aspirate have been compared to almost every graft with more success found in the treatment groups receiving bone marrow. What many orthopedic surgeons did not understand in the past was that bone marrow aspirate is not only useful for healing bone, but also for other tissues. We published a paper about our treatment with bone marrow aspirate concentrate of a 56-year-old woman with Achilles tendonopathy and a partially torn Achilles tendon that limited her ability to participate in daily activities that involved walking or wearing shoes other than sandals.[47] To our knowledge, she was the first Achilles tendonopathy patient treated with bone marrow aspirate. Previously an active tennis player, she hadn't been on the court in ten years due to her injury. She had seen multiple physicians over the years and followed standard conservative treatment involving stretching and anti-inflammatory medications. She had opted out of steroid injections and the standard surgery for the injury, but when presented with the possibility of an ultrasound-guided bone marrow aspirate concentrate injection of her own bone marrow, a non-invasive procedure that takes fewer than 60 minutes, she was interested.

Just six weeks after the procedure, the patient reported significantly less pain upon rest and while walking. The knot in her Achilles tendon decreased to 50 percent of its original size and was no longer tender to the touch. She was finally able to put on heels and walk over uneven surfaces without pain. And best of all, she returned to the court to play tennis for the first time in years. An MRI done ten weeks after the procedure showed that her heel looked almost indistinguishable from her other heel, which was not injured. A regeneration of tissue health such as this is not seen with other treatment types. Recovery time for the standard surgical procedure for her injury would have taken at least six months, but would not have restored her tendon as the bone marrow aspirate did, as evidenced by the MRI. Recovery like this simply doesn't happen with surgery.

Our rationale for treating this woman's Achilles tendonopathy came from our success with using bone marrow concentrate with Achilles tendon grafts in ACL (anterior cruciate ligament) tear repairs of the knee. ACL injuries are one of the most common injuries and often involve removing part of the patient's own tendon from below the kneecap to replace the ACL. This repair takes 369 days to heal, at which point it looks normal on an MRI. Unfortunately, the tendon that is removed from below the kneecap often does not heal properly, sometimes resulting in tendonitis or a shortening of the tendon, both of which affect the placement of the kneecap and can lead to arthritis. Orthopedic surgeons at RMI use a sterilized graft of an Achilles heel taken from a cadaver, which can be better tailored to the size of the new ACL without needing to remove the patient's own tendon. They inject bone marrow concentrate at the site of the injury, and healing time is fewer than 24 weeks, which is about half the time of the conventional treatment. Patients are able to avoid the complications of conventional treatment and get back to their normal lives sooner.

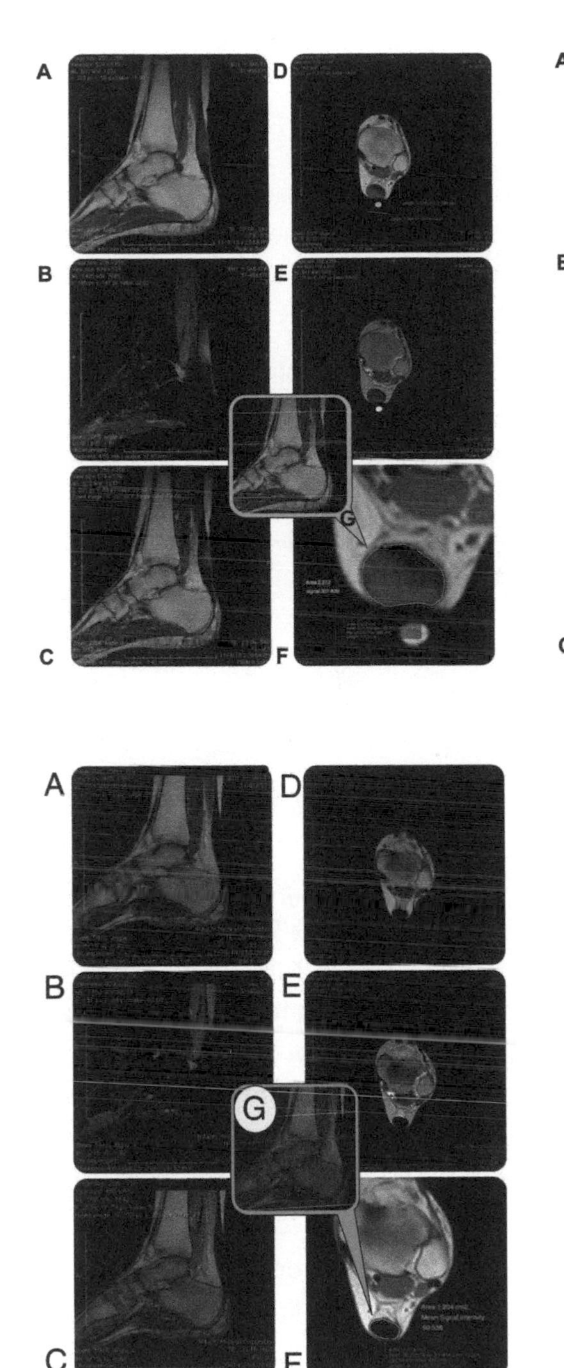

The patient's heel on MRI before treatment, 10 weeks after treatment, and 32 weeks after treatment. There is near complete healing of the affected tendon. The affected area decreased from 2.272 cm^2 to 1.204 cm^2.

Hyaline vs. Fibrocartilage

Cartilage is a connective tissue formed by cells called chondrocytes that are stacked within a collagen-based matrix. There are no blood vessels in this structure; nutrients are absorbed via the matrix, resulting in a limited capacity for regeneration. Cartilage may be classified into three types: hyaline cartilage, fibrocartilage, and elastic cartilage.[20]

Elastic cartilage is found in the ear and throat and is the most pliable of the three types. Fibrocartilage is designed to bear tension and compression, and as such it is a strong type of cartilage present in the vertebral discs of the spine, in the meniscus, at the end of tendons, and in the callus structure of the bones. Hyaline cartilage may be found in the rib area and in the more mobile articular joints (wrists, elbows, shoulders, hips, knees, etc.) where synovial fluid reduces friction in the space between the bones. The matrix of hyaline

Teresa Hamrick is a registered nurse from Tallahassee, FL. In 1983 she was injured in a bike accident but brushed off the injury and continued to walk around as normally as possible for as long as possible. Knee pain eventually brought her to the doctor two years later, where she was told that she had degenerative joint disease and needed to have both knees replaced. The cartilage in her knees was non-existent, and her femur heads were worn after being ground away by bone chips. Her doctors recommended that she find a new line of work that allowed her to sit. She went back to school and got a degree in management. Her orthopedic surgeon told her that if she proceeded with total knee replacement, she would need to repeat the surgeries about seven years later due to the wear and tear of her usual rate of activity. She opted out of the surgery and was soon bound to a motorized scooter.

Twelve years later, at age 50, Teresa experienced her first heart attack. She recovered and slowly began working out with a trainer to help prevent further heart problems. But in July 2011 she had a massive heart attack and was forced to retire due to the state of her heart. She was left with not much hope at that point. Her medical background spurred her interest in finding cartilage is formed by collagen type II, whereas fibrocartilage is made up of collagen type I. There are fewer chondrocytes in fibrocartilage than in hyaline cartilage, as well as fewer proteoglycans and glycoproteins. Under the microscope, cells in hyaline cartilage are rounded and cluster in small groups as they are scattered within the matrix, encased by the perichondrium, a supporting structure. Cells in fibrocartilage lie in rows and are surrounded by bundles of collagen fibers that give it an array-like appearance.

A particular concern[21,22] when treating cartilage defects in the joints is that the tissue that regrows might contain fibrocartilage instead of hyaline cartilage, leading to stiffness in a previously mobile joint and a loss of normal function. In some cases, hyaline-like tissue does form successfully, but fibrocartilage[23] and type I collagen[24] can appear in up to 40 percent of cases.[25]

a solution. She read scientific articles and clinical trials about her condition and possible options. She eventually decided to try autologous bone marrow stem cell therapy for her heart. After treatment her ejection fraction went from 12 to 30 percent in three months.

Fast forward to early September 2013. Her heart was in good shape—ejection fraction was 40 percent, and she was up to walking, albeit with some trouble, a mile and a half a day. One day she was walking down a hill and she felt a rip on the side of her knee. That injury put her back in the motorized scooter, only able to walk up to ten or fifteen feet on her own. She saw an orthopedic surgeon who recommended total knee replacement of both knees. Not a big fan of surgery or drugs, she went online to find out if anyone was doing stem cell treatments for knees. She learned about the International Stem Cell Symposium to be held in the Bahamas in September 2014. A year before, I had met an orthopedic surgeon at a conference in Florida organized by the same group. At the Bahamas symposium, he was scheduled to present his results on treating patients in his orthopedic practice. Teresa booked a ticket to the Bahamas to learn more about his work. She was impressed with his presentation and met him after his talk. They arranged for her to come back to Texas for treatment. In March, the orthopedic surgeon evaluated her knees and determined that she still needed a total knee replacement for the left knee, but only a partial for the right. He performed the surgery along with BMAC and amnion injections. Amnion is a human amniotic membrane product, derived from the lining of the amniotic sac from a healthy, live birth.

With age, the number of stem cells inside bone marrow steadily declines. By the time a human reaches skeletal maturity, the number of mesenchymal stem cells in bone marrow has declined by 90 percent. The doubling time of cells, which is an indication of their robustness, also declines with age. In older patients with chronic orthopedic conditions, the Riordan Medical Institute augments bone marrow concentrate with amnion. When exposed to the amnion, the cells of the bone marrow concentrate actually alter in such a way that makes them appear and behave like bone marrow concentrate cells from a younger individual.

Four weeks later, Teresa was able to fly home. The following September she came back for a right partial knee replacement and more BMAC and amnion injections. "No one ever thought I would get back to my current functional status after scootering and limping for 30 years and then being in a wheelchair for six months. I have been working out with a trainer again. I have been walking one to three miles every day. On X-ray my knees are perfectly aligned and there is a nice uniform spacing between the bones. My treatments were extremely successful. I am thriving. I am over-the-moon happy with my outcome. I have my life back."

"No one ever thought I would get back to my current functional status after scootering and limping for 30 years and then being in a wheelchair for six months. I have my life back."

Jennifer Ziegler is an active 50-year old woman who injured the ACL of her knee during a skiing accident in January 2015. "I dove out of the way of another skier, heard a pop in my knee, and limped back down the mountain," she said. ACL injury is common, and like Jennifer, many people are stubborn and try to muscle through the injury. A few months later, in June, Jennifer reinjured the knee while gardening. "I felt the pain all over again. Getting in and out of the car was difficult. Walking my dogs was interesting. I never knew when my knee was going to give out."

After her husband convinced her to get an MRI, she visited her orthopedic doctor. He recommended the traditional autotransplant surgery, which involves the removal of part of the infrapatellar tendon at the front of the knee to replace the missing ACL. This type of procedure creates yet another injury and takes up to a year to heal, if it even heals at all. The idea of going through such a surgery made Jennifer uncomfortable. That's when she contacted me. I referred her to our clinic.

A few days later, she was on a plane to Texas. After examination, our surgeon recommended arthroscopy and injection of BMAC and amnion. Some of her ACL remained intact so he didn't feel she needed a more extensive procedure. She went through with the treatment, and six weeks later Jennifer was hiking and biking on vacation in Colorado. By January she was skiing again. "I wish everyone had the opportunity to choose a less invasive treatment. It should be covered by insurance. It should be something that everyone in the United States has the option to do," she said.

Jim Morello is a 70-year-old marathon runner who was experiencing what he called "bone on bone pain" in his knees while running. A friend of his had received stem cell treatment in Colorado and was happy with it, which prompted Jim to research different clinics. After speaking with our orthopedic surgeon, he decided to undergo stem cell treatment along with arthroscopy on both knees.

> ***I wanted my knees to be in good shape to stay active with my grandkids—that was my biggest impetus."***

"The experience was very positive," he said. "The staff there is awesome." The procedure occurred on Monday with a follow-up on Thursday, after which he

Bone Marrow Aspirate Concentrate (BMAC)

Bone marrow aspirate concentrate (BMAC) is the preferred source of stem cells for orthopedic injuries due to the improved focus of the stem cells toward skeletal healing. One peptide secreted by these cells, known as sox-9, is useful in the formation of cartilage. The high concentration of CD34+ stem cells in bone marrow concentrate is another reason why it's the stem cell source of choice. The CD34+ cells are focused on angiogenesis, or growth of new blood vessels, which are essential for healing orthopedic injuries that are already at a blood supply disadvantage. The bone marrow concentrate secretes what the body already knew it needed in order to heal.

Bone marrow aspiration is a procedure that extracts a small amount of bone marrow in liquid form. Well-tested harvesting techniques allow a simple and safe aspiration to be performed within the clinic under local anesthesia. Bone marrow may be obtained from bones in the leg or arm, or from the iliac crest (hip area). The extracted liquid (between 60 and 120 cc) is then concentrated down to 5 cc. This bone marrow aspirate concentrate is rich in mesenchymal stem cells (MSCs), endothelial progenitor cells (EPCs), and other proteins and factors secreted by these cells, such as CD133+ and CD34+.

As discussed elsewhere, MSCs have anti-inflammatory properties, promote blood vessel growth, and are able to modulate the immune system.[26] It has recently been shown that the secretions stimulated by MSCs are responsible for their therapeutic potential,[27] including for cartilage repair.[28] In particular, vascular endothelial growth factor (VEGF) stimulates blood-forming cells (endothelial progenitor cells, or EPCs) to grow new blood vessels in the injured or inflamed area. This process provides nutrients more efficiently and promotes faster healing.

BMAC treatment has been safely used in animal models. Goats that received BMAC showed significant improvements in the damaged joints, with almost complete recovery of the cartilage.[29] Similarly, when treatment was enhanced with BMAC, the cartilage of horses showed greater healing.[30] Horses that received bone marrow-derived MSCs after meniscal damage arthroscopy showed an improvement in ability to return to work compared to those receiving surgery alone.[31] Similarly, rats receiving human bone marrow-derived MSCs as a complement to rotator cuff repair surgery showed early improvements.[32]

BMAC has also been used in clinical settings with no adverse effects[33] and with positive results. Patients who received BMAC after knee surgery showed higher improvement in all measured scores, with healthy cartilage covering the injured areas in a two-year follow-up.[34] BMAC was also shown to be beneficial in the treatment of bone defects,[35] bone grafts,[36] tendon injuries,[37,38] and arterial disease in the lower limbs.[39] A recent review reports excellent overall outcomes with the use of BMAC for osteoarthritis and cartilage injuries.[40]

PRP and BMAC have been used together to treat a football athlete following complications of a hip arthroscopy, with significant improvements in physical activity as well as in the appearance of tendons under magnetic resonance imaging (MRI).[41] Treatment with BMAC to complement rotator cuff arthroscopy was shown to be safe and to enhance tissue quality in affected tendons after a one-year follow-up.[42]

Probably the most compelling argument for the use of BMAC in orthopedics, both from a patient-centric perspective and also from an economic perspective, is a 2014 article by Hernigou, et al.[43] It documented the results of ten-year study—a follow-up of rotator cuff repair in two groups of patients, one that received BMAC and another that did not. The group receiving BMAC had a 100 percent healing rate at six months, compared to 67 percent in the non-BMAC group. Ten years later only 13 percent of the patients who received BMAC had failure in their rotator cuff compared to 66 percent of the patients who did not. Given the high costs of rotator cuff repair surgery for an insurance company, it becomes readily apparent that paying for a single BMAC procedure would be more cost effective for insurance companies, as well as patients.

returned home to Tulsa. "I was able to start running a little bit over time. I ran a race, carefully, three months later. I had some MRIs done, which showed new growth between the bones—good news after spending the money." One year after treatment he ran a race that qualified him to be up front in the next Tulsa Run. "I wanted my knees to be in good shape to stay active with my grandkids—that was my biggest impetus," Jim said. "The stem cell outcome was very positive. I've recommended a number of people to go."

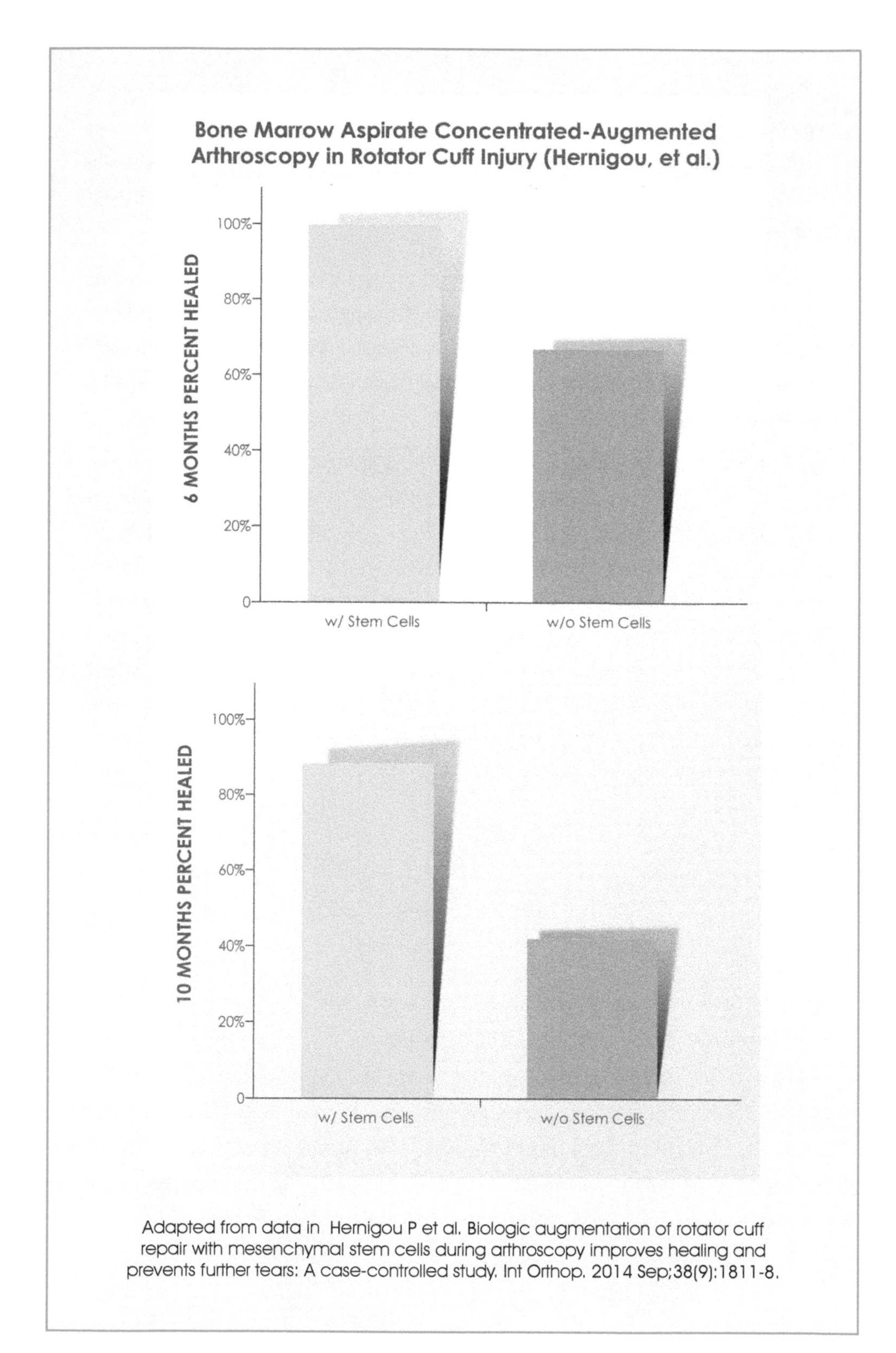

Adapted from data in Hernigou P et al. Biologic augmentation of rotator cuff repair with mesenchymal stem cells during arthroscopy improves healing and prevents further tears: A case-controlled study. Int Orthop. 2014 Sep;38(9):1811-8.

There are currently several clinical trials registered on ClinicalTrials.gov to investigate the effects of treatment with MSCs as an aid to arthroscopic procedures, such as umbilical cord MSCs for ACL (anterior cruciate ligament) arthroscopy,[44] BMAC for rotator cuff arthroscopy,[45] and BMAC for ankle arthroscopy.[46]

David Crumpton, DDS happens to be the dentist for one of our former physician's family. One day David reached over to lift an object, and with nothing more than a slight amount of pressure, his bicep detached from the bone and tore some of the tendon. He came to Southlake for treatment. Our orthopedic surgeon reattached the bicep and injected BMAC and amnion to help it heal. "The way I think about it is, something tore in my arm so that I could learn how to fix my back," he said. While his bicep was healing, the pressure he put on his left arm to compensate for his right bicep aggravated an old back injury. As a dentist, Dr. Crumpton is always bent at the waist, which left him with a chronic backache, especially after his bicep injury. He had pinched and injured discs in his lumbar spine that caused a lot of discomfort. Our doctor first referred him to another physician to try epidurals, but when those didn't work, he recommended a discogram to determine which discs were affected, and then injected BMAC and amnion into three discs. The procedure was done on a Thursday; he experienced some soreness on Friday and Saturday and was back to work on Monday. "Immediately after the surgery the pain went away, and over the next six months it continued to improve week by week. Today I am probably the best I have ever been in 30 years. I feel so great about what I did."

> ***"Today I am probably the best I have ever been in 30 years."***

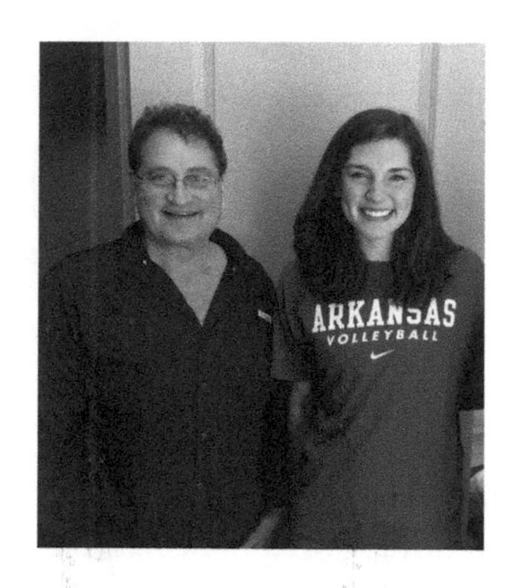

Elizabeth Fortado, a twenty-one-year-old Division 1 volleyball player for the University of Arkansas, tore all the ligaments in her ankle playing the sport in Europe during her sophomore year. She visited two prominent orthopedic specialists who both told her she needed surgery and that the recovery would be at least eight months. That meant she would not be able to play volleyball that year. Elizabeth's father was familiar with our surgeon, being a sales representative for orthopedic devices, so he brought Elizabeth in for a consultation. "We would lose two months undergoing this treatment, but we were already going to lose her entire season if she had to have surgery."

They decided to go ahead with the procedure and Elizabeth was injected with BMAC and amnion in 2015. Eight weeks later she started training again. "I immediately noticed the difference with my ankle," she said. "It felt so much stronger than it did before. It was amazing. Before the procedure I had so much popping in the ankle that was extremely painful. I have no popping anymore." Ten weeks later she started her first volleyball game, achieving her highest hitting percentage ever. Then, in her second game, she experienced her all-time career high. "As a high-level athlete trying to get back into the game, to come back and compete at a stronger position than she ever had, it made such an unbelievable difference," her father added. "Everyone was skeptical about the procedure—her orthopedic surgeons at the school, her trainers— everyone handled her with kid gloves. It blew everyone's mind that

"I immediately noticed the difference with my ankle," she said. "It felt so much stronger than it did before. It was amazing."

she could come back from such a severe injury. They see those injuries in volleyball and never see people return like that." Elizabeth experienced a strengthening and improvement in range of motion in her ankle that surpassed even her uninjured ankle. She later returned for another injection of BMAC and amnion to continue to fortify her ankle. "Now my bad ankle at the time is my good ankle, and my good ankle is my bad ankle," she said.

Billy Minick is a 77-year-old bull rider from Texas. One of the world's top four professional bull riders in his youth, he has spent his life riding bulls, roping steer, and running Billy Bob's Texas, a bull riding arena and country club in Fort Worth that he eventually purchased along with three friends. He married his wife, Pam, in 1983 and ran the company with her until 2013 when they both retired. Pam is extremely active with a number of charities and is well known throughout Fort Worth, Texas.

While roping a calf one day, Billy's arm went limp. "His arm turned blue," Pam said. He put off a doctor's visit for a few days, in true cowboy style, but his pain pushed him to consult an orthopedic specialist who recommended a reverse rotator cuff arthroplasty, the most drastic surgery for this type of injury. Billy had seen Pam suffer tremendously for eight months from a lesser surgery two years prior for her own rotator cuff tear. "It was months before I didn't call my doctor a four-letter word," she said. Billy was reluctant to undergo a major surgery because he didn't want to suffer as Pam had, so he sought a second opinion. The next doctor recommended a much more conservative treatment—physical therapy alone.

"My colleagues tend to be at extreme ends of the spectrum," said a surgeon at RMI. "Mr. Minnick had been told that his shoulder was so chronically injured that he was no longer a candidate for a traditional shoulder replacement, but that he would need a reverse arthroplasty—where they reverse the cup and ball because of the lack of rotator cuff—due to the significant and chronic nature of his tear. At the other end of the spectrum, the second doctor told Mr. Minick that there was nothing that could be done other than physical therapy to try to get back some deltoid function. I didn't think either was the best option for Mr. Minick. Reverse arthroplasty is the most significant shoulder intervention that can be accomplished surgically. The problem with this surgery is that there are no good fallback procedures—if it doesn't work out, nothing can be done. It basically burns your bridges. There is nowhere to go after that. The surgery is fairly new, and for patients like Mr. Minick, who do not have significant humeral arthritis, its popularity is beginning to wane."

Billy's close friend had been treated with BMAC and amnion with excellent results, and recommended that Billy visit the clinic. Billy had no strength or use of his right arm at the time. Moving his arm was painful and difficult. He decided to pay us a visit. "Mr. Minick had significant weakness of the upper extremity and couldn't really raise his arm to get his elbow to the level of his chest," said our doctor. "He had no significant rotator cuff tissue left. He had a complete retraction of the most important muscle of his rotator cuff. His shoulder was basically dislocated—we call it cephalad migration—the bone of his humerus was riding up underneath the bones of his shoulder blade because he had no muscle or tendon of the rotator cuff to keep it in place."

"After significant discussion of what I thought were his options, I did not think he was a good candidate for stem cell therapy alone. I also did not think he was a good candidate for a total reverse shoulder arthroplasty. I recommended a combination of cell therapy, using injections of his own BMAC along with amnion, and a minimally invasive partial arthroplasty of the shoulder." After some consideration, Mr. Minick decided to proceed with our surgeon's recommendations. The doctor was able to clean up the loose pieces and debris in his shoulder with arthroscopy, remove the bone spurs, and insert a partial shoulder that would reduce pain and help improve range of motion. The cell therapy would help increase cellular volume to increase the strength of his deltoid muscle.

Billy's pain after the procedure was so minimal that he took only one pain pill. "I never had any pain amount to anything other than soreness," he said. Within several weeks Billy was out of his arm sling and working on range of motion with physical therapy.

"What amazed me," said the surgeon, "was that even at 77 years old and with little function in his arm at the time of his exam, Mr. Minick was anxious to get back to roping. I told him that our goal was to see how much function, strength, range of motion, and pain relief we could get for him. Even getting a wallet out of his pocket or putting on a seatbelt was difficult at the time. But sure enough, eight months after the procedure, Mr. Minick was roping again."

"It wasn't pretty, but I got him," Billy said. "The strength part has been a slow process, but I am more than satisfied. It is getting better and better every week. The pain relief was the greatest thing." Between Pam and some of Billy's friends who had undergone similar surgeries without cell therapy, their recoveries took much longer than Billy's. "I credit the stem cells personally," he said.

"Without cell therapy, this type of surgery—even though it's minimally invasive—in this age group can still result in significant pain relief but doesn't really result in improvements of range of motion or strength," said the surgeon. "With cell therapy, within two months he was able to fully elevate his shoulder. Repopulating the areas of atrophy, the cellularity is restored and the patient heals and has less pain and more function."

Our goal is to use BMAC and amnion to turn big surgeries into small surgeries and small surgeries into simple injections. In-office injections are currently used for conditions such as osteoarthritic or inflamed joints, partial and full thickness tears, and chronic, painful, partial tearing. Minimally-invasive surgeries are augmented with BMAC and amnion.

I have computed the savings to insurance companies, extrapolated from published data,[48] of the inclusion of autologous BMAC to rotator cuff injury surgery. Assuming a surgical cost of $25,000 and a bone marrow kit cost of $2,500, roughly $4.8 billion would be saved by insurance companies annually due to surgical failures and revision surgeries for shoulders alone. That number does not include any of the lost time at work, or the increased aftercare due to follow-up surgeries that would be saved by employers and employees.

A notable effect of bone marrow concentrate treatment is that patients who undergo orthopedic surgeries may experience a lower infection rate when they receive bone marrow concentrate than they would without it. At least one surgeon has been able to dramatically lower infection in surgeries that typically have around a three to five percent infection rate. One explanation for this is likely due to the highly antimicrobial peptide known as LL-37, secreted by mesenchymal stem cells found in bone marrow concentrate. Another explanation for reduced infection is the faster healing rate of the wound due to greater mobility of the patient, which increases blood flow to the wound site and reduces swelling.

Chapter Thirteen

AUTISM—PROGRESS, NOT REGRESSION

At our clinic in Panama we treat many people who have chronic conditions that their doctors have told them they have little hope of curing, but none of these diseases engages my heart the way autism does. Many people who come down with chronic diseases are shattered by how it changes their lives and rearranges plans for the future. Unlike diseases that come late in life, with autism the shattering is often more brutal and almost always affects the entire family.

Many parents of autistic children realize their child is different early on—typically between one and two years of age—and end up receiving a diagnosis from their family physician. However, there is a subset of families with an autistic child that have an entirely different story: the child is happy and healthy, making all his developmental milestones, and then suddenly one day it all stops. He is limp, unresponsive to the smiles and hugs of his parents and, in many cases, fills his days with repetitive behaviors that are disturbing to watch, such as rocking back and forth, repeating the same phrases, or doing the same activity with blocks or cars over and over again.

For families living with autism, the pain is so much stronger because of the loss of hope. When you are stricken with a chronic condition at the age of 50, you've already lived a large part of your life and made some good memories. When a small child is diagnosed with a condition as persistent as autism, the future looks bleak. Parents can't help but worry about how their child will survive as an adult and what special care he will need after they have gone.

Unfortunately, autism is widespread, and the number of children diagnosed with it is increasing. Today one in every 68 children is diagnosed with autism, making it more prevalent than childhood cancer, juvenile diabetes, and childhood AIDS combined. And government statistics suggest that the number of children diagnosed with autism is increasing at a rate of between 10 and 17 percent annually. This might be because we are getting better at diagnosing it, or it may be due to an increase of whatever is causing it—be it environmental influences or the result of multiple genetic factors. Other research points to the mother having been exposed to viral infections or chemical insults. Some evidence collected over the last 30 years suggests that autism may be caused by inflammation of the central nervous system. This is where, we have found, stem cell therapy can help because of stem cells' ability to help mediate inflammation.

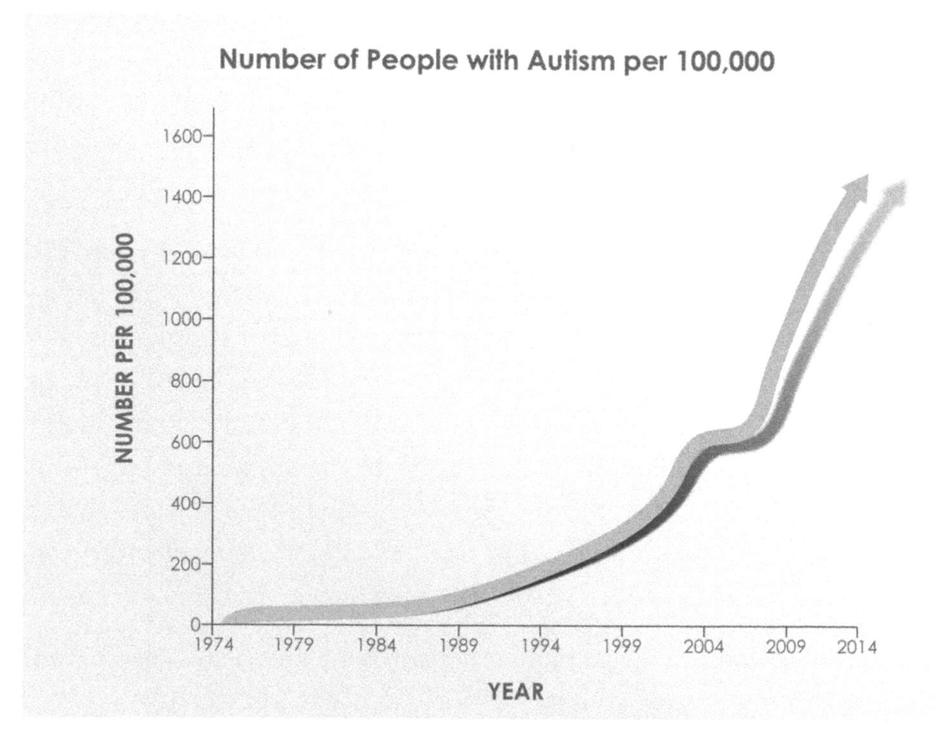

From data found in Centers for Disease Control and Prevention (CDC) website at https://www.cdc.gov/ncbddd/autism/data.html

Mesenchymal Stem Cells for Treatment of Autism

Autism spectrum disorder (ASD) refers to a group of brain development disorders that affect communication skills and social interaction to varying degrees of intensity, with significant impact on the patient, his or her family, and society. The mechanisms that cause ASD have not been completely determined,[7] and there is currently no cure. Treatment is focused on behavior management; medical intervention usually targets symptoms, for example with antipsychotic medication in certain cases.[8] There is a pressing need for different therapeutic approaches,[9] especially those focused on what is known so far about the biological processes associated with ASD.

Recent studies have found that there may be a link between ASD, the immune system, and inflammation. Children with ASD have higher measures of certain chemokines (signaling proteins secreted by cells, in this case MDC and TARC) that are expressed locally by inflamed tissues, with higher levels in those with more severe ASD symptoms.[10] Likewise, children with ASD have been found to have significantly higher inflammatory Th1 cytokine (IL-12 and IFN-γ) levels in their blood compared to similar-aged children.[11] Proteins that are involved in binding white blood cells to blood vessel walls (an important step of inflammation) have been found in significantly high levels in children with ASD.[12] After a 26-week treatment with the dietary supplement luteolin, a subset of children with ASD showed a reduction in levels of inflammatory cytokines TNF-α and IL-6, which was strongly associated with an improvement in behavior.[13] As in this trial, we are finding that response to treatment varies by subset of ASD children. Detecting biomarkers to identify such subsets is key in treating children with this disorder.

Children with autism have immune dysregulation and increased inflammation. Because the immune and nervous systems are closely interconnected, several immunological abnormalities have been detected in the nervous system of autistic children. Inflammatory compounds have been found in the brains and bloodstream of autistic children.[1,2,3] And children with autism have an autoimmune-like condition that several lines of reason suggest might play a causative role.[4] First, several types of autoantibodies have been found in autistic children. Second, family members of autistic children are more likely to have autoimmune conditions. And third, autism has been

About 20 percent of children with ASD have gastrointestinal symptoms, with greater symptom severity in those with ASD measures of irritability, anxiety, and social withdrawal.[14] High sensitivity (hypersensitivity) to stimulus (auditory, visual, touch) is a common trait of ASD; a study of 2,973 children with ASD found a highly significant rate of over-responsivity to sensory stimulus in those who had gastrointestinal symptoms.[15] Inflammation in both the upper and lower intestinal tract has also been reported,[16] and a test for certain genes along with markers for inflammation were able to correctly identify ASD in 83 percent of cases.[17] This level of constant inflammation originating in the gut might cause alterations in the structure of the brain; it has been shown that cerebral white matter is disproportionately larger in children with ASD[18] and that neuroinflammation and enlarged white matter of the brain likely co-occur.[19] Recent reviews have highlighted growing evidence of neuroinflammation in children with ASD[20] and that the mechanisms of said inflammation may contribute to ASD,[21] stressing the need for treatments targeting this aspect of the condition. Our group has been proposing since 2007[22] that the characteristics of mesenchymal stem cell (MSCs) make them a viable treatment option to address the inflammatory and immunological issues associated with ASD—a double-blind, placebo-controlled trial of MSC treatment in children with ASD would be ideal to demonstrate this.

The anti-inflammatory effects of mesenchymal stem cells and their secretions[23] have been demonstrated for several inflammatory conditions,[24,25,26,27] making MSC therapy a very promising treatment for ASD patients.[28] Clinical trials have already demonstrated that treatment with MSCs is safe for ASD.[29] Children treated with a combination of umbilical cord MSCs and other umbilical cord cells showed significant differences in visual, emotional, and intellectual responses and nonverbal communication among other measures.[30] In another study, children with ASD were treated with cells derived from bone marrow, including MSCs; global improvements were observed for 96 percent of patients, including behavior patterns (66 percent), social relationships (90.6 percent), and speech, language, and communication (78 percent).[31]

Several clinical trials are currently approved and ongoing on ClinicalTrials.gov to treat ASD with bone marrow MSCs, adipose-derived MSCs, and umbilical cord MSCs.[32,33,34,35,36]

associated with an autoimmune-like bowel condition similar to Crohn's disease. And not only do children with autism have more inflammation and immune imbalance, but they also produce fewer anti-inflammatory compounds,[5,6] which only adds to their already excessive inflammation.

Our team wrote a scientific journal article (referenced above) about the rationale for using umbilical cord stem cells for autism in 2007. It was published in the *Journal of Translational Medicine* and it is one of the most accessed and cited articles—accessed more than 74,000 times.

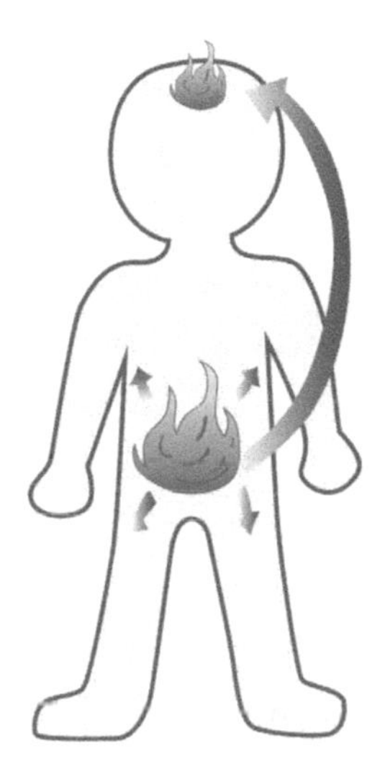

Inflammation in the gut affects inflammation in the brain.

If inflammation and immune dysregulation are a cause of the symptoms of autism, then treating this inflammation might help to ease symptoms. We speculated that if we could inject mesenchymal stem cells into children who suffered with autism, those cells would secrete factors that quell inflammation and help to balance the immune system. If the cells worked, as they had done with so many other conditions, it was possible that we could really help these children and their families battle against this punishing condition and live more normal lives, as we did with Anthony.

Anthony Guerriero was developing normally. He talked and walked before his first birthday and met all of his developmental and behavioral milestones—that is, until about 18 months. He suddenly stopped trying to interact and became difficult to engage. He wouldn't look when his name was called and slowly lost all the vocabulary he had gained. He was officially diagnosed with autism at age two. "He didn't know who he was or who we were. He was mute for two years. It was difficult," said John Guerriero, Anthony's dad.

Anthony became hyperactive, climbing on furniture, bouncing, jumping—even walking on countertops. It was like he was trying to escape something he didn't have the words to describe. "He wasn't comfortable in his own skin," John said.

The reason doctors use the word *spectrum* is to acknowledge that there is a wide range of behaviors that fall under the umbrella diagnosis of autism. With most diseases, you either have it or you don't. With autism, a child can be highly functioning and able to talk freely and socialize but still have some significant delays in processing the stimuli that bombard him every day. Or a child can be severely affected by the condition—withdrawn, uncommunicative, and lost in his own world. One common aspect of the condition, no matter where the child is on the spectrum, is that the earlier the parents establish therapy to help the child, the more effective that therapy is in the long run. They call this the *autism window*, the time between the ages of two and seven when the various therapies available for speech, motor skills, and socialization can have the biggest impact on correcting the condition.

Anthony underwent a wide range of therapies—behavioral, occupational, physical, speech, biomedical, and dietary—as most autistic children do. While he made progress and gained some speech, he still struggled with processing and expressive language, and he continued to have sensory challenges, digestive issues, and allergies.

Anthony's parents first heard about stem cell treatment from a prominent autism doctor, but when they looked into it, the cost seemed prohibitive. But when it was mentioned again by the parents of another autistic child, and again by a family member, they decided to do some research. They reached out to a mother on Facebook who had taken her child—who had symptoms and behaviors similar to Anthony—down for treatment. They were so impressed by her child's improvements that they decided to try to raise money for the treatment. When the mayor of their town heard about their intentions, he offered to hold a fundraiser for them, which allowed them to come down for treatment in 2015.

After his first treatment, his parents noticed right away that his skin became much softer, "like he had found the fountain of youth," said his dad. The positive changes continued when they arrived back home. Anthony began asking for new foods that he normally didn't eat. Before his treatment, he would only eat a few foods because most foods brought him digestive pain. "He put on so much weight and filled out. He's so healthy," noted his father.

His behavior also changed. He stopped climbing on furniture inappropriately. "He does normal boy stuff now. And he's super calm," John said. He was able to sit in one place for his sister's two-and-a-half-hour dance recital—an impossibility just the year before. "Last year he would have lasted one minute, and it would've been a rough day for all of us!"

Anthony's best improvement was his new connection to his brother and sister. "Now he's talking to us and his siblings. Before treatment he didn't have a relationship with his brother. He was off in his own world. Now they are best friends. The three of them are inseparable."

I've seen how powerful these cells can be in causing a dramatic turnaround in children who seemed so closed off and isolated from the world. Time after time, if the parents are willing to come back for a second treatment with stem cells, they report back that their child has made huge leaps forward toward being just a normal kid with the same issues and challenges as his or her peers.

Anthony came back for a second treatment. We saw with Anthony the same behavior we've seen with so many autistic kids who return for subsequent treatment—they actually look forward to it. First-time treatments for autistic children can be difficult. With their heightened sensitivities, need for routine, and young age, blood draws and injections can be intimidating. That's why we have partnered with autism experts from around the world to help us design an autism treatment room specially dedicated to comforting these kids. From the colors of the walls to the added touches of ambiance, the autism treatment room is designed from the ground up to help make the treatment easier for autistic children. But for subsequent treatments we often find the children eager and ready, holding out their arms to us for injections because they know it means they will feel better soon. When

Anthony returned for his second treatment, on the day of his first injection he woke up asking for stem cells.

Shortly after returning home from his second treatment, Anthony asked that his harness be removed when he rode the bus. Before treatment he had to be harnessed to his seat because he would spontaneously try to escape the bus when it stopped or even jump into the bus driver's lap while he was driving. But Anthony felt ready "to be a big boy." He no longer had trouble sitting still on the bus without his harness.

Within about a month of his second treatment Anthony's speech and conversation really took off. He engaged in imaginative play for the first time ever. And he became able to communicate when he wasn't feeling well, which makes the job of his parents so much easier. Autistic children are often suffering from ailments they do not have the ability to describe. When Anthony's molars were loose, he was able to say, "My teeth hurt here," something most parents take for granted.

Eight weeks after his second treatment his parents were calling him "blabber mouth" while remembering a time when they wondered if he would ever make a single sound again. He began telling jokes and poking fun at his dad. "This is going to be the best year of our lives," John said.

Six months after his second treatment he asked to go back to speech therapy, something he had previously asked to be taken out of because it was so stressful for him. "I can't make this stuff up—looks like it may be time for speech therapy again," John said.

Kenneth Kelley's story began a bit differently than Anthony's. When he was six months old his mother took him with her to a dental appointment where she was having her amalgam fillings removed. He slept on the floor in his carrier during the procedure, unknowingly inhaling the vaporized mercury fumes. The next day, they came back for another round. By his next doctor appointment, he had fallen off the growth chart and was having trouble nursing. He seemed weaker and his babbling never progressed. His first birthday came and went and he was no closer to walking or talking than he had been months before. His pediatrician didn't see a problem. Nor did the next few doctors his parents consulted. They finally found a doctor who listened to their concerns, and at the age of two Kenneth was diagnosed with autism. His parents set him up with the conventional behavioral and speech therapy, but by the age of four he still had no vocabulary. The doctors said, "Maybe he's a late speaker."

At age five, Kenneth received 38 vaccinations over an eight-week period so that he could catch up with the vaccine schedule required for him to attend school. That's when his behavior took a turn for the worse. "His autism escalated probably 100-fold," said Marty Kelley, his mother. He became aggressive. When meeting new people, he would show off, shout and scream, demand attention, jump on furniture, throw things, crawl on the floor, take off his clothes. He would yell, "shut up," to his family or to strangers. He would try to run away sometimes and would carry his baby sister with him out into the road. Some days he would scream from morning until night. He could not dress himself and would put up a fight when his parents dressed him. He was still in diapers. There was very little he had mastered by that age. He needed to be shown how to do everything.

His parents went to work researching options for their son. They learned about biomedical treatments and dietary methods. It wasn't until Ken tested for mercury that his parents realized what had happened. Those two days in the dental office inhaling mercury had taken their toll. The doctors had never seen a mercury level so high. Kenneth underwent therapy to help remove the mercury, and at the age of five and a half, he began hyperbaric oxygen therapy, which helps to bring more oxygen to areas of the brain that are hypoperfused, or not getting enough oxygen, a common feature in children with autism. The therapy did help him develop some speech and become calmer, but Kenneth still had a long way to go.

Kenneth's parents continued with a range of biomedical treatments, visiting some of the top autism doctors in the world. They spent $300,000 on treatments and implementation of different protocols. Some treatments and therapies helped to a degree, and others made him worse. After two years of hyperbaric oxygen therapy—the therapy his parents felt had worked best—his improvements did not increase.

At age eight he still couldn't answer "who, what, where, when, why" questions. "What was left to do? We had done it all," Marty said. He was on the severe end of the autism spectrum and had also been diagnosed with severe mental retardation. "There is nothing you're going to be able to do with this child," the doctors told them.

Kenneth's parents became aware of stem cell therapy at that time when they saw a news story about another autistic boy who had been treated at our clinic—our first autistic patient, in fact. They talked to the boy's father and followed his progress. "I didn't believe the results they were getting at first," Marty said. But they were so impressed with his progress and knew they needed a new approach, so they decided to apply for stem cell treatment at our clinic.

Fewer than one hundred patients had used stem cells for autism at that time. "We knew that we would be out a lot of money if it didn't work. We also knew we would always wonder 'What if?' if we didn't try." Kenneth came to our clinic in Costa Rica in 2009 at age eight.

At the time, he had the vocabulary of a four-year-old, the body of a five-year-old, and he was still in diapers. "Do you know what it is like for your child to not be able to speak to you? To not be able to tell you how his day was? What he wants to be when he grows up? What his favorite color is?" Kenneth's mom summed up what it's like to live as a parent of an autistic child.

Within days of his stem cell treatment he began talking more and using more common sense, but his parents were hesitant to attribute the changes to stem cells. A week later he brought up an event from the past—something he had never done before. It stopped his mother in her tracks. Within two weeks of treatment his speech improved by 20 percent.

Within six months of his first treatment Ken began to read, his abstract thinking had improved, he exhibited more self-control, spoke more clearly, was more aware, could do math problems and write simple sentences—and finally, he no longer needed to wear diapers. His screaming and inappropriate behavior stopped. "He has emerged daily before our eyes," said his mom.

A year later, the Kelleys returned for a second treatment, this time to our clinic in Panama, hoping to see even more gains. And they did. He continued to improve his reading, speech, and behavior. By the next year, at age ten, his conversational skills were on par for his age. And he returned for a third treatment.

"Kenneth is a miracle," said Marty. "I never want to go back to autism before stem cells." After his third treatment she said, "The results from stem cells can be seen every day in his amazing thoughts and vast imagination. Watching my son play today, it's hard to believe where he was just a few short years ago."

Marty has become so comfortable with travel to Panama that she comes alone with her son. "Panama was awesome. I'd love to live there. It's very safe there. The clinic is amazing, the doctors are the best I've ever met. The clinic is clean—it's not third world. Seeing the lab just blows you away. I wish more Americans knew about this. I wish that we had it here in the United States," she said.

"To have someone be severely autistic and then become normal, that just doesn't happen. Every day I wake up I'm amazed by him. It's hard to believe it really happened."

Four years after his first treatment, "Ken is pretty much normal. His conversations are interesting and engaging. His mind is always thinking—in a serene, methodical way. He has a million ques-tions and loves to do schoolwork and history. He is the epitome of perfection—perfect manners, helpful to his father, full of happiness and life." His IQ has risen from 52 at age six to 98 by age 13. Not bad for a boy once diagnosed with mental retardation. "To have someone be severely autistic and then become normal, that just doesn't happen. Every day I wake up I'm amazed by him. It's hard to believe it really happened."

Ken was followed by a neurologist over the years and underwent quantitative electroencephalography (qEEG) brain scans. The results of Kenneth's qEEG scans before and after stem cell treatment were remarkably different. In 2007 his scan showed borderline seizure activity, while the scan in 2013, after six stem cell treatments, showed normal functioning in many areas of the brain.

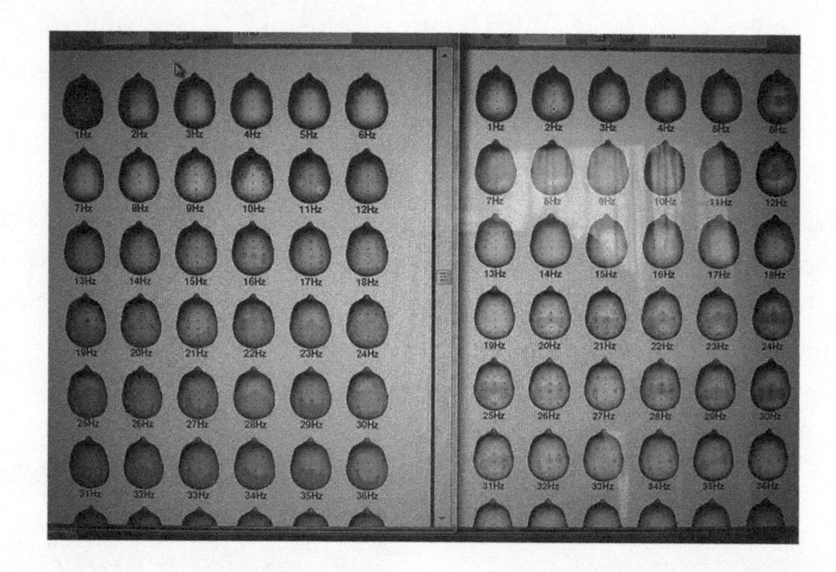

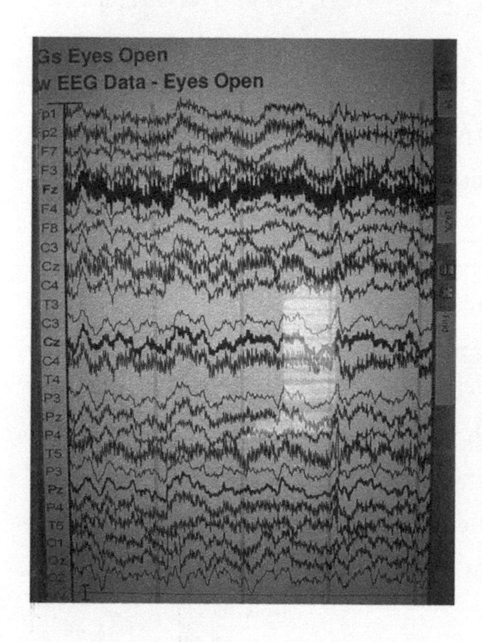

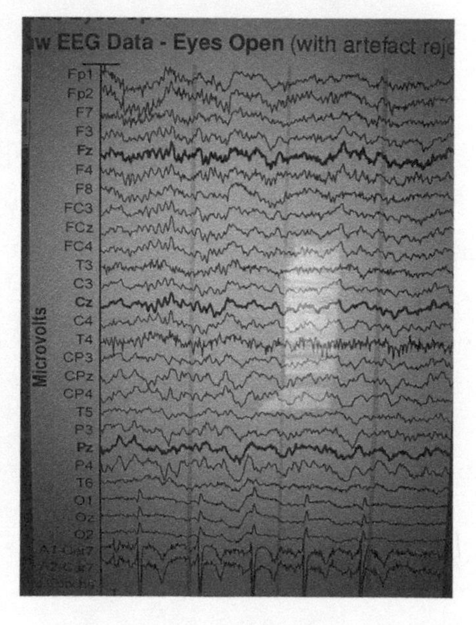

Ethan Collins was assessed at age two and found to have a severe developmental delay. He loved to spin the wheels of his cars and propellers of his airplanes. He held socks in front of his face and repeatedly slapped. He played inappropriately with toys—he would take them apart or smash them. At age four he was diagnosed with pervasive personality disorder not otherwise specified (PDDNOS), which is on the autism spectrum, and attention-deficit hyperactivity disorder (ADHD). The psychiatrist prescribed some heavy medications, but his parents refused them.

Ethan was eventually pulled out of public school because his behavior and flight tendencies were too high of a risk. Ethan's mother Sarah happened to be the special education teacher at his school, but she quit when he changed schools. "I couldn't take care of everyone else's special needs children when I felt like I couldn't take care of my own," she said. Ethan was placed into a self-contained school for autistic children.

They began to look into stem cell treatment, and found Marty Kelly's story of Kenneth. After speaking with her, Ethan's parents decided to come down for treatment. Ethan was eight years old. "Instantly, things started to change for him," Sarah said. There was a pool at the condo they stayed in during their visit. Swimming lessons—or any sports, for that matter—had always been an issue. Ethan would become so disruptive that sports were not an option. The first two days in the pool in Panama were no different—Ethan was panicked, screaming, "I'm drowning! I'm going to die!" But on day three, he said, "I feel really good," as he slid into the pool and began to swim with no problem. "We couldn't believe the difference in him that quickly," Sarah said.

Later that week they went out to eat and expected Ethan to opt for his usual chicken nuggets and French fries, but when asked if he saw anything he wanted to try, Ethan asked for a new food. "This is a kid who would literally vomit if you

> ***"He's doing amazingly well. He's adapting, learning how to do new things. He manages his classes, makes his own breakfasts, dresses himself—he's a normal kid."***

tried to get him to eat something that wasn't in his regular diet," Sarah said. "We were so excited. We couldn't believe that he was eating something different and that it had vegetables in it."

On their way home to Arizona, Ethan was full of conversation. He even remembered the name of his teacher's dog, which says a lot considering he usually couldn't even remember his teacher's name. Once home, he visited his psychiatrist, who likened Ethan's progress to the clearing of a fogged mirror. He was amazed. "We eventually stopped seeing him because Ethan was able to come off of all five heavy medications he had been taking," Sarah said. Ethan's tics, teeth grinding, constipation, and aggression all stopped.

Ethan is now twelve and attends regular seventh-grade classes. "He's doing amazingly well. He's adapting, learning how to do new things. He manages his classes, makes his own breakfasts, dresses himself—he's a normal kid," his mom says.

Victoria's son was diagnosed with autism at 19 months of age. By the time he was nine years old, after having tried a wide array of therapies and treatments, her son hadn't made much progress. He was violent and attacking his family daily. "I had bruises and scratches all over my arms," Victoria said. Because of his explosive and dangerous behavior and the fact that they had a younger daughter in the home, his parents were faced with the heartbreaking decision to place him in a residential program for children like him, but his mother feared the consequences. "My son was very close to me. He needed to be near me at all times. His biggest rages were when I left him to go to the bathroom. My family was falling apart because of it."

Victoria had heard about stem cells from another family who told her the treatment might help her son. "I thought it was bogus at first. But I'd heard stories of remarkable improvements and I knew that we were at a crossroads. I didn't want to send my son away, but something had to change in him because he was putting my daughter at risk." When she became pregnant with her third child, Victoria decided to try stem cell treatment.

"Before stem cell therapy, my son was miserable. No test could tell me whether he was in pain, but he was angry all the time. I just wanted my son to smile."

The first four weeks after treatment, her son got worse. "At first I thought, 'What did I do?'" Stem cell treatment does not always work right away as it did for Anthony and Kenneth. Sometimes the body needs time to adjust to the changes going on inside. "At the sixth week he started getting happy, and his behaviors got better." Even his team of therapists agreed that it was the stem cells that had finally made a difference.

> ***"If this treatment hadn't been an option, I don't know what my life would be like right now."***

He started having regular bowel movements—no more fecal impaction. He slept at night like he hadn't been able to before. His learning improved. And most importantly, he stopped attacking his family. He no longer needed to be placed outside the home. "I have my happy son back, and that was all I wanted. Everything else is bonus. If this treatment hadn't been an option, I don't know what my life would be like right now."

We are currently analyzing data on a prospective analysis of a 33-case series of autism patients who were treated with umbilical cord MSCs. The patients were treated on four occasions, three months apart, with four infusions of stem cells. Data are being analyzed on the suppression of inflammatory cytokines commonly elevated in autistic patients, EEG scans, Childhood Autism Rating Scale scores, and Autism Treatment Evaluation Checklist scores. The study will be published in the next couple years, after patients have been followed for at least one year after treatment.

The Marcus Foundation has funded stem cell research at Duke University and the University of Miami for children with autism. They are currently recruiting for their second clinical trial, a phase II clinical trial that will examine the effect of both donor and the patients' own umbilical cord stem cells in autistic children. Bernie Marcus, founder of the Marcus Foundation, believes that once the results of these clinical trials are published, parents of autistic children will push legislators to pass bills that make stem cell research available to this population of children who are in desperate need of an effective treatment. I agree with him. "I have been a real advocate for stem cells, starting with Panama, trying to get some of these things past the FDA. We're hoping to prove the point that none of this is placebo effect," said Marcus.

Chapter Fourteen

ULCERATIVE COLITIS—AUTOIMMUNITY IN THE GUT

At the age of 15, Henry's life dramatically changed. Bloody diarrhea and abdominal cramping left him doubled over in pain and unable to eat many of the foods he once enjoyed. He was diagnosed with ulcerative colitis, a form of inflammatory bowel disease that involves an autoimmune response in which the immune system mistakes food, bacteria, and other substances in the large intestine as foreign invaders, and mounts an inflammatory response that damages the lining of the intestines.

Normally, the body's immune response to the content of the intestines is dampened. The inside of the digestive tract, although housed within the body, can actually be considered outside the body. Only when digested food passes through the digestive lining can it be considered within the body. In a healthy person, the immune system does not mount much of an immune response along the lining of the digestive tract. In patients with ulcerative colitis, however, the immune system does mount an attack at this critical interface, leading to a chronic state of inflammation and intestinal damage.

Henry was treated with the anti-inflammatory drug mesalamine, which worked for a while. But soon he needed to add prednisone to the medication to keep his symptoms in check. Later his doctor switched his mesalamine for sulfasalazine, and his prednisone for another steroid, budesonide. "The prednisone would keep me in remission, but brought horrible side effects including stretch marks, water retention, weak bones, insomnia, and changes in mood," Henry said. He tried biological treatments such as Remicade, Simponi, and Entyvio, but these brought little relief. He tried antibiotics such as Flagyl and Xifaxan, which only helped his irritable bowel symptoms. Mercaptopurine and methotrexate only worsened his condition. He even tried Chinese medicine, which helped with bleeding but only for a short time.

I have seen major improvement with my colitis symptoms after the treatment, amazingly better than any medicine I have ever taken," he said. "I feel a lot happier, free, and with more energy in my life now."

It seemed as though he had tried everything, but still he suffered with symptoms, until one day his mother told him about a treatment she had heard about—stem cell therapy. Henry came down for umbilical cord MSC treatment at our clinic in Panama and began to experience relief after the second IV infusion. His abdominal pain subsided and he was visiting the bathroom less frequently. He continued to improve, so much so that he no longer needs to take any medication to control his disease. "I have seen major improvement with my colitis symptoms after the treatment, amazingly better than any medicine I have ever taken," he said. "I feel a lot happier, free, and with more energy in my life now."

A significant percentage of ulcerative colitis patients are like Henry—refractory to therapy. They continue to worsen despite treatment. Altered diet, frequent and unpredictable bowel movements, and chronic pain leave ulcerative colitis patients feeling like they cannot participate in regular social events. They may lose weight and have low energy levels. And for many, medications are only somewhat effective. The chronic inflammation in the gut eats away at the intestinal lining so much so that the intestine is no longer useful. Surgery to remove part or all of the colon is common in patients with ulcerative colitis, often necessitating the insertion of a colostomy bag. To properly address disease progression in patients with ulcerative colitis, the underlying immune dysfunction, which compromises the integrity of the intestinal lining and leads to symptoms, must be treated.

Mesenchymal Stem Cells for Ulcerative Colitis

Mesenchymal stem cell (MSC) treatment for patients with ulcerative colitis has been under investigation. In 2010, a group of researchers from Russia published a study on the first use of bone marrow-derived donor MSCs in ulcerative colitis patients.[1,2] The MSCs reduced the autoimmune inflammation and stimulated the reparative process in the intestinal lining, increasing duration of remission while reducing recurrence of disease and hospitalization frequency in 72.7 percent of patients. MSC treatment allowed most of the patients to discontinue or reduce steroid use. The same Russian group studied MSCs in combination with the standard anti-inflammatory treatment in a group of patients experiencing an acute disease flare-up, finding that bone marrow-derived donor MSCs increased the effect of anti-inflammatory treatment.[3]

Researchers from Brazil assessed whether intravenous or intraperitoneal (into the abdominal cavity) infusion is best for ulcerative colitis, finding IV infusion to be most effective for reducing colon inflammation in an animal model of colitis.[4] This study demonstrates the ability of MSCs to home to the area of damage, especially when introduced via the bloodstream. Another colitis animal model showed an accumulation of MSCs in the inflamed region of the colon after IV injection.[5] The use of umbilical cord MSCs has been studied in animal models of colitis and found to diminish severity of disease, reduce inflammatory cytokines and oxidation activity, as well as reduce intestinal permeability and beneficially alter immune balance.[6,7,8] A clinical trial using umbilical cord MSCs for ulcerative colitis is currently underway to further establish safety and determine clinical response and control of inflammation.[9]

Chapter Fifteen

DIABETES— A PARADIGM SHIFT

We currently do not treat diabetes in Panama, but it's a very interesting area of potential treatment. Diabetes affects 29.1 million people in the United States, or 9.3 percent of the U.S. population.[1] Of those, 8.1 million are undiagnosed. Prediabetes, the precursor to diabetes type 2, affects 37 percent of adults aged 20 years or older and 51 percent of those aged 65 years or older. That means 86 million more Americans are prediabetic. Diabetes is the seventh leading cause of death[2] and accounts for more than $245 billion in estimated costs—$176 billion in direct medical costs and $69 billion in reduced productivity.[3] On average, the health care costs for diabetes type 2 patients are approximately $13,700 annually, 2.3 times higher than what expenditures would be in the absence of diabetes.

There are two main forms of diabetes: type 1 and type 2. In diabetes type 1, also known as insulin-dependent diabetes mellitus (IDDM), or juvenile diabetes, the patient's pancreas produces little or no insulin, believed to be in part the result of an autoimmune attack on the insulin-producing beta cells in the pancreas. Diabetes type 1 is one of the most costly chronic diseases of childhood and one that is widely considered to never be outgrown.

Patients with diabetes type 1 must take multiple insulin injections daily or continually infuse insulin through a pump, and test their blood sugar by pricking their fingers six or more times per day. Since numerous factors such as stress, hormones, growth, physical activity, medications, illness/infection, and fatigue affect insulin utilization, even a strictly monitored program of insulin administration does not mimic the endogenous functions of the pancreas, and as a result numerous complications can develop. Ketonemia, excessive ketones in the blood, can result from the loss of insulin-secreting capacity and may lead to ketoacidosis, a buildup of acids in the blood, which if untreated may result in diabetic coma. Ultimately, diabetics with type 1 disease can suffer from all of the problems associated with long-term high blood sugar including heart and blood vessel disease, kidney disease, blindness, poor circulation, amputations, and shortened life span (11 years shorter for men and 13 years for women).

Diabetes type 2, also known as non-insulin-dependent diabetes mellitus (NIDDM) and formerly adult-onset diabetes before it began showing up in children, is associated with impairment of peripheral tissue response to insulin. In other words, in healthy people, cells respond to insulin by letting glucose (sugar) into the cells from the bloodstream, but in people with diabetes type 2 cells become resistant to insulin and no longer let in glucose, leaving it to accumulate in the bloodstream. As a result of the obesity epidemic, substantially younger patients are beginning to be diagnosed with this condition.

In the United States, diabetes type 1 affects about five percent of all diabetes patients.[4] Diabetes type 2 is far more common, at 90 to 95 percent. Diabetes type 1 affects 15 to 30 million people globally and 1.4 million in the United States.[5,6] The incidence is increasing significantly in many populations, especially among young children. In general, most people are diagnosed with diabetes type 1 before the age of 30. Not only will these people be insulin dependent for life, but devastating life-limiting and life-shortening complications can occur. Insulin is the primary method of controlling diabetes by regulating blood glucose levels, but it may not reverse or prevent disease progression.

Because the beta cells are the target of attack in diabetes type 1, attention has been on trying to replace islets, groups of cells including beta cells, in the pancreas to treat or cure the disease. Common thinking has always been that once the immune system has attacked the islets and destroyed the beta cells, there is no turning back disease progression. We were taught in medical school that once the immune attack starts, it is only a matter of time before all or most of the beta cells are destroyed. The period of time before their destruction and before complete reliance on insulin injections is called the "honeymoon period."

The paradigm is shifting, however. In the past few years new information has become available that suggests that type 1 diabetes can not only be treated, but also cured, using cells that are not simply replacements for the beta cells or the islets but that stimulate their regeneration.

Old Paradigm: Diabetes type 1 is an irreversible short-term autoimmune disease that destroys all of the insulin-producing cells in the pancreas.

New Paradigm: Diabetes type 1 is a chronic autoimmune disease that, when corrected, allows the insulin-producing cells of the pancreas to regenerate.

The first evidence comes from Riccardo Calafiore, MD from Italy. He was the first person to inject islets into the abdominal cavity of humans.[7] In order to do this, he first needed to protect the introduced islets from an immune attack by the recipient. He coated the islets in alginate, an inert substance obtained from seaweed and used to protect the cells from immune attack. He then placed the islets into the abdomens of people with diabetes type 1. The islets survived for a period of time and helped to control the blood sugar until they eventually died. The patients were not retreated.

What Dr. Calafiore did next changes everything. He implanted neonatal pig Sertoli cells, which are very much like mesenchymal stem cells (MSCs), into the abdomens of mice with type 1 diabetes.[8] Sertoli cells are normally found in the testicles, oftentimes referred to as nurse cells because they nourish and protect immature sperm cells. These cells were again encapsulated in alginate and injected into the mice. Sertoli cells do not secrete insulin, but like MSCs they do secrete immune-modulating molecules, and when injected into animals with other types of autoimmune diseases they have been found to suppress the immune system through their secretions.[9] In Calafiore's second study, 81 percent of non-obese diabetic treated mice became non-diabetic as a result of a single injection into the abdomen.

What is truly amazing, and contrary to prior beliefs, is that the inflammation of the pancreas in these treated mice subsided, and the islets and beta cells regenerated. There was also a significant increase in the number of T regulatory cells in the circulation of the treated animals compared to the controls. T regulatory cells have a profound ability to modulate and even suppress immunity in the body. They can "turn off" the white blood cells that are activated (trained) to kill beta cells. The pancreases of the treated animals had normal islets with normal production of pancreatic molecules, including insulin, glucagon, and somatostatin.

More evidence of regeneration comes to us from a study in China.[10] In this study white blood cells were harvested from twelve patients using a machine similar to a dialysis machine. Instead of harvesting the waste products from the blood, as in dialysis, the machine harvests the white blood cells in a procedure that takes two to three hours. Once harvested, the white blood cells were mixed with hundreds of millions of umbilical cord MSCs. The MSCs were placed into a "box" they deemed the "Stem Cell Educator." The box was comprised of many layers onto which the mesenchymal cells were attached. The researchers then placed the patients' white blood cells into the Stem Cell Educator box, and placed the box into an incubator for between two and three hours to allow the cells to co-mingle.

Stem Cell Re-education

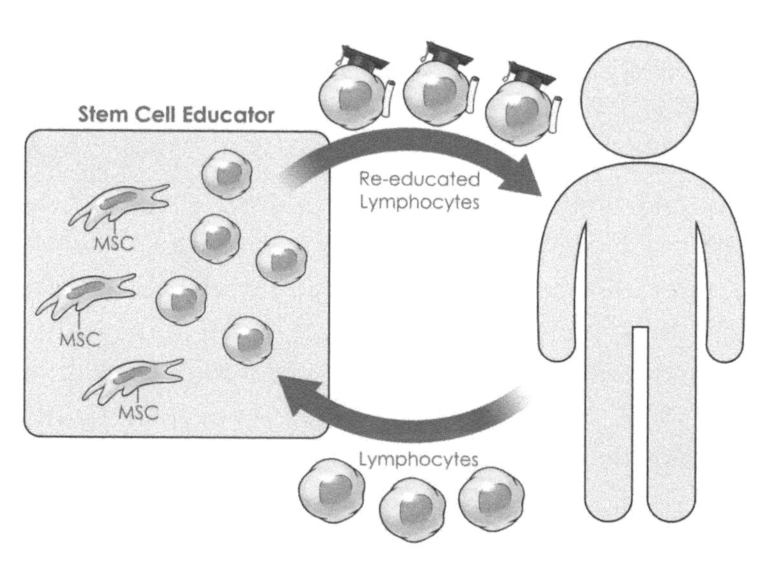

The patient's lymphocytes are re-educated through contact with human umbilical cells, to aid in the regeneration of islet beta cells and blood sugar control.
Adapted from Zhao Y et al. Reversal of type 1 diabetes via islet β cell regeneration following immune modulation by cord blood-derived multipotent stem cells. BMC Med. 2012 Jan 10;10:3

One of the beautiful things about MSCs is their ability to sense and respond to the environment in which they are placed. After the cells co-mingled, the white blood cells were rinsed out of the box and infused back into the patients. The results were impressive. This one-day procedure resulted in blood sugar control and increased production of C-peptide, a marker of insulin production. (When a molecule of insulin is produced, so is a molecule of C-peptide. Since the test for insulin can't determine whether the insulin was injected or produced in the body, C-peptide is the best way to measure how much insulin the pancreas is producing.) Of particular note is that these patients had already passed the honeymoon period before the procedure. Their bodies were no longer producing enough insulin on their own. The median time since diagnosis in these patients was eight years—it had been quite some time since their pancreases had produced enough insulin. Before treatment improvements, half of those patients were secreting some C-peptide (or producing some insulin) while half were secreting none (or producing zero insulin).

A recent article describes a safety study in diabetes type 2 patients given intravenous umbilical cord MSCs. The study, a phase I/II, 36-month, randomized, controlled trial was conducted at Qingdao University by Hu Jianxia, MD, et al.[11] Two intravenous infusions were given four weeks

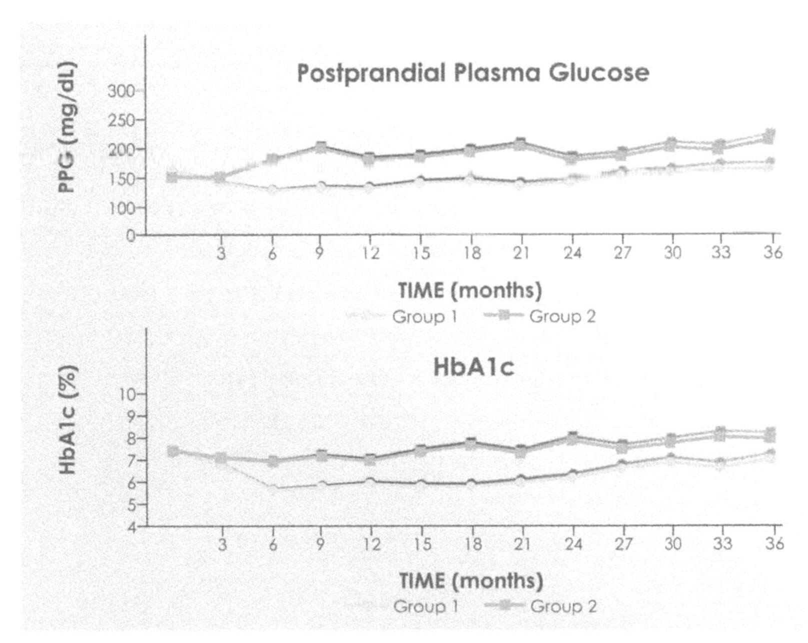

Improvements in blood sugar control in diabetes type 2 patients treated with umbilical cord MSCs (in blue). Adapted from Hu J, Wang Y, Gong H, et al. Long term effect and safety of Wharton's jelly-derived mesenchymal stem cells on type 2 diabetes. Exp Ther Med. 2016 Sep;12(3):1857-1866. Epub 2016 Jul 26.

apart. Not only were there no adverse events in the treatment group of 31 subjects, but there were significant improvements in blood sugar control, and diabetes-related complications decreased. For example, significant improvements were seen in the treatment group in postprandial glucose (blood sugar levels after eating), hemoglobin A1C levels (a marker of long-term blood sugar control), C-peptide (surrogate for endogenous insulin production), C-peptide-to-glucose ratio, and HOMA β (homeostasis model assessment of pancreatic islet beta cell function). There was no improvement for fasting glucose or in HOMA IR (homeostasis model assessment of insulin resistance). The improvements seemed to peak between 15 and 21 months after treatment, supporting a rationale for retreatment before 15 months.

The first safety and feasibility results of clinical trials using MSCs to treat diabetes types 1 and 2 are just coming out from Sweden and India.[12,13] Similar treatments are being investigated in the United States,[14] and more are sure to follow. As Hao Wu, PhD and Ram Mahato, PhD from the University of Nebraska Medical Center noted in 2014, current treatment for diabetes with insulin injection or islet transplantation addresses the reduction of hyperglycemia.[15] If the underlying autoimmunity, which destroys beta cells in the first place and will continue to do so if not addressed, is not quelled, the diabetes will likely return. Through transdifferentiation and immune modulation, MSCs can relieve autoimmunity and regenerate islets to resolve the hyperglycemia.

In summary, I believe the easiest treatment for diabetes type 1 will be intravenous infusions of umbilical cord MSCs. Reducing or removing the immune inflammation component is key. We need to get the immune attack rock over the mountain. For persistent and refractory diabetes type 2, MSCs have already been shown to be a useful treatment, albeit in a relatively small study. The highest level of benefit in that study was between 12 and 21 months. So ideally, a study design with multiple infusions six to 12 months apart would potentially yield even more significant benefits.

Chapter Sixteen

LUPUS— AN OPPORTUNITY IN AUTOIMMUNE HEALTH

Lupus is the common name for lupus erythematosus, of which there are four types. One type, systemic lupus erythematosus (SLE), is the most common and serious form. SLE is a chronic autoimmune disease in which the immune system attacks the body's own tissues and organs—any area of the body can be affected, including the joints, skin, kidneys, heart, lungs, blood vessels, and the brain. Sometimes called "the great imitator" because of the many body systems affected and varying symptoms, lupus can mimic other conditions, making it difficult to diagnose. Common symptoms, which tend to come on slowly, include pain or swelling in the joints, muscle pain, fever with no known cause, red rashes—especially on the face, chest pain, hair loss, poor circulation in the fingers or toes, sun sensitivity, swelling in the legs or around eyes, mouth ulcers, swollen glands, and fatigue.

I became interested in lupus after learning about the research of Lingyun Sun, MD, a doctor in China who was researching the use of mesenchymal stem cells for lupus. He began with a mouse model of lupus and then treated a series of four people who were not responding to six months of antibiotic and steroid treatment.[1] Both the mice and humans received donor bone marrow MSCs. The humans were slowly weaned off of the antibiotic over the next six months while maintaining a low dose of the steroid medication. The patients' kidney function, survival, and disease remission improved. Dr. Sun also cultured the patients' own bone marrow MSCs to study their robustness. They were found to have an impairment in their ability to form bone. This deficiency comes along with impaired ability to produce T-regulatory cells, key for keeping the immune system in check. These cells are often decreased in patients with autoimmune diseases.

Dr. Sun's next study followed 15 patients with severe lupus who were also treated with bone marrow MSCs.[2] There were no serious side effects of the treatment, and their disease activity scores improved after one, three, 12, and 24 months; protein in the urine improved, and so did the amount of circulating T-regulatory cells. Next, Dr. Sun used umbilical cord MSCs from healthy donors instead of bone marrow MSCs in patients with lupus who were not responding to treatment and who had life-threatening organ involvement.[3] "Significant reduction in disease activity was achieved in all patients, and there has been no recurrence to date and no treatment-related deaths."

In yet one more study, four patients with a lupus-derived severe lung complication that has a 50 percent mortality rate, meaning that 50 percent of patients with this condition do not survive it, were treated with umbilical cord MSCs.[4] The four patients not only survived but improved dramatically. In his latest article, Dr. Sun's team summed up four years of treating 87 patients with severe SLE.[5] The complete clinical remission rate at one year was 28 percent, 31 percent at two years, 42 percent at three years, and 50 percent at four years. Overall relapse rate was 23 percent. No transplantation-related adverse events were observed.

Despite Dr. Sun's success with treating severe and refractory lupus with MSCs, research into the use of MSCs for lupus has been scant. I am extremely excited to recently have seen a six-university trial using umbilical cord mesenchymal stem cells for the treatment of lupus. This study has been a long time coming and is historic, I believe, for the research of these cells in the United States. It is sponsored by the Medical University of South Carolina, one of the trial locations.[6] Additional sites are Cedars-Sinai Medical Center in Los Angeles, the University of North Carolina at Chapel Hill, the University of Rochester Medical Center, Northwestern University in Chicago, and Emory University in Atlanta.

This trial will evaluate umbilical cord MSCs along with standard of care treatment as compared to a placebo infusion along with standard of care in adults with SLE. The potential for treating this difficult condition with MSCs, especially in severe cases, is huge. I hope that more researchers and doctors pay attention to Dr. Sun's research and to the clinical trial currently underway so that more patients will eventually have access to this treatment.

We have not treated patients with lupus at the Stem Cell Institute largely because of my early ignorance before learning about Dr. Sun's research. You see, in medical school we learn that the immune system has two branches that act in balance—when one side is dominant, the other is dampened. I am referring to the Th1 and Th2 immune responses. People with rheumatoid arthritis or multiple sclerosis have a strongly exaggerated Th1 response, which stem cells help to quell. Because it was understood that lowering a Th1 response would potentially raise the Th2 response, and that people with lupus experience an exaggerated Th2 response, I wrongfully assumed that stem cells would not benefit people with lupus because they would favor a Th2 immune response. It was a counterintuitive treatment, so it was off the table. But Dr. Sun's research, as well as the discovery that the Th1-Th2 immune responses are also balanced by Th3 as well as Th17, and probably most importantly by increasing the number of T-regulatory cells, the "mothering cells of the immune system," has changed my opinion about treating lupus with stem cells.

Chapter Seventeen

MAGIC JUICE—THE ELIXIR OF LIFE?

Most people don't want to live forever, but everyone wants to feel as young as possible for as long as they can. Unfortunately, our bodies don't cooperate. We start to slow down in many ways. We just can't get the energy to jump up and do the things we used to do. And when we do get up, those movements and thought processes sometimes make us feel as though we are moving through molasses—and in many cases, molasses full of broken glass.

Scientists have been researching for centuries what happens to the body to cause this change in energy and pace, hoping to unlock the secret to the Fountain of Youth. You probably won't be surprised by the following assertion: the secret lies within your stem cells.

> ***A key bodily process that declines with age is its production of stem cells.***

Scientists know that as you age your body starts producing cells more slowly. The body is constantly replenishing itself, replacing the cells that die off with new ones. This happens quickly when you are young but slows considerably as you age—just notice the contrast between the chubby pink cheeks of babies and the considerably dryer and less vibrant cheeks of the elderly. A key bodily process that declines with age is its production of stem cells.

When you need to catch a vase before it falls off the bookshelf, your mind tells your body to leap up, run across the room, and thrust your arm forward to rescue it before it shatters. If you're sixteen, no problem. Thinking about leaping and leaping up from the couch are one and the same function.

But as you edge toward sixty, you think about getting up, place your hand on the arm rest, and hoist yourself to standing while your heart labors to pump more blood to support you in the effort of getting to your feet. By the time this whole sequence is complete, the vase is shattered on the floor.

The optimal performance period for an Olympic athlete is between the ages of 22 and 24. It's not a coincidence that that is the time of life when they have peak coordination, judgment, and practice—and, not to mention, the largest number of stem cells. Their cells regenerate quickly and, if they get injured, their stem cells rush to the site of inflammation and manage the repair.

As discussed throughout this book, adult stem cells, and mesenchymal stem cells in particular, work by stimulating the body itself to regenerate rather than by regenerating themselves—a fact that caused the father of the MSC, Arnold Caplan, PhD, to want to rename MSCs *medicinal signaling cells.* Their magic lies not in their ability to become and replace different tissues and cells, but in their production of trophic factors, bioactive molecules produced in response to the environment in which the cells find themselves. These chemicals aid in the repairing of tissue and the recruitment of new blood vessels to support nutrient flow to the area and decrease inflammation. So it's not the cells themselves that work their magic. It's what the cells secrete that has such medicinal potential.

Stem cells secrete a wide range of cellular products, molecules, exosomes, and microvesicles that act in different ways to stimulate the body's healing process. Growth factors, cytokines, hormones, and cellular mitochondria and RNA are among the secreted bioactive molecules and cellular material that characterize the wide range of activities carried out by MSCs. When considering that the main function of MSCs lies in their secretome—the bioactive molecules they secrete—rather than in the ability of the cells to differentiate into new tissue, isolating these trophic factors separate from the cells offers an intriguing mode of treatment.

When we harvest stem cells from a patient in our clinic, we culture them to make a plentiful supply. Not only do we want to have plenty on hand for treatments, but we also place some in storage for future treatments, should they be necessary. We grow them in a broth that is rich in nutrients, designed to encourage them to divide at a healthy rate. When we have a large enough batch, we rinse and purify those cells carefully because some of the elements of the broth contain animal proteins that we don't want to introduce into the body of a patient. Then we place the cells into a broth that is free of antibiotics or animal proteins.

As the cells grow, they release trophic factors as part of their natural development. We then rinse off the chemically-derived broth, which is rich in trophic factors. I and others hypothesized that if we concentrated the broth and injected it into the body, all those trophic factors might give a boost to an aging body.

And what better aging body to try it on than mine? I still have aches in my knees and ankles, and pain in my neck from that time in my twenties when I had the severe case of the bends. I wondered if taking a shot of these concentrated trophic factors could offer me some relief, given the anti-inflammatory qualities these factors exhibit. So I tried it.

The first thing I noticed, within an hour of the first injection, was that I had the energy of a young kid, spinning around, ready for anything. I was at a casino playing blackjack that evening. Normally I would have shuffled up to the table and plopped myself down until either the money ran out or I declared myself the victor and cashed in my chips. But that night, every time the dealer paused to shuffle the six-deck shoe, I walked laps around the casino. I had more energy than I knew what to do with.

The next day, I noticed something else: all my pain was gone. The ache in my knees and my ankles—gone! The throbbing in my neck—disappeared!

The other effect was increased stamina. Remember when you were a kid and you played flag football with your friends? My friends and I used to do that every Sunday when I was younger. I'd get tackled in the gut, tossed to the ground, spun around, arm twisted. The next day, because I was a young guy, I might be a little sore but it wouldn't last more than a day. After injecting myself with these trophic factors, I went on a long overseas flight, which is the equivalent of getting beat up in football for a guy in his 50s, and I felt fine. I didn't even whine about jet lag.

For lack of a better name, I decided to call the serum we'd developed from rinsing off the stem cells we had cultured *magic juice*. Its effects typically last three to six days, and there have been no reported side effects.

I believe magic juice can be useful in regenerating the skin too. I gave some of it mixed in a face cream to my daughter Tierney when she was suffering from a particularly nasty flair of acne. A few days after applying magic juice topically, her acne disappeared.

One of the first patients treated with trophic factors in our clinic was a man in his 70s with polymyalgia rheumatica, an autoimmune disease that affects the muscles of the upper body and causes severe pain, headaches, and restriction of movement in the upper arms. He was injected with trophic factors into the muscles of his arm and his upper trapezius muscle. He received weekly treatments. Each week he called the clinic to report that he was feeling better and sleeping well. His muscle tension had decreased. By his third treatment his symptoms were 90 percent gone, and his inflammation had decreased by half.

Dr. Paz, our medical director, broke his large toe one night when his laptop fell squarely on it. On X-ray the bone was broken in four pieces. The orthopedic doctor told him he would need to be off of it for eight weeks. After a few injections of magic juice he was able to go back to his daily basketball game in just three weeks.

Dr. Paz has subsequently used the trophic factors in selective patients with ailments such as ligament injuries and tendonitis. Dr. Paz's wife was treated with trophic factors for an Achilles tendon injury, and by the next day she was no longer in pain. Two days later she was running again.

Another athlete with a bulging disc in her spine has been treated regularly with trophic factors and no longer experiences pain despite once having been recommended for spinal surgery.

Another patient with uveitis, an inflammation in the eye, had been to one of the best eye clinics in the United States yet her eye health continued to decline. She was told she would ultimately be blind in both eyes. She was treated for six weeks with trophic factors by a weekly injection into the muscle of her arm. Her blurred vision and pain diminished, and upon follow-up at the prestigious clinic, the U.S. doctors were perplexed that her exams showed she had complete regression of the disease. You may wonder how an injection in the arm could help the eyes. Uveitis is a disease of inflammation. The trophic factors and anti-inflammatory factors in the juice circulate throughout the body and stimulate regeneration and decrease inflammation. A few months before this writing, I saw the patient at a social event and, after a big hug, she told me her eyes are fine.

A local Panamanian baseball player was headed for the playoffs when Achilles tendonitis set in, preventing him from playing. He could barely walk when he came to the clinic. He was injected with trophic factors on either side of his Achilles tendon and three days later was in no pain. His team won the playoff series and went on to play in the equivalent of the World Series in Panama. After they won, Dr. Paz received a baseball signed by all the players, thanking him for getting their teammate back on the field.

Given the enormous need for a non-toxic, super anti-inflammatory, and enhanced regenerative capacity product, and its off-the-shelf qualities and relatively low cost to produce, I believe magic juice, or some iteration of it, will be in broad clinical use within a decade. In addition, the use of trophic factors derived from stem cells is one way to circumvent some regulatory hurdles that stem cells present. Trophic factors are not nuclear DNA-containing cells—they are simply cell products. Since there are no cells in the product, its use will likely be more easily accepted by regulatory bodies. Because the secretions of stem cells are really where their magic lies, the use of magic juice could lead to a huge leap forward for the field of regenerative medicine.[1]

Next-Generation Magic Juice —Personalized

There's a lot of evidence showing that MSCs exhibit an appropriate molecular response to the environment they are exposed to. For example, in the presence of a lot of the inflammatory protein TNF-alpha, MSCs will produce receptors that sop up the TNF-alpha. I wondered what would happen if the MSCs were put in contact with my own white blood cells, which produce inflammatory molecules, so I devised an experiment to see if co-culturing white blood cells with MSCs would produce a different product by simply collecting the wonderful array of trophic factors and anti-inflammatory molecules innately secreted by the MSCs in order to modulate the immune system.

Dr. Paz and I both donated two tubes of blood. Our white blood cells were purified and placed with mesenchymal stem cells in a culture for about 48 hours. Marialaura, our research director, then co-cultured our white blood cells with the MSCs for 48 hours. She took that mixture and centrifuged it and then sterile filtered it and measured the amount of PGE2, an anti-inflammatory molecule, in both of the samples. The PEG2 level of my cells in culture was more than double that of Dr Paz's, which makes sense given that Dr. Paz is much younger, and I would consider healthier because he plays basketball five days a week for an hour in the Panama heat. The most interesting thing came next. We injected 1 cubic centimeter (equivalent to about one tenth of everything produced) intravenously. The next day I woke up and I was completely pain free. The effects lasted approximately 30 days. This is in contrast to the magic juice that is not personalized for the individual's immune system, and for which the inflammatory effects typically last between three and six days. I believe this will be the next generation of magic juice—magic juice that is made for each person based on his or her own immune irregularities.

Chapter Eighteen

LIFESTYLE CHOICES—HOW TO PROTECT YOUR HEALTH

If stem cells are the body's way of retaining health and extending longevity, then how can we optimize the pool of stem cells we already have within us? Is there a way to reduce our loss of stem cells as we age or perhaps even increase our reserve of these regenerative cells?

The stem cells in our blood, also called circulating stem cells, are the tools our bodies use to repair damaged tissue and to keep us healthy. Aging, genetics, and poor lifestyle choices use up our supply of circulating stem cells. You can't stop aging, and you can't help genetics, but you can improve both areas by taking action with what you can change: your lifestyle choices. The harder you work to take care of the stem cells you have, and the less frequently you use them to repair damages you could have avoided with a healthy lifestyle, the more you are doing to protect what all the money in the world can't buy back once it's wasted: your own good health.

As I mentioned in Chapter 8, I like to think of our reserve of stem cells as a bank account. Depending on the day or the state of our health, our account may be replenished or depleted. There's a difference between taking calculated risks, making safe investments, and reckless gambling. If you want a good future, you don't gamble what you can't afford to lose, and the circulating stem cells in your body are the rescue team your body can't afford to lose. When we engage in healthy behaviors, our stem cells are able to multiply and remain robust. When we engage in unhealthy behaviors, our stem cells deteriorate—and we pay for it by depleting our store of cells.

There are two main types of stem cells that work together in lockstep and are particularly responsive to lifestyle factors:

- endothelial precursor cells (EPCs): primarily found in bone marrow and circulating throughout the bloodstream
- mesenchymal stem cells (MSCs): found in every tissue, attached to blood vessels

The total number of circulating EPCs determines the body's capacity to repair and heal the vascular system.[1] And the density of the vascular system determines the total number of MSCs. Promoting a healthy level of circulating EPCs, therefore, is very important for maintaining the body's store of MSCs. Without EPCs continually restoring our vasculature, it withers, and our number of MSCs declines. Professor Arnold Caplan once told me that the number of capillaries in the skin of a 75-year-old is merely two percent of that of a newborn.

The endothelium is the inner lining of the blood vessels. The health of this lining is crucial to healthy cardiovascular function. Normal endothelial function depends on the balance between the loss of endothelial cells and their regeneration by circulating EPCs released from the bone marrow. EPCs home to sites of endothelial injury and ischemia (low blood supply), where they proliferate, differentiate, and integrate into a healthy endothelial layer.[2] EPCs also exert a paracrine, or hormone, function by producing vascular growth factors, proteins that encourage the growth of blood vessels. Without the regenerative capacity of enough circulating EPCs, atherosclerosis occurs. Atherosclerosis is the most common form of cardiovascular disease, the number one cause of death in the United States.

Endothelial dysfunction leads to more than just atherosclerosis. It is a precursor to high blood pressure, stroke, heart attack, heart failure, migraine headaches, angina, peripheral artery disease, pre-eclampsia, dementia, erectile dysfunction, macular degeneration, sleep apnea, hearing loss, diabetes, kidney failure, and Raynaud's disease.

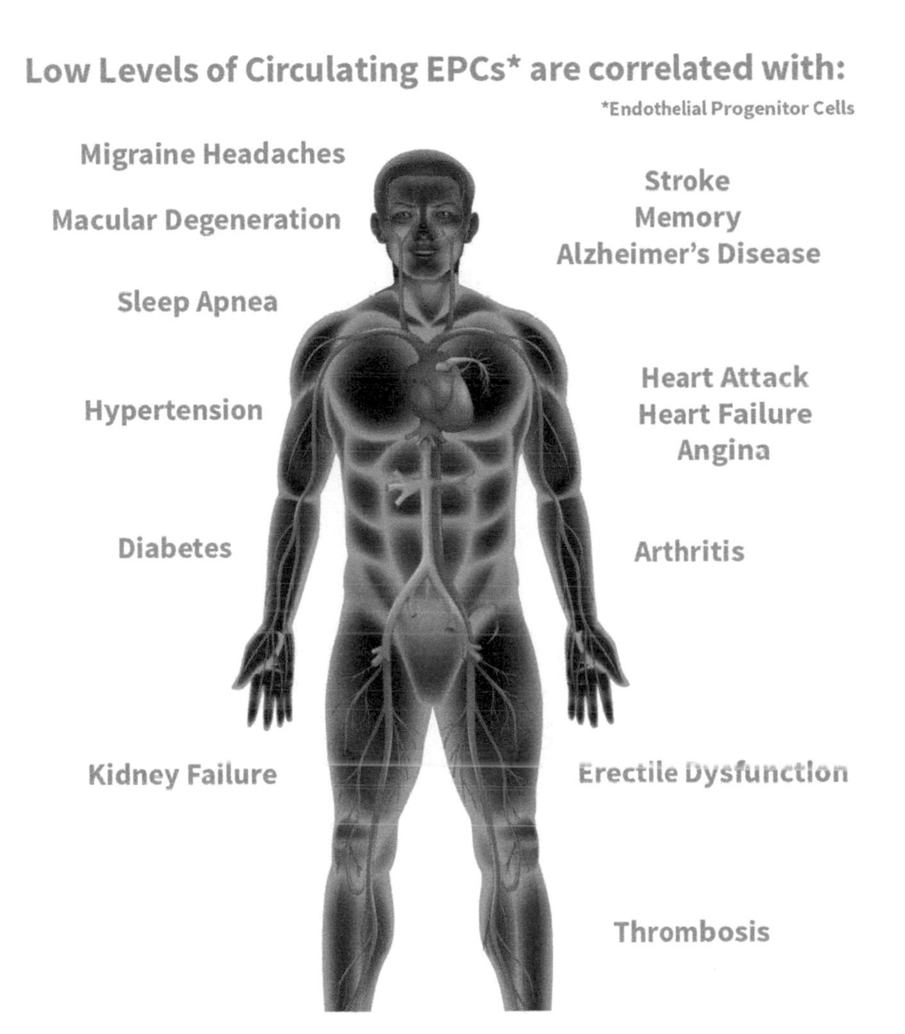

Circulating stem cells are closely related to health. Individuals with a higher concentration of circulating stem cells recover better from a stroke than those individuals with fewer circulating stem cells.[3] Increasing the number of circulating stem cells leads to a therapeutic effect in cardiac regeneration.[4] The body mobilizes EPCs in response to heart attack, which is an injury of the heart tissue.[5] Individuals with Alzheimer's disease have reduced levels of circulating stem cells, which is correlated with severity of the disease.[6] Patients with migraine headaches have decreased circulating stem cells.[7] And erectile and endothelial function are directly related to the number of EPCs in circulation.[8]

In addition, aging and many chronic diseases are associated with a decrease in vascular density, or the amount of blood vessels found within the body. Blood vessels are regenerated by EPCs, so a decrease in number of EPCs means a decreased ability for blood vessel growth. It also means a decrease in number of MSCs, which must adhere to capillaries.

What I have learned about the body's ability to regenerate and heal after receiving MSCs tells me that preserving or boosting the body's reserve of these cells—EPCs and MSCs—is beneficial. Ultimately, we're fighting a losing battle, but we can make lifestyle changes that help to slow the decline and possibly even reverse it. The following outlines some ways to help maintain a healthy reserve of stem cells in your body by optimizing your lifestyle.

Exercise

Circulating EPCs have been found to be significantly decreased in middle-aged and older men. However, a three-month training program of walking at moderate intensity increased circulating EPCs by 120 percent.[9] In another study of a three-month training program, both older and younger men were tested.[10] Interestingly, the older men had a higher increase in circulating EPCs than the younger men. But even in children, daily physical activity has been found to increase the number of circulating EPCs.[11]

Taking up a physically active lifestyle results in a markedly improved and biologically "younger" vascular lining—it won't turn back time, but if you've ever had a fitness instructor, coach, or PE teacher tell you that exercise "gets your blood moving," they were right. A sedentary lifestyle slows down our blood flow—it makes our blood and our bodies sluggish.

Cardiovascular workouts are the best way to keep up your cardiovascular health. Your body adapts to the life you lead, and if parts of you go unused for long stretches of time, your body (and your blood flow) will start to ignore those parts in favor of prioritizing the parts you do use. This is a survival mechanism, and it can keep you alive in extreme emergencies, but that's why you need to work with your body and not against it. If you're trapped under an avalanche of snow, your body will stop sending blood to your fingers and toes first because you can live without them. But you can't live without your vital organs. If you're in a life-or-death situation, shutting down circulation to some areas might save you, but your day-to-day life shouldn't be so extreme. Something as simple as taking the stairs can be breathtakingly hard when you're out of practice, and why? Your heart and lungs aren't used to doing the work they were made for often enough, and that connection begins to lapse over time without use.

Even without the time it takes to join a fitness class, get up early for yoga, or take weekend hikes, exercise can still be peppered throughout your daily routines. If you must be at a desk, alternate between standing and sitting. If you must sit, consider replacing your chair with a stability ball—it improves your balance and keeps your muscles active without you having to think about it. If you can go out for lunch, try picking a place close enough to walk to rather than drive—every single step will count, no matter how small.

Diet

You are what you eat, so the saying goes, and it's certainly true that what you take into your body affects and changes it. For blood health, the most important dietary factors are sufficient protein intake, the inclusion of plenty of anti-inflammatory foods, and maintaining low blood pressure and low blood sugar. Protein is crucial for building muscle and tissue, anti-inflammatory foods and low blood pressure reduce blood vessel damage, and low blood sugar decreases inflammation and reduces heart disease.

A diet with adequate protein, whether vegetarian or meat-containing, is crucial for rebuilding your body's tissues. Proteins break down into amino acids, the body's building blocks. Choose a variety of high-protein foods, including fish, meats, eggs, beans, and, if tolerated, dairy. Fish such as salmon, sardines, and herring will give you an added anti-inflammatory boost due to their high omega-3 content, while also being low in the heavy metal mercury, commonly found in many fish. Grass-fed meats and pasture-raised eggs also contain omega-3. Organic beans and dairy, when available, will help to minimize potentially damaging pesticide and growth hormone residues while leaving a cleaner footprint on the environment.

In conjunction with a high-protein diet, minimizing carbohydrates, especially in the form of grains, potatoes, and sugars, will help you maintain a healthy blood sugar level and reduce inflammation. A diet high in carbohydrates raises blood sugar and inflammation. Pairing high-protein foods with plenty of vegetables is a great way to plan your meals. Aim for five to nine servings of vegetables and low-sugar fruits daily to give your body a wide array of beneficial phytonutrients that help to control blood pressure, reduce blood sugar, lower inflammation, and improve digestion while you're at it. Replace mashed potatoes with cauliflower, French fries with sweet potato fries, rice with salad, and try to cut out bread and sweets altogether.

The Japanese, known for their longevity, have a high vegetable intake. A 2009 study found that a diet high in Okinawan vegetables, which are rich in antioxidants, increased circulating EPCs in healthy young women, which coincided with decreased homocysteine levels.[12] Homocysteine is known to accelerate cell senescence, or wearing out, and reduces the proliferation of EPCs. It is well known that homocysteine levels can be lowered by eating more vegetable matter.

For a long time, a low-sodium diet was recommended for lowering blood pressure, but new research shows that a diet too low in sodium can actually have adverse effects on blood pressure. A diet with moderate sodium levels is ideal. You don't have to forgo your seasoning or salty treats, but be sure not to go overboard. Moderation is key.

Certain foods and dietary supplements are known to protect your fund of circulating stem cells. Add the following to your diet regimen:

- Blueberries – contain potassium, calcium, and magnesium (good for decreasing blood pressure), as well as fiber, folate, vitamin C, and vitamin B6 (good for healthy cholesterol levels and improving heart health)

- Goji berries – contain vitamin C, vitamin A, iron, beta-carotene (for skin health), and antioxidants that protect cells from breaking down, plus their seeds contain fiber
- Green tea extract – contains antioxidants including the compound EGCG, which helps control blood sugar and is helpful for cancer, neurodegenerative diseases, and atherosclerosis
- Astragalus – has shown promise in stimulating the immune system, lowering blood sugar, and promoting healthy cardiovascular function
- Carnosine – a protein building block that naturally occurs in the body and is found in the muscles, heart, and brain; helps with complications from diabetes, eye disorders, and kidney problems
- Red wine (primarily resveratrol) – resveratrol is the component in the skin of red grapes that reduces oxidation, prevents damage to blood vessels, and helps prevent blood clots
- Folate – a B vitamin that has been found to stimulate stem cell proliferation[13]
- Vitamin C – promotes the production of collagen in the basement membrane just below the endothelium, improving the structure of the blood vessels

One of my companies, Aidan Products, created a dietary supplement called Stem-Kine™, which contains ellagic acid, a polyphenol antioxidant found in numerous vegetables and fruits; vitamin D3, which has been shown to mildly increase circulating progenitor cells; beta 1,3 glucan, which has been shown to mobilize stem cells; and a ferment of the bacterium *Lactobacillus fermentum* with green tea and goji berry extracts and astragalus root. There are three published studies on the use of Stem-Kine for increasing circulating stem cells in humans.[14,15,16]

Caloric restriction, or the reduced intake of daily calories over an extended period of time, has been found to extend life in animal models. Reducing calorie intake by 40 percent extended average life span by 36 percent and maximum life span by 20 percent when compared to an unrestricted diet.[17] Investigators have been studying caloric restriction for longevity in animals since the 1930s. The National Institute on Aging has begun preliminary studies of a 25 percent calorie restriction in humans.[18]

My father used to ask the question, "What is the most important nutrient?" After the audience replied, "Vitamin C," "Magnesium," or "Zinc," he would correct them. "No. It's the nutrient you are lowest in." I learned from my dad that it's important to know your nutrient status. A recent study found that a diet deficient in the essential amino acid valine depleted the population of stem cells.[19] Scientists are likely to discover more nutrients that affect stem cell function and number as this area of investigation expands. Replenishing nutrients creates a healthy environment in which stem cells can thrive. In the meantime, it may make sense to find out what your most important nutrients are by having your blood tested at a place like the Riordan Clinic. Visit www.riordanclinic.org for more information.

Smoking

One of the main purposes of circulation is to get oxygen to all areas of your body. If you're smoking, your oxygen intake is impaired, and all the improvements made to your blood flow won't matter much if you're poisoning the air you take in.

We all know smoking causes health problems, but it's not just from the dangerous ingredients in mass-produced cigarettes—the cancer-causing chemicals, toxic metals, and poisonous gases. The smoke itself is doing damage to your lungs, blackening what was once pink and healthy, and essentially replacing oxygen with soot. Smokers have impaired circulating stem cells, which increase upon quitting and decrease when smoking is resumed.[20] Again, modifying habits can be the first step toward changing them. Quitting smoking altogether will increase your life expectancy and quality of life.

Living at Higher Altitude

If you live at higher altitude, you may be setting up your body for a health boost. An interesting study of 11 healthy volunteers who spent one week at moderate altitude (5,525 feet above sea level) in Oberlech, Austria found that levels of circulating EPCs increased, which they determined may be due to the body's response to decreased availability of oxygen at higher altitude.[21] While these individuals were also physically active, the degree of daily activity did not correlate with the stem cell increase. The Harvard Initiative for Global Health did a study that revealed seven out of the top 10 longest-living U.S. counties were all in the Colorado mountains, having an average life span of 81.3 years.[22]

Hyperbaric Oxygen Therapy

Hyperbaric oxygen therapy is the application of higher atmospheric pressure—100% oxygen—delivered inside a chamber to help the body carry more oxygen in the blood to organs and tissues. High oxygen concentrations stimulate angiogenesis, or the growth of blood vessels, which aids in the delivery of nutrients, growth factors, and circulating stem cells to a tissue or organ. A 2006 study found that circulation of CD34+ stem cells doubled after a single two-hour exposure to hyperbaric oxygen, and 20 treatments increased these cells eightfold while not raising white blood cell counts.[23] A 2014 study confirmed these results, finding 2.5 atmosphere of air pressure absolute (ATA), or two and a half times normal pressure, for two hours to be the ideal oxygen dosage.[24]

Statins

Statin drugs are one of the most widely prescribed medications for patients with certain risk factors for heart disease. Statins lower cholesterol, which has been touted for many years as the main reason for their cardiovascular benefit. Recently, however, studies have found that they also exhibit an anti-inflammatory effect, which may better explain how they help protect against heart disease in certain populations. Interestingly, statins also increase circulating EPCs. A study of 14 patients with heart disease who took 40 mg of atorvastatin for four weeks experienced a 1.5 increase in circulating EPCs after one week and a threefold increase after four weeks.[25] Perhaps the beneficial anti-inflammatory effect of this medication is due to an increase in circulating stem cells. More research is needed to work out the details.

Sage Advice

Circulating stem cells are the tools our bodies use to repair damaged tissue and to keep us healthy. Aging, genetics, and poor lifestyle choices decrease our number of circulating stem cells. The best advice probably comes from your grandmother: Eat your vegetables and go out and play (read: exercise).

Chapter Nineteen

CONTROVERSY AND LEGALITY

Legality

I have spent decades working with stem cells in hopes that my work—and the work of diligent stem cell researchers around the world—will one day be more widely available. Currently, the United States regulatory policy is lagging behind this critical field of scientific advancement. At the time of this writing, the only pathway toward stem cell use in the United States is the costly $1.2 billion route leading to new drug approval. Since stem cells come from the human body, they are not patentable, and so pharmaceutical companies are not interested in spending billions of dollars to bring a product to market they cannot exclusively own. It's simply not profitable. It's a catch-22, and the millions of patients in this country with chronic diseases that might benefit from stem cell treatment are the real victims. The FDA's overreach in the area of regenerative medicine is stifling the United States' progress in this important frontier of medicine.

The use of amnion, a human amniotic membrane product, is the perfect example. Amnion has been in use since 1910, but every ten years or so the FDA further restricts its use. They also want to regulate the use of your own stem cells from fat. Taking stem cells from fat out of your body and reinjecting it—within the very same procedure—is a currently accepted practice in the United States, but the FDA is trying to regulate this simple procedure as well. What is behind all this regulation? You may have guessed that the pharmaceutical industry, which lines the pockets of many lawmakers, unfortunately, is behind it. Smaller companies and medical practitioners who are trying to make life-saving treatments more readily available to the patients who desperately need them are continually overshadowed by the big money and influence of gigantic pharmaceutical companies that have the resources to persuade lawmakers to write laws that pad their bottom lines while patients wait decades for treatments they will possibly never be able to afford. It's a strong opponent to face, but like David and Goliath, a worthwhile endeavor, however small a step our progress gains us. Stem cell therapy has the potential to eliminate the need for a wide range of very expensive medications. If stem cell treatments become everyday medicine, pharmaceutical companies stand to lose a whole lot of money. If they can't make money off of it, and if they stand to lose money because of it, you can be sure they will do all they can—and they can—to make sure the treatment isn't approved. The FDA is predominately funded through payments from pharmaceutical companies that are run by former FDA employees. It's a vicious cycle of influence.

Currently in the United States, the regulatory path for stem cell treatment outside of a clinical trial is the path we took with Ryan Benton—investigational new drug (IND) use. This application process cost us $700,000. And that is just for IND use; that doesn't include the long and expensive path involving phase I, II, and III clinical trials that will take years, possibly decades, and over a billion dollars to complete. Contrast this cost with our costs in Panama. Our spinal cord injury patients receive our most extensive and costly treatment. For under $38,000 they receive about 15 IV injections and eight spinal injections, in addition to lab workup, follow-up, physical therapy, and transportation to and from the clinic and the airport. If you amortize our budget, this same treatment, not including transportation, would cost $300,000 in the United States. The cost of medicine in the United States has become prohibitive. The current regulatory state is not working. This is why I believe it's so important that stem cell treatment be regulated as the practice of medicine and not as a drug. It will greatly lower the cost of the treatment and make it more available to the millions of people suffering from chronic diseases these cells can treat.

I have operated clinics outside of the United States because it's the only way to advance this area of research without the debilitating and incredibly slow process currently required in the United States. People need this treatment now, not twenty years from now. When I decided upon Panama as the location for our current clinic, it was because of two laws that were already in effect. The first basically states that embryonic stem cells cannot be used in research or treatment. I had no interest in working with embryonic stem cells and did not want the government or the population to confuse my work with that of embryonic stem cells. The second law allows for the use and expansion of tissue derived from umbilical cords from newborns for the treatment of patients under consent. It was the perfect combination of laws for us to establish our work. I was interested in using umbilical cord stem cells donated from healthy, live births, which have the best safety profile and provide the most robust cells. Panama was the perfect place to provide this treatment.

Japan is ahead of the stem cell research curve and provides a great example of how we might model our stem cell regulation here in the United States. In 2014, the Japanese Congress introduced laws that grant conditional approval of stem cell products after their safety has been demonstrated. Companies then have seven years to gather efficacy data while their products are in use. South Korea, Taiwan, and Germany are about to pass similar legislation. Legislation such as this allows stem cell therapies that have been demonstrated as safe to be used clinically, allowing companies to fund further research while providing the treatment to patients who need it most.

Patients who have undergone stem cell treatment—and their doctors—are speaking up about its life-changing effects. Some legislators in the United States are starting to listen. Texas Congressman Joe Barton is one such politician trying to carve out a legacy as a regenerative medicine supporter. He is attempting to introduce a bill that would amend the Federal Food, Drug, and Cosmetic Act such that autologous stem cells—those harvested from the patient's own body—can be isolated, expanded, and used under the practice of medicine rather than as a drug. Currently, bone marrow transplants and organ transplants are regulated similarly. Bone marrow and organs are not considered to be "drugs" since they come from the body, and so can be transplanted under the practice of medicine. Consider that organ transplants contain millions of stem cells. Organ transplants are, in a sense, stem cell transplants. State medical boards ensure that these procedures are carried out safely, and patients are able to receive life-saving treatments. Stem cell treatments could proceed in the same way. If Joe Barton's bill is passed, patients in the United States will have access to stem cell therapy using their own stem cells. This is an important first step toward making stem cells available to the population at large.

Former Senator Mark Kirk, Senator Joe Manchin, and Senator Susan Collins introduced another bill, the REGROW Act, in March of 2016 that is quite similar to Japan's law, but requires a five-year period for efficacy studies to be concluded, compared to Japan's seven-year period. Many academics that I admire are behind the REGROW Act, but after discussing it with my FDA counsel, I don't think it has a good chance of making it through the Senate. It has already been kicked back for changes.

As I have already mentioned, regulating stem cell therapy by state medical boards as medical therapy is the best way to manage this field of medicine. State medical boards do a fine job regulating surgery, bone marrow and organ transplants, blood transfusions, and a wide range of treatments that involve the transplant of cell materials from one body to another. Complicating stem cell therapy by requiring researchers, who do not have billions of dollars, to follow the drug development pipeline is greatly inhibiting the potential reach of stem cell therapy.

Berkley Bedell, a six-time Iowa Congressman from 1975–1987, is a strong proponent of stem cell therapy, in part because he has experienced the benefits himself. After his run with Congress he set up the Foundation for Alternative and Integrative Medicine in an effort to identify breakthrough complementary and alternative therapies

> ***"It's heartbreaking that we can't have these treatments available to our people."***

Congressman Joe Barton on Stem Cells

NEIL RIORDAN: Do you believe the U.S. is at a competitive disadvantage in the regenerative medicine space given current regulations?

JOE BARTON: A fine line exists between proper regulation and forward-leaning advances in regenerative medicine. I believe we must always continue to explore new treatments, while also approving and assuring safety in health care in our great nation.

NR: How did you first learn about adult/postnatal stem cell treatment?

JB: I was contacted by stakeholders in Texas who are helping many patients with various health care needs. I was very pleased to learn of these patients' success and became interested in the topic.

NR: Do you think the American public understands the difference between embryonic stem cell treatment and adult/postnatal stem cell treatment?

JB: I believe stem cell therapy is complex and scientific and many people are not educated on these therapies and treatments. Stakeholders and advocates could do a better job to educate the general public on stem cell treatments.

and to research and report on their effectiveness. He later became involved by trying to influence Congress to write legislation for stem cell therapy. He introduced some of our patients who have had amazing results to former Senator Tom Harkin, who served as chairman of the Senate Committee on Health. Unfortunately, he had trouble making any headway because of the FDA involvement in the subcommittee and their reluctance to consider the therapy. The FDA is heavily dependent on the pharmaceutical industry for its revenue. "They're just partners, really," Bedell said. "It's heartbreaking that we can't have these treatments available to our people." When I asked him what he thinks it would take for Congress to make a change, he replied, "Money controls things now. We have to take it out. When I first ran for Congress, I spent about $80K to run my campaign. Today it costs a million dollars to run a campaign, and most of that money comes from the top one percent of the wealthy. And every member knows he has to run again in two years, so they are beholden to the large donations they depend on."

NR: Do you have any personal experience with anyone who has received adult stem cells for a particular condition?

JB: I have interacted with many patients that have benefited from stem cell treatments.

NR: What are you doing to help move this research and treatment forward?

JB: I am very interested in introducing a bill that would allow individuals to use their own stem cells for treatment without the FDA requiring these stem cells to go through the drug approval process.

NR: What are the biggest obstacles to passing this legislation?

JB: Unfortunately, the legislative calendar is our biggest obstacle at this time. We only have a handful of legislative days left in the 114th Congress. The complexity of this issue does not yield quick legislative results, but with a thoughtful strategy we will prevail.

NR: What do you hear from your constituents about adult/postnatal stem cell treatment?

JB: I have heard from many Texans about the remarkable results they have had.

NR: What are your thoughts on the potential impact of adult stem cell treatments regarding the treatment of chronic diseases?

JB: I believe that adult stem cells could be the answer to many of the health care mysteries we still have today. The specific cases that I am aware of show magnificent and groundbreaking results. If the science continues to show great results, I think there will be a lot less suffering in this world.

NR: What are your thoughts on the potential impact of adult stem cell treatments on the cost of health care?

JB: I believe this treatment could help many patients stay healthy and lower health care costs.

Controversy

In 2010, 60 Minutes aired an episode about a particular stem cell business led by a gentleman in California with no medical background. Unfortunately, this gentleman made farfetched claims about the treatments to two men suffering from amyotrophic lateral sclerosis (ALS), sometimes called Lou Gehrig's disease, who posed as potential patients. Undercover cameras revealed fabricated claims made by the gentleman, who charged $125,000 for treatment. He claimed to have successfully treated ALS patients, reversing their condition and taking them from wheelchair to walking, a claim that was later refuted once he was confronted by 60 Minutes. The man claimed to be working with the FDA and the University of Texas, claims that were also refuted by 60 Minutes. The stem cell treatments were performed in Mexico by a partner, a man who claimed to be medical doctor licensed in the United States to practice medicine, but who actually had a fraudulent medical degree. This television special has painted stem cell therapy as a whole in a terrible light. While there are many clinics throughout the world operating as these gentlemen do, I take exception to the press grouping all stem cell therapy under the same umbrella.

Scrutiny has also come down upon clinics in the United States that use autologous (self-derived) fat tissue stem cell therapy. The practice has come under question by the FDA. The removal and same-day reinjection of minimally manipulated cells is legal in the United States. But some clinics have been expanding the cells, which takes a few days, and then reinjecting the cells, calling into question their legal use of the procedure. Many clinics have also been making unsubstantiated claims about the stem cell activity of their treatments and about what diseases they treat. Such clinics are still widespread in the United States, but the FDA is trying to further define and regulate the procedures.

In many cases, the removal of fat tissue and the reinjection of stromal vascular fraction (fat tissue) derived from said tissue during the same procedure is not the most effective treatment in my opinion. We learned early on in Panama that time is needed after liposuction for inflammation to subside in the body. Stem cells migrate to areas of injury, so reinjecting stromal vascular fraction the day it is removed is likely not going to give the same benefits as waiting for the inflammation to subside. We have also learned that not all MSCs are alike. Some people have less robust MSCs, which would limit the therapeutic benefits of an autologous treatment. But we need to start somewhere. If legislators are comfortable with autologous treatment, then we must do our best to administer the treatment safely and in the best interest of our patients.

The 60 Minutes special isn't the only bad press stem cell treatments have received. *The New York Times* recently reported on a case report that was published in the *New England Journal of Medicine* about a man who had received stem cells from China, Mexico, and Argentina to treat his ischemic stroke. The man developed a non-cancerous tumor in his spine that paralyzed him from the neck down. After reading the article, anyone would conclude that stem cell treatment is dangerous. Unfortunately, the journalists did not emphasize the fact that the stem cells used in these treatments were fetal stem cells, which have a greater potential to differentiate into different tissues and can be tumorigenic. While they are not embryonic cells, they are much closer to embryonic cells than adult stem cells. We do not use fetal stem cells in our clinic for this very reason.

Articles in the press such as these—and there are others—remind me of our experience with the press in the Bahamas. They implied that we were using embryonic stem cells, the public believed it, and so we were forced out of the country on baseless claims that our treatments were dangerous.

At our clinic in Panama, we don't overpromise, and we don't overcharge. Our most expensive treatment is $38,000. In fact, we operated as a non-profit for the first six years. I am doing everything I can to make these treatments available to as many people as possible, but I can't do it alone. The path to providing these treatments in the United States requires the input of patients, legislators, doctors, researchers, and the community at large.

Experience

Roberta Shapiro, DO, is a physiatrist, board certified in physical medicine and rehabilitation, affiliated with New York-Presbyterian University Hospital of Columbia, and working in New York City with an impressive list of patients. Her focus is on musculoskeletal pain management and pediatric rehabilitation. "About 20 years ago I hit a wall with the available treatment options for my chronic pain patients. I theorized that there was an inflammatory pathology to their disease processes, but I had very few options for treating them." She began to investigate inflammatory diseases and their treatment options. "We're very limited in the United States; non-steroidals, steroids, immunoglobular therapy—that was as far as I could take it. I was really frustrated that I wasn't getting anywhere." She found steroids to be particularly ineffective for long-term use, some of which caused symptoms to come back with a vengeance. "These were not options for me," she said.

She dove into the scientific literature and found that stem cells were another possible treatment of inflammatory and autoimmune disease. "It was foreign to me when I first read about it," she said. She decided to travel the world to learn more about stem cell treatments. In the meantime, she began collecting data on her patients using advanced testing of inflammatory cytokines and interleukins. She brought the raw data to Israel, where she met with the head of a bone marrow transplant unit and asked him if he thought she was crazy to think that stem cells might be the answer. He reassured her as he described how his treatment for all post-cancer autoimmune patients involved the use of bone marrow-derived autologous stem cells that had been expanded in culture. "This doctor selected the most potent cells, expanded them, and reinjected them back into his patients. He had been doing it for years and swore that it stopped the autoimmune disease in its tracks."

Dr. Shapiro began to research stem cell clinics around the world. That's when she found our clinic in Panama. She attended one of my seminars and became excited when she learned about how stem cells work. She traveled to our clinic in Panama as well as to other clinics in Mexico, Germany, and Switzerland. "One of the things that amazed me about the Stem Cell Institute in Panama was the transparency of your clinic, which was not available to me in any other facility. They told me, 'No, you can't see the lab,' or 'You can't see the charts. You can't talk to the patients.' In Panama they told me, 'Sure! Let's go to the lab and talk to the lab director and technicians. Let's talk to the doctors. Ask any patient in the waiting room if you want.' There was nothing withheld. That made a huge statement to me."

Her confidence in our clinic was also cemented when she had the opportunity to sit next to Arnold Caplan, the father of the MSC, on a flight back from Panama. "He literally said to me, 'This is a world-class lab, and I would trust it for my own family.' That gave me an additional level of confidence," Dr. Shapiro said.

Dr. Shapiro now treats, almost exclusively, people with chronic pain who have inflammatory disorders. She began recommending stem cell treatment to her patients, offering to accompany them to Panama. Since then she has brought over 60 patients and recommended even more go on their own. Most of her colleagues at Columbia thought she was crazy, but they are starting to ask about her successes with the treatment.

Of the many patients Dr. Shapiro has brought to Panama for stem cell treatment, one stands out as exceptional. A woman with mild emphysema and abnormal pulmonary function, which her highly respected pulmonologist had told her was abnormal and irreversible, received one week of stem cell treatment and felt fantastic within days. Upon return, her pulmonary function test was completely normal, causing her pulmonologist to incorrectly conclude that she must have had a respiratory infection during the last test.

"Every single patient I have sent to the Stem Cell Institute experienced some improvement, even if it was not as dramatic as normalized test results. It has been so refreshing for me, because I was about to close my doors because I was so frustrated with the practice of

Every single patient I have sent to the Stem Cell Institute experienced some improvement, even if it was not as dramatic as normalized test results. It has been so refreshing for me, because I was about to close my doors because I was so frustrated with the practice of medicine in the United States, but now I feel that I am making a difference in people's lives, and in my own life."

—Roberta Shapiro, DO, MD

medicine in the United States, but now I feel that I am making a difference in people's lives, and in my own life."

Indeed, Dr. Shapiro is herself a patient of ours. "I have a history of autoimmune disorders in my family. Lyme disease kicked off one of the worst cases of menopause I have ever seen. I was diagnosed with osteoporosis at age 40, and for 15 years my numbers did not budge. I had developed hypertension. After stem cell treatment, my bone density score actually bumped up, which is significant since I am now postmenopausal so my numbers are expected to go down. I think that is a significant improvement. I am also on half the dose of blood pressure and thyroid medication. My energy is better; I lost 15 pounds; my hair, skin, and nail quality is better. I have seen the benefits in my own life."

Research in animals backs up the results Dr. Shapiro has experienced with stem cell treatment for her osteoporosis. In combination with parathyroid hormone, injected MSCs were found to migrate to the site of bone injury, and increased new bone formation when compared to standard or no treatment.[1]

CONCLUSION

I hope this book has answered some questions and more importantly has whet your appetite for learning more about the potential benefits of adult stem cells, MSCs in particular. I hear from people every day who now have hope when there was none before. That has been my prime motivation throughout my stem cell journey, and that feedback is what drives our team of now 60 employees in Panama.

Some people have asked me, "If these cells work so well and all of these people are getting better, why is it not on CNN?" My answer is, "Just wait." I don't believe we'll have to wait too long. PBS has already done a piece on what we do in Panama. It is now being aired around the country. It is an episode in the series *Natural Health Breakthroughs with Brenda Watson*. Last week I heard from Sanjay Gupta's people, and they are planning on doing a piece in May of this year. So, I think it's coming. As I've mentioned earlier, there has been a concerted effort to not have information out there about the benefits of a technology that will, when broadly accepted, massively disrupt the economics of not just the pharmaceutical industry but also medicine in general. They way medicine is practiced will be changed forever when these cells are widely available.

If this is such cutting-edge science, why isn't it part of the mainstream research in the United States? Why do I have to do business offshore in Central America?

The answer is what you would expect: money. The big pharmaceutical companies are scared to death of stem cells.

Think of how a drug enters the marketplace. Big Pharma determines which diseases are the most widespread and therefore present the biggest market for new drugs. Teams of well-paid scientists spend years in their laboratories trying to devise a special molecule that will help alleviate the symptoms of these diseases. Whatever they come up with, by its very nature, will not be something necessarily tolerated easily by the human body. In fact, it could have some pretty horrible side effects. Expensive clinical trials must begin, and many drugs don't make it past that stage. Some that do are later recalled by the government.

All of these necessary steps add significant cost to the price of drugs. Manufacturers say that they are only attempting to recoup the investment they made in developing the drug. When patients pick up their drugs for the first time, the sticker shock, even with insurance, can cause them to decline to take the course of medicine. They'd rather suffer, as Marian D'Unger did. She refused to buy an injectable form of methotrexate and pay $1,584 a month when she knew the drug would only make her arthritis slightly better.

The market for these drugs is in the billions of dollars. People with diabetes pay about $73.5 billion a year for anti-diabetic medicine, supplies, and prescriptions that treat diabetic complications. Nearly 30 million Americans today have diabetes, and 86 million more have prediabetes, according to the American Diabetes Association.[1] The top seven arthritis medications brought in $16 billion a year for their manufacturers in 2008, with huge growth potential.[2] The market for those drugs increased from between 14 and 91 percent in a single year. Big Pharma looks positively on the notion of such a rapidly expanding market for its drugs as the country's population ages.

The last thing the big drug companies want is for stem cell treatments to advance in popularity. After all, when a drug company comes out with a new drug, it is patented and no one else has the right to use it for the life of the patent. For decades, that company has the exclusive right to the proceeds of that chemical compound. If the mechanism for healing you of your disease comes from the cells of your body, no drug company can make a nickel from that. Our cells are not patentable.

A good example of drug companies blocking advances in healing is the discovery that *H. pylori* bacteria cause ulcers. For decades, doctors believed that the cause of ulcers was stress and eating spicy food. In fact, there was a billion-dollar drug industry centered on relieving the horrible pain ulcer sufferers experienced. Those who had ulcers saw the condition as a lifelong curse because most drugs on the market offered them little or no relief from their symptoms.

In 1979 Australian researchers Dr. Barry Marshall and Dr. Robin Warren discovered *Helicobacter pylori*, the bacteria that cause ulcers. At the time, this went counter to everything science thought about the mechanism of the stomach and digestion. The widespread opinion was that stomach acid was so strong, no bacteria could survive in the gut. When Marshall and Warren found the spiral-shaped bacteria, they had trouble culturing it so that they could present it in a scientific paper. Luck prevailed in the form of a mistake. By accident, the doctors left the Petri dishes incubating over a five-day Easter holiday. When they returned to the lab, they found the dishes teeming with *H. pylori*.

Even though they were able to put up slides that showed the unique spiral-shaped bacteria and could tie it to bacteria cultured in other mammals such as dogs, the doctors were shunned by the scientific community. When they would present their findings at big research conferences, other scientists who were on the payroll of the big drug companies would stand up and walk out of the room when the Australians began their talks. They were threatening a $5 billion-a-year segment of the drug industry.

In frustration, one day in the lab Warren decided he had had it with the doubters who maintained that *H. pylori* was not the cause of ulcers, but merely a bystander. He drank a beaker of solution that contained the bacteria, and within days he came down with gastritis. A culture of the contents of his stomach revealed the presence of *H. pylori*, which had not been there before.

Eventually, the Australian analysis of the cause of ulcers prevailed. In fact, in 2005 Marshall and Warren won the Nobel Prize in medicine for their research. Now doctors treating ulcers prescribe antibiotics, which are much more effective than antacids in fighting the true cause of ulcers.

The blockages that stand in the way of more widespread use of stem cells to treat chronic diseases are a good corollary to the saga of the doctors from Australia. Warren and Marshall's work killed off a profitable portion of the drug manufacturing industry, as will widespread treatments with people's own stem cells. I know it is inevitable. Patients talk to other patients. Augment that with the blinding speed of the Internet, and eventually everyone will understand. Stem cell medicine is not snake oil, and it's not a scam. There are certainly more than a few unscrupulous people and businesses taking advantage of this industry, which is in its infancy. Despite the challenges that lay ahead, stem cell medicine is here to stay, and we should welcome it when done by responsible people in a responsible way.

Some groups do criticize the stem cell industry by using the argument that if you're able to treat so many things with one drug it must be snake oil or quackery. I'd like to address that here. Given that these cells are potently anti-inflammatory, are able to modulate and even fix a broken immune system, and secrete molecules that stimulate regeneration, it only makes sense that they're able to treat conditions in which those particular processes are out of whack. For example, autism is really an inflammatory disease, as witnessed by elevated inflammatory blood markers. Autoimmune diseases are a not only a dysfunctionality of the immune system, but upstream of that, also a dysfunctionality or depletion of the mesenchymal stem cells. In spinal cord injury, the problem is a lack of MSCs secreting molecules that stimulate regeneration. In these three very disparate conditions the underlying mechanism is addressed by the MSCs. And that goes for every condition that we treat and that has been described in this book. There's a common thread of not enough regeneration going on, too much inflammation, or a dysfunctional immune system.

Another misconception is that what we are doing is extremely high-tech. Our work is actually quite low-tech. We're taking what nature has given us in abundant supply—immune-privileged, genetically hard-wired medicinal signaling cells that have the ability to stimulate regeneration, reduce inflammation, and modulate the immune system—selecting for the best ones, expanding them, and giving them to people with inflammation, immune dysfunction, or lack of regeneration.

It's taken us centuries of research to understand how the body heals itself and, in many ways I think we're just getting started in terms of comprehending the complex interplay of those forces. Still, with our research into the various kinds of stem cells, we're making rapid progress. In a few decades, I believe we will look back on some of the poisonous drugs and invasive and destructive treatments we've been using to treat chronic illnesses and they will seem as crude and barbaric as when we think of doctors 200 years ago using heavy metals to cure disease.

At a time when the country is in turmoil about the high cost of medical care, stem cells offer tremendous potential. These treatments, once they become more commonplace, will offer effective therapy at greatly reduced cost. My hope is that through persistence on my part and the part of others who are working in this line of research, some day many chronic conditions that ruin lives will be only a memory. We can live in a world where children don't suffer from muscular dystrophy; those who have spinal cord injuries can walk again; people with heart disease, multiple sclerosis, and arthritis can return to active lives; and diabetes patients don't have their legs amputated. It's only a matter of time—and some hard work from scientists—and these diseases can truly be things of the past.

But being a pioneer is typically not an easy road. There's an old saying, "You know how you can spot a pioneer? They have arrows in their backs." I've had my share of arrows. When I was wounded by one particularly large arrow, my brother Brian perked me up by saying, "If you don't have a few arrows in your back you are one boring guy."

On a hopeful note, in a recent meeting with Congressman Joe Barton, Vice-Chairman of the Committee on Energy and Commerce, he said to me, "You'll prevail in the end because what you're saying and doing is the truth."

I was also speaking recently with Representative Tan Parker, who represents the Flower Mound area of Texas in the Texas Legislature. Representative Parker has introduced a bill into the House of Representatives that would allow for the use of adult stem cells for the treatment of people with either a terminal illness or a chronic illness who don't have any other good treatment options. I asked Tan what his rationale was for introducing this bill—a bill, by the way, that would fly in the face of FDA regulations and would put the state at odds with the federal government. It would be very much like the situation in Colorado with marijuana, in which the Secretary of State would actually have to sue the federal government. If it comes to pass, it's going be a particularly contentious environment between Texas and the federal government.

When I asked Representative Parker why he created this bill, he told me he had several friends and family members with chronic conditions who had travelled out of the country to get these treatments and had seen success. He said that for most people, travelling out of the country is too onerous and costly, and that he wrote the bill for Texans to have the liberty to choose their medical care. I found that to be very poignant. Life, liberty, and the pursuit of happiness—those are the tenets upon which this country was founded. I feel that our liberty to choose our medical treatments has been increasingly diminished. Medical treatment should be between a doctor and a patient. A doctor, too, should have liberty to provide a patient with the treatment he or she believes to be the best for the patient's condition. In conclusion, I believe that we need to restore the premises of life, liberty, and the pursuit of happiness to our country. This Texas bill will, if passed, go a long way toward restoring that freedom.

Epilogue

BY ROGER NOCERA, MD

I remember the day Dr. Neil Riordan told me about mesenchymal stem cells for the first time, though since then they have been the topic of so many wonderful conversations between us. It was early on before we had treated many patients in Costa Rica. At the time, we were using umbilical cord-derived CD34 cell expansion culture progeny. Neil called me and said, "Roger, boy, if you ever remember anything, remember these words: mesenchymal stem cells."

Neil went on, "MSCs are multipotent for cellular transdifferentiated reproductive progeny derived from all three embryonic germ layers. MSCs transdifferentiate into all the known monopotent sentinel stem cells in organ tissues, such as type 2 pneumocytes in lung tissue, satellite cells in muscle tissue, oval cells in liver tissue, epidermal basal cells in the skin, and other progenitor cells—providing the rationale to label MSCs as master healing cells.

Mesenchymal stem cells are ubiquitous because they cling to blood vessels, positioning them at all possible tissue injury sites. They regulate each step of the complex cellular homeostasis process (healing), from inflammatory wound debridement to injured cell and matrix replacement processes. MSCs downregulate metabolically active cell production of inflammatory cytokines (such as TNF-alpha and interleukin 1) and upregulate the production of anti-inflammatory cytokines (such as interleukin 10), and we know overstimulation of inflammation is an ubiquitous obstacle to healing chronic disease processes, especially autoimmunity, which is more common than previously thought.

MSCs are universal donor cells endowed by nature with immune privilege as demonstrated by the universality of maternal microchimerism. They are immunomodulatory and can even trigger tolerogenesis for autoantigens. MSCs have healed lab animals paralyzed by femoral artery and nerve transection, among many other benefits supported by peer-reviewed evidence."

On and on he went, like an encyclopedia of future medicine. Soon thereafter, in typical Dr. Riordan style, he didn't just talk about it, he started treating patients with mesenchymal stem cells in Costa Rica, and immediately the results were enormously promising. The rest is now early twenty-first century medical history—a written history in which Neil has played a major role over the past decade.

As a doctor and a medical diagnostician myself, I predict this book will become the classic medical text on adult stem cell therapeutics. I would not be surprised if it became mandatory reading for all physicians, regardless of specialty, because I believe in the very near future doctors will begin practicing adult stem cell therapy in the United States (once the U.S. Food and Drug Administration finally catches up to the trail Dr. Riordan has provided in his extraordinary contributions to the field).

The story of how I first met Dr. Neil Riordan is very telling of who he is. I met him around 2003, at first indirectly, while I was working in my diagnostic imaging center in Phoenix, Arizona. There, my technologists performed diagnostic scans with high-tech computerized equipment, magnetic resonance imaging (MRI), computed axial topography, and real-time and Doppler ultrasound, which I would routinely interpret. One day I came upon a fascinating case of a middle-aged woman with widespread metastatic malignant melanoma diagnosed several months earlier. Her CT scan showed "cannonball"-sized tumors in the liver, lungs, and bones, with massive retroperitoneal adenopathy. My job was to evaluate the results of her therapy over the past four months with a second series of CT scans.

At first I was confused because the follow-up scan was clean, no tumors. They were gone. Something was not right; I knew this disease, and there was no treatment I knew of that had the required efficacy to produce this extraordinary result. After rechecking, I concluded that the tumors were indeed gone. Moreover, the referring doctor was a naturopath. So what exactly was he giving this patient? I recognized the name of the referring doctor, as he was one of my students when I taught a class on clinical medical diagnostics at a naturopathic medical school in Phoenix. I called him to ask what he had used to treat this patient with metastatic malignant melanoma. This young, relatively recently graduate proceeded in the most confident tone, waxing poetic in conventional medical terms a most erudite explanation of dendritic cell therapy. He explained that he worked with Dr. Neil Riordan, who at the time was using a process whereby he extracted the dendritic blood cells of cancer patients by apheresis and presented to them attenuated melanoma tumor cells, which then processed tumor antigen, because that is what dendritic cells do. The antigen-activated dendritic cells were then expanded in number exponentially in cytokine cell culture and reintroduced into the patients' blood, after which they found their way to lymph nodes where they presented the molecular antigenic memory to T helper cells; T helper cells activate T killer cells, which in turn target and kill the malignant melanoma cells. When I presented this story to my friends at the Mayo Clinic Oncology Department, they said dendritic cell therapy was so new and complex to them at the time, and they were making plans to conduct some cases in the future. All I knew was that Dr. Neil Riordan was ahead of the Mayo Clinic.

Shortly thereafter, I had the opportunity to meet Neil formally while he was raising funds to start Medistem, Inc., one of the first publically traded American adult stem cell biotechnology companies at the time. We became fast friends because I immediately recognized Dr. Riordan's medical intellect. I knew upon speaking with him about many clinical issues that he had an extraordinary fund of both macroscopic and microscopic medical knowledge. We eventually found ourselves heading for Costa Rica to interview doctors to run the lab and clinic where Neil's umbilical cord-derived CD34 cells would be administered to patients with diseases that conventional medicine had failed to effectively and efficiently treat in the United States.

Throughout the next decade, first in Costa Rica and later in Panama, Neil devised some of the first adult stem cell therapy protocols for treating multiple sclerosis, rheumatoid arthritis, non-ischemic dilated myocardiopathy, autism, dermatomyositis, Duchenne muscular dystrophy, overwhelming psoriatic arthritis, and more. Countless lives were improved and hope given where previously there was none. Dr. Riordan's simple, elegant, and clinically powerful approach to stem cell medical science adds profound clarity to the field.

As our friendship developed over the years, I was not surprised to learn that Neil came from a family of brilliant medical pioneers. His father, Dr. Hugh Riordan, who was thought by many to be the grandfather of alternative and orthomolecular medicine, worked closely with three-time Nobel Laureate Dr. Linus Pauling. The Riordan family worked with other medical giants as well, including Gladys McGarey, MD—often called the Mother of Holistic Medicine—and Elisabeth Kübler-Ross, MD, who through her groundbreaking book, *On Death and Dying*, informed a generation of the need for hospice care in the United States.

Within Neil's book, he presents a decade of innovative clinical work with compelling success in treating a broad range of difficult-to-treat diseases, with results unequaled in conventionally offered traditional allopathic therapies. Neil learned early that the healing abilities of MSCs are tissue-source dependent. This is because of the inherent epigenetics of the tissue source (tissue milieu) and its influence on interference ribonucleic acids (RNA-i) and other gene function determinants within the realm of the same cell surface marker determined by MSC phenotype population. I remember fondly how, during my tenure as chief medical officer at Medistem, we proudly sent Dr. Thomas Ichim (our chief scientific officer at the time) to London to receive for Medistem a first-prize award from the worldwide PubMed organization for Neil's seminal peer-reviewed discovery of an endometrial tissue-derived, epigenetically endowed, "sub-phenotype" of MSCs that are super angiogenic: endometrial regenerative cells (ERCs). That article won first prize out of over 30,000 other competing scientific professionally published research papers. Within it are the seeds of the future of medical practice and an important part of the unfolding of twenty-first century medical history. Neil also discovered that human umbilical cord mesenchymal stem cells derived from Wharton's Jelly are better for treating myocardiopathies than MSCs derived from elsewhere, especially if treated alongside high IV doses of vitamin C.

I talk about Dr. Riordan in the beginning of my book, *Cells That Heal Us From Cradle To Grave: A Quantum Leap In Medical Science*, published in 2011, and the words are just as true today: "A special thanks to my colleague, partner, and dear friend Dr. Neil Riordan, a brilliantly skilled clinician, a medical genius, and a modern-day embodiment of Dr. Edward Jenner—the father of immunology. Dr. Riordan is one of the world's most important medical scientists living today, is the person who taught me everything I know about stem cells and who has done much to sow the seeds to important medical advance in this century, as did his famous late father in the latter half of the twentieth century, Hugh Riordan, MD, whose written trilogy of history's medical mavericks has inspired much of this book."

Roger M. Nocera, MD is a world leader in stem cell therapy research. He received his medical degree from the University of Massachusetts Medical School and has been in practice for more than 35 years.

References

BY CHAPTER

Chapter One

1. Vieira NM, Valadares M, Zucconi E, et al. Human adipose-derived mesenchymal stromal cells injected systemically into GRMD dogs without immunosuppression are able to reach the host muscle and express human dystrophin. Cell Transplant. 2012;21(7):1407-17. doi: 10.3727/096368911X.
2. Muntoni F, Torelli S, Ferlini A. Dystrophin and mutations: one gene, several proteins, multiple phenotypes. Lancet Neurol. 2003;2(12):731-740.
3. Spuler S, Engel AG. Unexpected sarcolemmal complement membrane attack complex deposits on nonnecrotic muscle fibers in muscular dystrophies. Neurology. 1998;50(1):41-46.
4. Skuk D, Vilquin JT, Tremblay JP. Experimental and therapeutic approaches to muscular dystrophies. Curr Opin Neurol.2002;15(5):563-569.
5. Balaban B, Matthews DJ, Clayton GH, Carry T. Corticosteroid treatment and functional improvement in Duchenne muscular dystrophy: long-term effect. Am J Phys Med Rehabil.2005;84(11):843-850.
6. Ricotti V, Ridout DA, Scott E, et al. Long-term benefits and adverse effects of intermittent versus daily glucocorticoids in boys with Duchenne muscular dystrophy. J Neurol Neurosurg Physchiatry.2013;84(6):698-705.
7. Ginn SL, Alexander IE, Edelstein ML, Abedi MR, Wixon J. Gene therapy clinical trials worldwide to 2012 - an update. J Gene.Med.2013;15(2):65-77.
8. Aggarwal S, Pittenger MF. Human mesenchymal stem cells modulate allogeneic immune cell responses. Blood.2005;105(4):1815-1822.
9. Caplan AI. Adult mesenchymal stem cells for tissue engineering versus regenerative medicine. J Cell Physiol.2007;213(2):341-347.
10. Chamberlain G, Fox J, Ashton B, Middleton J. Concise review: mesenchymal stem cells: their phenotype, differentiation capacity, immunological features, and potential for homing. Stem Cells.2007;25(11):2739-2749.
11. Bachrach E, Perez AL, Choi YH, et al. Muscle engraftment of myogenic progenitor cells following intraarterial transplantation. Muscle Nerve. 2006;34(1):44-52.
12. Bailo M, Soncini M, Vertua E, et al. Engraftment potential of human amnion and chorion cells derived from term placenta. Transplantation.2004;78(10):1439-1448.
13. Pelatti MV, Gomes JP, Vieira NM, et al. Transplantation of human adipose mesenchymal stem cells in non-immunosuppressed GRMD dogs is a safe procedure. Stem Cell Rev. 2016;12(4):448-53. doi: 10.1007/s12015-016-9659-3.

14. Vieira NM, Valadares M, Zucconi E, et al. Human adipose-derived mesenchymal stromal cells injected systemically into GRMD dogs without immunosuppression are able to reach the host muscle and express human dystrophin. Cell Transplant. 2012;21(7):1407-1417. doi: 10.3727/096368911X.

15. Rodriguez AM, Pisani D, Dechesne CA, et al. Transplantation of a multipotent cell population from human adipose tissue induces dystrophin expression in the immunocompetent mdx mouse. J Exp Med. 2005;201(9):1397-1405.doi: 10.1084/jem.20042224.

16. Ichim TE, Alexandrescu DT, Solano F, et al. Mesenchymal stem cells as anti-inflammatories: implications for treatment of Duchenne muscular dystrophy. Cellular Immunol. 2010;260(2):75-82.doi: 10.1016/j.cellimm.2009.10.006.

17. Acibadem University. Efficacy of Umbilical Cord Mesenchymal Stem Cells in Duchenne Muscular Dystrophy. In: ClinicalTrials.gov [Internet]. Bethesda (MD): National Library of Medicine (US). 2000- [cited 2016Jul]. Available from: https://clinicaltrials.gov/ct2/show /NCT02285673 NLM Identifier: NCT02285673.

18. Allogeneic human umbilical cord mesenchymal stem cells for a single male patient with duchenne muscular dystrophy (DMD). ClinicalTrials.gov NCT02235844.

19. Neurogen Brain and Spine Institute. Stem cell therapy in duchenne muscular dystrophy. In: ClinicalTrials.gov [Internet]. Bethesda (MD): National Library of Medicine (US). 2000- [cited 2016Jul]. Available from: https://clinicaltrials.gov/ct2/show/NCT02241434 NLM Identifier: NCT02241434.

20. University of Gaziantep; Alper Dai. Efficacy of stem cell therapy in ambulatory and non-ambulatory children with duchenne muscular dystrophy - phase 1-2. In: ClinicalTrials.gov [Internet]. Bethesda (MD): National Library of Medicine (US). 2000- [cited 2016Jul]. Available from: https://clinicaltrials.gov/ct2/show/NCT02484560 NLM Identifier: NCT02484560.

21. Chaitanya Hospital, Pune; Sachin Jamadar. Study safety and efficacy of bone marrow derived autologous cells for the treatment of muscular dystrophy. In: ClinicalTrials.gov [Internet]. Bethesda (MD): National Library of Medicine (US). 2000- [cited 2016Jul]. Available from: https://clinicaltrials.gov/ct2/show/NCT01834066 NLM Identifier: NCT01834066.

Additional References

Markert CD, Atala A, Cann JK, et al., "Mesenchymal stem cells: emerging therapy for Duchenne muscular dystrophy." *PM R.* 2009 Jun;1(6):547-59. doi: 10.1016/j.pmrj.2009.02.013.

Chapter Two

1 Creagan ET, Moertel CG, O'Fallon JR, et al. Failure of high-dose vitamin C (ascorbic acid) therapy to benefit patients with advanced cancer. A controlled trial. N Engl J Med. 1979 Sep 27;301(13):687-90.

2 Hoffer LJ. Proof versus plausibility: rules of engagement for the struggle to evaluate alternative cancer therapies. CMAJ. 2001;164(3):351-3.

3 Padayatty SJ, Levine M. New insights into the physiology and pharmacology of vitamin C. CMAJ. 2001;164(3):353-5.

4 Riordan NH, Riordan HD, inventors; The Center for the Improvement of Human Functioning Int'l, Inc., assignee. Therapeutic method for the treatment of cancer. US patent 5,639,787. June 17, 1997.

5 Casciari JJ, Riordan NH, inventors; The Center for the Improvement of Human Functioning Int'l, Inc., assignee. Treatment of cancer using lipoic acid in combination with ascorbic acid. US patent 6,448,287. September 10, 2002.

[6] Mayland CR, Bennett MI, Allan K. Vitamin C deficiency in cancer patients. Palliat Med. 2005;19(1):17-20.

[7] Cieslak JA, Cullen JJ. Treatment of pancreatic cancer with pharmacological ascorbate. Curr Pharm Biotechnol. 2015;16(9):759-70.

[8] Lillberg K, Verkasalo PK, Kaprio J, Teppo L, Helenius H, Koskenvuo M. Stressful life events and risk of breast cancer in 10,808 women: a cohort study. Am J Epidemiol. 2003;157(5):415-23.

[9] Head JF, Wang F, Elliott RL, McCoy JL. Assessment of immunologic competence and host reactivity against tumor antigens in breast cancer patients. Prognostic value and rationale of immunotherapy development. Ann N Y Acad Sci. 1993;690:340-2.

[10] Riordan NH, Riordan HD, Meng X, Li Y, Jackson JA. Intravenous ascorbate as a tumor cytotoxic chemotherapeutic agent. Med Hypotheses. 1995;44(3):207-13.

[11] Houghton J, Stoicov C, Nomura S, et al. Gastric cancer originating from bone marrow-derived cells. Science. 2004;306(5701):1568-71.

Chapter Three

[1] Mayordomo JI, Zorina T, Storkus WJ, et al. Bone marrow-derived dendritic cells pulsed with synthetic tumour peptides elicit protective and therapeutic antitumour immunity. *Nat Med.* 1995;1(12):1297-302.

[2] Nair SK, Snyder D, Rouse BT, Gilboa E. Regression of tumors in mice vaccinated with professional antigen-presenting cells pulsed with tumor extracts. Int J Cancer. 1997;70(6):706-15.

[3] Hsu FJ, Benike C, Fagnoni F, et al. Vaccination of patients with B-cell lymphoma using autologous antigen-pulsed dendritic cells. Nat Med. 1996;2(1):52-8.

[4] Murphy GP, Tjoa BA, Simmons SJ, et al. Phase II prostate cancer vaccine trial: report of a study involving 37 patients with disease recurrence following primary treatment. Prostate. 1999;39(1):54-9.

[5] Nestle FO, Alijagic S, Gilliet M, et al. Vaccination of melanoma patients with peptide- or tumor lysate-pulsed dendritic cells. Nat Med. 1998;4(3):328-32.

Chapter Four

1. Pai M, Spalding D, Xi F, Habib N. Autologous bone marrow stem cells in the treatment of chronic liver disease. Int J Hepatol. 2012;2012:307165. doi: 10.1155/2012/307165.
2. Li B, Cohen A, Hudson TE, et al. Mobilized human hematopoietic stem/progenitor cells promote kidney repair following ischemia reperfusion injury. Circulation. 2010; 121(20): 2211–2220.
3. Mendonça MV, Larocca TF, de Freitas Souza BS, et al. Safety and neurological assessments after autologous transplantation of bone marrow mesenchymal stem cells in subjects with chronic spinal cord injury. Stem Cell Res Ther. 2014;5(6):126.doi: 10.1186/scrt516.
4. Jiang PC, Xiong WP, Wang G, et al. A clinical trial report of autologous bone marrow-derived mesenchymal stem cell transplantation in patients with spinal cord injury. Exp Ther Med. Jul 2013;6(1):140-146.
5. Caplan AI. New era of cell-based orthopedic therapies. Tissue Engineering Part B: Reviews. 2009;15(2):195–200.

6. Hernigou P, Flouzat Lachaniette CH, Delambre J, et al. Biologic augmentation of rotator cuff repair with mesenchymal stem cells during arthroscopy improves healing and prevents further tears: A case-controlled study. Int Orthop. 2014;38(9):1811–1818.doi: 10.1007/s00264-014-2391-1.
7. Emadedin M, Ghorbani Liastani M, Fazeli R, et al. Long-term follow-up of intra-articular injection of autologous mesenchymal stem cells in patients with knee, ankle, or hip osteoarthritis. Arch Iran Med. Jun 2015;18(6):336-344.doi: 012157/AIM.0010.
8. Bonab MM, Sahraian MA, Aghsaie A, et al. Autologous mesenchymal stem cell therapy in progressive multiple sclerosis: an open label study. Curr Stem Cell Res Ther.2012;7(6):407-414.
9. Connick P, Kolappan M, Patani R, et al. The mesenchymal stem cells in multiple sclerosis (MSCIMS) trial protocol and baseline cohort characteristics: An open-label pre-test: Post-test study with blinded outcome assessments. Trials. 2011;12(1).
10. Connick P, Kolappan M, Crawley C, et al. Autologous mesenchymal stem cells for the treatment of secondary progressive multiple sclerosis: an open-label phase 2a proof-of-concept study. Lancet Neurol.2012;11(2):150-156.
11. Yamout B, Hourani R, Salti H, et al. Bone marrow mesenchymal stem cell transplantation in patients with multiple sclerosis: a pilot study. J Neuroimmunol. 2010;227(1-2):185-189.oi: 10.1016/j.jneuroim.2010.07.013.
12. Sharma A, Sane H, Badhe P, et al. A clinical study shows safety and efficacy of Autologous bone marrow mononuclear cell therapy to improve quality of life in muscular dystrophy patients. Cell Transplant. 2013;22(1):127–138.doi: 10.3727/096368913X672136.
13. Saito F, Nakatani T, Iwase M, et al. Spinal cord injury treatment with intrathecal autologous bone marrow stromal cell transplantation: the first clinical trial case report. J Trauma. 2008;64(1):53–59. doi: 10.1097/TA.0b013e31815b847d.
14. Karamouzian S, Nematollahi-Mahani SN, Nakhaee N, Eskandary H. Clinical safety and primary efficacy of bone marrow mesenchymal cell transplantation in subacute spinal cord injured patients. Clin Neurol Neurosurg. 2012;114(7):935–939.doi: 10.1016/j.clineuro.2012.02.003.
15. Mendonça MV, Larocca TF, de Freitas Souza BS, et al. Safety and neurological assessments after autologous transplantation of bone marrow mesenchymal stem cells in subjects with chronic spinal cord injury. Stem Cell Res Ther. 2014;5(6):126.doi: 10.1186/scrt516.
16. Jiang PC, Xiong WP, Wang G, et al. A clinical trial report of autologous bone marrow-derived mesenchymal stem cell transplantation in patients with spinal cord injury. Exp Ther Med. 2013;6(1):140-146.
17. Syková E, Homola A, Mazanec R, et al. Autologous bone marrow transplantation in patients with Subacute and chronic spinal cord injury. Cell Transplant. 2006;15(8):675–687.
18. Geffner LF, Santacruz P, Izurieta M, et al. Administration of Autologous bone marrow stem cells into spinal cord injury patients via multiple routes is safe and improves their quality of life: Comprehensive case studies. Cell Transplant. 2008;17(12):1277–1293.
19. Yoon SH, Shim YS, Park YH, et al. Complete cord injury treatment using autologous bone marrow cell transplantation and bone marrow stimulation with granulocyte macrophage-colony stimulating factor: phase I/II clinical trial spinal. Stem Cells. 2007;25(8):2066–2073.
20. Orozco L, Munar A, Soler R, et al. Treatment ofknee osteoarthritis with autologous mesenchymal stem cells: a pilot study. Transplantation.2013;95(12):1535-1541.doi: 10.1097/TP.0b013e318291a2da.
21. Emadedin M, Ghorbani Liastani M, Fazeli R, et al. Long-term follow-up of intra-articular injection of autologous mesenchymal stem cells in patients with knee, ankle, or hip osteoarthritis. Arch Iran Med. 2015;18(6):336-344.doi: 012157/AIM.0010.

22. Davatchi F, Abdollahi BS, Mohyeddin M, Shahram F, Nikbin B. Mesenchymal stem cell therapy for knee osteoarthritis. Preliminary report of four patients. Int J Rheum Dis. 2011;14(2):211–215. doi: 10.1111/j.1756-185X.2011.01599.x.

23. Centeno CJ, Busse D, Kisiday J, et al. Increased knee cartilage volume in degenerative joint disease using percutaneously implanted, autologous mesenchymal stem cells. Pain Physician. 2008;11(3):343–53

24. Fisher SA, Brunskill SJ, Doree C, et al. Stem cell therapy for chronic ischaemic heart disease and congestive heart failure. Cochrane Database Syst Rev. 2014.;(4):CD007888. doi: 10.1002/14651858. CD007888.pub2.

25. Ichim TE, Solano F, Lara F, et al. Combination stem cell therapy for heart failure. Int Arch Med. 2010;3(1):5.doi: 10.1186/1755-7682-3-5.

26. Perin EC, Dohmann HF, Borojevic, R et al. Transendocardial, autologous bone marrow cell transplantation for severe, chronic ischemic heart failure. Circulation. 2003;107(18):2294–2302.

27. Mathiasen AB, Qayyum AA, Jørgensen E, et al. Bone marrow-derived mesenchymal stromal cell treatment in patients with severe ischaemic heart failure: A randomized placebo-controlled trial (MSC-HF trial). Eur Heart J. 2015;36(27):1744–1753.doi: 10.1093/eurheartj/ehv136.

28. Patel AN, Geffner L, Vina RF, et al. Surgical treatment for congestive heart failure with autologous adult stem cell transplantation: A prospective randomized study. J Thorac Cardiovasc Surg. 2005;130(6):1631–1638.e2.

29. Pätilä T, Lehtinen M, Vento A, et al. Autologous bone marrow mononuclear cell transplantation in ischemic heart failure: A prospective, controlled, randomized, double-blind study of cell transplantation combined with coronary bypass. J Heart Lung Transplant. 2014;33(6):567–574.doi: 10.1016/j.healun.2014.02.009.

30. Falanga V, Iwamoto S, Chartier M, et al. Autologous bone Marrow–Derived cultured Mesenchymal stem cells delivered in a fibrin spray accelerate healing in murine and human cutaneous wounds. Tissue Eng. 2007;13(6):1299–1312.

31. Yoshikawa T, Mitsuno H, Nonaka I, et al. Wound therapy by marrow mesenchymal cell transplantation. Plast Reconstr Surg. 2008;121(3):860–877.doi: 10.1097/01.prs.0000299922.96006.24.

32. Jain P, Perakath B, Jesudason MR, Nayak S. The effect of autologous bone marrow-derived cells on healing chronic lower extremity wounds: Results of a randomized controlled study. Ostomy Wound Manage. 2011; 57: 38–44.

33. Sharma A, Gokulchandran N, Chopra G, et al. Administration of autologous bone marrow-derived mononuclear cells in children with incurable neurological disorders and injury is safe and improves their quality of life. Cell Transplant. 2012;21 Suppl1:S79-90. doi: 10.3727/096368912X633798.

34. Sharma A, Gokulchandran N, Sane H, et al. Autologous bone marrow mononuclear cell therapy for autism: an open label proof of concept study. Stem Cells Int. 2013;2013:623875. doi: 10.1155/2013/623875.

35. Gobbi A, Karnatzikos G, Scotti C, et al. One-step cartilage repair with bone marrow aspirate concentrated cells and collagen matrix in full-thickness knee cartilage lesions: results at 2-year follow-up. Cartilage. 2011;2(3):286-299.doi: 10.1177/1947603510392023.

36. Centeno C, Busse D, Kisiday J, Keohan C, Freeman M, Karli D. Increased knee cartilage volume in degenerative joint disease using percutaneously implanted, autologous mesenchymal stem cells. Pain Physician. 2008;11(3):343–53.

37. Stein BE, Stroh DA, Schon LC. Outcomes of acute Achilles tendon rupture repair with bone marrow aspirate concentrate augmentation. Int Orthop. 2015;39(5):901-905.doi: 10.1007/s00264-015-2725-7.

38. McKenna RW, Riordan NH. Minimally invasive autologous bone marrow concentrate stem cells in the treatment of the chronically injured Achilles tendon: a case report. CellR4. 2014;2(4): e1100.

39. Ellera Gomes JL, da Silva RC, Silla LM, Abreu MR, Pellanda R. Conventional rotator cuff repair complemented by the aid of mononuclear autologous stem cells. Knee Surg Sports Traumatol Arthrosc. 2011;20(2):373–377.

40. Hernigou P, Flouzat Lachaniette CH, Delambre J, et al. Biologic augmentation of rotator cuff repair with mesenchymal stem cells during arthroscopy improves healing and prevents further tears: A case-controlled study. Int Orthop. 2014;38(9):1811–1818.doi: 10.1007/s00264-014-2391-1.

41. Campbell KJ, Boykin RE, Wijdicks CA, et al. Treatment of a hip capsular injury in a professional soccer player with platelet-rich plasma and bone marrow aspirate concentrate therapy. Knee Surg Sports Traumatol Arthrosc. 2013;21(7):1684-1688.doi: 10.1007/s00167-012-2232-y.

42. Umemura T, Nishioka K, Igarashi A, et al. Autologous bone marrow mononuclear cell implantation induces angiogenesis and bone regeneration in a patient with compartment syndrome. Circ J. 2006; 70: 1362-1364.

43. Hernigou P, Poignard A, Beaujean F, Rouard H. Percutaneous autologous bone-marrow grafting for nonunions. Influence of the number and concentration of progenitor cells. J Bone Joint Surg Am. 2005;87(7):1430.

44. Giannotti S, Trombi L, Bottai V, et al. Use of Autologous human mesenchymal Stromal cell/fibrin clot constructs in upper limb non-unions: long-term assessment. PLoS ONE. 2013;8(8):e73893. doi: 10.1371/journal.pone.0073893.

45. Ripa RS, Haack-Sørensen M, Wang Y, et al. Bone marrow derived mesenchymal cell mobilization by granulocyte-colony stimulating factor after acute myocardial infarction: results from the stem cells in myocardial infarction (STEMMI) trial. Circulation. 2007;116(11_suppl):I–24–I–30.

46. Lamirault G, de Bock E, Roncalli J, et al. Sustained quality of life improvement after intracoronary injection of autologous bone marrow cells in the setting of acute myocardial infarction: Results from the BONAMI trial. Qual Life Res. July 2016.

47. Chen SL, Fang WW, Ye F, et al. Effect on left ventricular function of intracoronary transplantation of autologous bone marrow mesenchymal stem cell in patients with acute myocardial infarction. Am J Cardiol 2004; 94:92–95.

48. Choudry F, Hamshere S, Saunders N, et al. A randomized double-blind control study of early intra-coronary autologous bone marrow cell infusion in acute myocardial infarction: The REGENERATE-AMI clinical trial. Eur Heart J. 2015;37(3):256–263.doi: 10.1093/eurheartj/ehv493.

49. Peng L, Xie DY, Lin BL, et al. Autologous bone marrow mesenchymal stem cell transplantation in liver failure patients caused by hepatitis B: Short-term and long-term outcomes. Hepatology. 2011;54(3):820–828.doi: 10.1002/hep.24434.

50. Mohamadnejad M, Alimoghaddam K, Bagheri M, et al. Randomized placebo-controlled trial of mesenchymal stem cell transplantation in decompensated cirrhosis. Liver Int. 2013 Nov;33(10):1490-6. doi: 10.1111/liv.12228.

51. Amer ME, El-Sayed SZ, El-Kheir WA, et al. Clinical and laboratory evaluation of patients with end-stage liver cell failure injected with bone marrow-derived hepatocyte-like cells. Eur J Gastroenterol Hepatol. 2011;23(10):936–941.doi: 10.1097/MEG.0b013e3283488b00.

52. Venkataramana NK, Kumar SK, Balaraju S, et al. Open-labeled study of unilateral autologous bone-marrow-derived mesenchymal stem cell transplantation in Parkinson's disease. Transl Res. 2010;155(2):62–70.doi: 10.1016/j.trsl.2009.07.006.

53. Geffner L, Montenegro X, Bassanini M, et al. Transplant of autologous bone marrow stem cells into Parkinson's disease patients is safe and may improve their quality of life. XVIII World Federation of Neurology Congress on Parkinson's Disease and Related Disorders. Parkinson's Disease and Related Disorders. 2009;15(S2):124.

54. Bhansali A, Asokumar P, Walia R, et al. Efficacy and safety of autologous bone marrow-derived stem cell transplantation in patients with type 2 diabetes mellitus: a randomized placebo-controlled study. Cell Transplant. 2014;23(9):1075–1085.

55. Wu Z, Cai J, Chen J, et al. Autologous bone marrow mononuclear cell infusion and hyperbaric oxygen therapy in type 2 diabetes mellitus: An open-label, randomized controlled clinical trial. Cytotherapy. 2014;16(2):258–265.doi: 10.1016/j.jcyt.2013.10.004.

56. Mesples A, Majeed N, Zhang Y, Hu X. Early immunotherapy using autologous adult stem cells reversed the effect of anti-pancreatic islets in recently diagnosed type 1 diabetes mellitus: preliminary results. Med Sci Monit. 2013;19:852–857.doi: 10.12659/MSM.889525.

57. Park SS, Bauer G, Abedi M, et al. Intravitreal autologous bone marrow cd34+ cell therapy for ischemic and degenerative retinal disorders: preliminary phase 1 clinical trial findings. Invest Ophthalmol Vis Sci. 2014;56(1):81–89.doi: 10.1167/iovs.14-15415.

58. Weiss JN, Levy S, Benes SC. Stem cell ophthalmology treatment study (SCOTS) for retinal and optic nerve diseases: a case report of improvement in relapsing auto-immune optic neuropathy. Neural Regen Res. 2015;10(9):1507.doi: 10.4103/1673-5374.165525.

59. Mazzini L, Ferrero I, Luparello V, et al. Mesenchymal stem cell transplantation in amyotrophic lateral sclerosis: a phase I clinical trial. Exp Neurol. 2010;223(1):229–237.doi: 10.1016/j.expneurol.2009.08.007.

60. Duijvestein M, Vos AC, Roelofs H, et al. Autologous bone marrow-derived mesenchymal stromal cell treatment for refractory luminal Crohn's disease: results of a phase I study. Gut. 2010;59(12):1662–1669.doi: 10.1136/gut.2010.215152.

61. Ciccocioppo R, Bernardo ME, Sgarella A, et al. Autologous bone marrow-derived mesenchymal stromal cells in the treatment of fistulising Crohn's disease. Gut. 2011;60(6):788–798.doi: 10.1136/gut.2010.214841.

62. Benedict XVI. Address to the participants in the Symposium on the topic: "Stem Cells: what is the future for therapy?" organized by the Pontifical Academy for Life. September 16, 2006.<http://w2.vatican.va/content/benedict-xvi/en/speeches/2006/september/documents/hf_ben-xvi_spe_20060916_pav.html >Accessed August 2016.

63. Congregation for the Doctrine of the Faith. Instruction Dignitas Personae on Certain Bioethical Questions. September 8, 2008; 32.< http://www.vatican.va/roman_curia/congregations/cfaith/documents/rc_con_cfaith_doc_20081208_dignitas-personae_en.html> Accessed August 2016.

64. Benedict XVI. Address of His Holiness Benedict XVI to participants in the International Conference promoted by the Pontifical Council for Culture. November 12, 2011. < https://w2.vatican.va/content/benedict-xvi/en/speeches/2011/november/documents/hf_ben-xvi_spe_20111112_stem-cells.html > Accessed August 2016.

65. Los Angeles Times. Vatican signs deal to collaborate on adult stem cell research. October 20, 2011. <http://articles.latimes.com/2011/oct/20/business/la-fi-vatican-stem-cells-20111020> Accessed August 2016.

66. Ichim T, Riordan NH, Stroncek DF. The king is dead, long live the king: entering a new era of stem cell research and clinical development. J Transl Med. 2011;9:218. doi: 10.1186/1479-5876-9-218.

67. Henning RJ, Abu-Ali H, Balis JU, Morgan MB, Willing AE, Sanberg PR. Human umbilical cord blood mononuclear cells for the treatment of acute myocardial infarction. Cell Transplant. 2004;13(7-8):729-39.

68. Stone LL, Xiao F, Rotshafer J, et al. Amelioration of ischemic brain injury in rats with human umbilical cord blood stem cells: Mechanisms of action. Cell Transplant. 2016 Mar 18.[Epub ahead of print]

69. Riordan NH, Ichim TE. Immune privilege of cord blood. In: Bhattacharya N, Stubblefield P, eds. Regenerative Medicine Using Pregnancy-Specific Biological Substances. New York, NY: Springer;2010:307-319.

Chapter Five

1 Stelnicki EJ, Chin GS, Gittes GK, Longaker MT. Fetal wound repair: where do we go from here? Semin Pediatr Surg. 1999;8(3):124-30.

2 Caplan AI. Mesenchymal stem cells. J Orthop Res. 1991 Sep;9(5):641-50.

3 Hristov M, Erl W, Weber PC. Endothelial progenitor cells: mobilization, differentiation, and homing. Arterioscler Thromb Vasc Biol. 2003;23(7):1185-9.

4 Urbich C, Dimmeler S. Endothelial progenitor cells: characterization and role in vascular biology. Circ Res. 2004;95:343-353.

5 Watt SM, Gullo F, van der Garde M, et al. The angiogenic properties of mesenchymal stem/stromal cells and their therapeutic potential. Br Med Bull. 2013;108:25-53. doi: 10.1093/bmb/ldt031.

6 Caplan AI. Why are MSCs therapeutic? New data: new insight. J Pathol. 2009;217(2):318-24. doi: 10.1002/path.2469.

7 Alt EU, Senst C, Murthy SN, et al. Aging alters tissue resident mesenchymal stem cell properties. Stem Cell Res. 2012 Mar;8(2):215-25. doi: 10.1016/j.scr.2011.11.002.

8 Chang HX, Yang L, Li Z, Chen G, Dai G. Age-related biological characterization of mesenchymal progenitor cells in human articular cartilage. Orthopedics. 2011;34(8):e382-8. doi: 10.3928/01477447-20110627-06.

9 Stolzing A, Jones E, McGonagle D, Scutt A. Age-related changes in human bone marrow-derived mesenchymal stem cells: consequences for cell therapies. Mech Ageing Dev. 2008;129(3):163-73. doi: 10.1016/j.mad.2007.12.002.

10 Riordan NH, Ichim TE, Min WP, et al. Non-expanded adipose stromal vascular fraction cell therapy for multiple sclerosis. J Transl Med. 2009;7:29. doi: 10.1186/1479-5876-7-29.

11 Rodriguez JP, Murphy MP, Hong S, et al. Autologous stromal vascular fraction therapy for rheumatoid arthritis: rationale and clinical safety. Int Arch Med. 2012;5:5. doi: 10.1186/1755-7682-5-5.

12 Ichim TE, Harman RJ, Min WP, et al. Autologous stromal vascular fraction cells: a tool for facilitating tolerance in rheumatic disease. Cell Immunol. 2010;264(1):7-17. doi: 10.1016/j.cellimm.2010.04.002.

13 Makary MA and Daniel M. Medical error—the third leading cause of death in the US. BMJ. 2016;353:i2139. doi: 10.1136/bmj.i2139.

14 O'Donoghue K, Chan J, de la Fuente J, et al. Microchimerism in female bone marrow and bone decades after fetal mesenchymal stem-cell trafficking in pregnancy. Lancet. 2004;364(9429):179-82.

15 Johnson, KL, Samura O, Nelson JL, McDonnel M d WM, Bianchi DW. Significant fetal cell microchimerism in a nontransfused woman with hepatitis C: Evidence of long-term survival and expansion. Hepatology. 2002 Nov;36(5):1295-7.

16 Khosrotehrani K and Bianchi DW. Multi-lineage potential of fetal cells in maternal tissue: a legacy in reverse. J Cell Sci. 2005 15;118(Pt 8):1559-63.

17 Turco AE, Bambara LM. Pregnancy, microchimerism and autoimmunity: an update. Lupus. 2004;13(9):659-60.

18 Guthrie KA, Dugowson CE, Voigt LF, Koepsell TD, Nelson JL. Does pregnancy provide vaccine-like protection against rheumatoid arthritis? Arthritis Rheum. 2010;62(7):1842-8. doi: 10.1002/art.27459.

19 McArdle PF, Pollin TI, O'Connell JR, et al. Does having children extend life span? A genealogical study of parity and longevity in the Amish. J Gerontol A Biol Sci Med Sci. 2006;61(2):190-5.

20. Han X, Meng X, Yin Z, et al. Inhibition of intracranial glioma growth by endometrial regenerative cells. Cell Cycle. 2009;8(4):606-10.

21. Ganta C, Chiyo D, Ayuzawa R, et al. Rat umbilical cord stem cells completely abolish rat mammary carcinomas with no evidence of metastasis or recurrence 100 days post-tumor cell inoculation. Cancer Res. 2009;69(5):1815-20. doi: 10.1158/0008-5472.CAN-08-2750.

22. Lalu MM, McIntyre L, Pugliese C, et al. Safety of cell therapy with mesenchymal stromal cells (SafeCell): a systematic review and meta-analysis of clinical trials. PLoS One. 2012;7(10):e47559. doi: 10.1371/journal.pone.0047559.

Chapter Six

1. Grayson J. Microcirculation: Blood-vessel interactions systems in special tissues 1. Oxygen Supply to the Spinal Cord and Its Autoregulation. Erdmann W et al. Springer Science & Business Media; 2012;13.5

2. Purves MJ. The physiology of the cerebral circulation. CUP Archive; May 25, 1972.

3. Fausto N, Campbell JS, Riehle KJ. Liver regeneration. Hepatology. 2006 Feb;43(2 Suppl 1): S45-53.

4. Michalopoulos GK. Liver regeneration: alternative epithelial pathways. Int J Biochem Cell Biol. 2011 Feb;43(2):173-9. doi: 10.1016/j.biocel.2009.09.014.

5. Thron AK. Vascular anatomy of the spinal cord: Radioanatomy as the key to diagnosis and treatment. Springer;2016.

6. Hagg T, Oudega M. Degenerative and spontaneous regenerative processes after spinal cord injury. Journal of neurotrauma. 2006;23(3-4):264-280.

7. Simpson LA, Eng JJ, Hsieh JT, et al. Spinal Cord Injury Rehabilitation Evidence Scire Research T. The health and life priorities of individuals with spinal cord injury: a systematic review. JNeurotrauma. 2012;29(8):1548-1555.

8. Kang KS, Kim SW, Oh YH, et al. A 37-year-old spinal cord-injured female patient, transplanted of multipotent stem cells from human UC blood, with improved sensory perception and mobility, both functionally and morphologically: a case study. Cytotherapy. 2005;7(4):368–373

9. Li HJ, Liu HY, Zhao ZM, et al. [Transplantation of human umbilical cord stem cells improves neurological function recovery after spinal cord injury in rats]. Zhongguo Yixue Kexueyuan Xuebao. Acta Academiae Medicinae Sinicae. 2004;26(1):38–42.

10. Zhao ZM, Li HJ, Liu HY, et al. Intraspinal transplantation of CD34+ human umbilical cord blood cells after spinal cord hemisection injury improves functional recovery in adult rats. Cell Transplant. 2004;13(2):113-22.

11. Nishio Y, Koda M, Kamada T, et al. The use of hemopoietic stem cells derived from human umbilical cord blood to promote restoration of spinal cord tissue and recovery of hindlimb function in adult rats. Journal of neurosurgery. J Neurosurg Spine. 2006 Nov;5(5):424-33.

12. Cízková D, Rosocha J, Vanický I, Jergová S, Cízek M. Transplants of human mesenchymal stem cells improve functional recovery after spinal cord injury in the rat. Cell Mol Neurobiol. 2006 Oct-Nov;26(7-8):1167-80.

13. Saito F, Nakatani T, Iwase M, et al. Spinal cord injury treatment with intrathecal autologous bone marrow stromal cell transplantation: the first clinical trial case report. J Trauma. 2008 Jan;64(1):53-9. doi: 10.1097/TA.0b013e31815b847d.

14. Geffner LF, Santacruz P, Izurieta M, et al. Administration of autologous bone marrow stem cells into spinal cord injury patients via multiple routes is safe and improves their quality of life: comprehensive case studies. Cell Transplant. 2008;17(12):1277-93.

15. Yang CC, Shih YH, Ko MH, Hsu SY, Cheng H, Fu YS. Transplantation of human Umbilical Mesenchymal stem cells from Wharton's jelly after complete transection of the rat spinal cord. PLoS One. 2008;3(10):e3336. doi: 10.1371/journal.pone.0003336.

16. Kim JW, Ha KY, Molon JN, Kim YH. Bone marrow-derived mesenchymal stem cell transplantation for chronic spinal cord injury in rats: comparative study between intralesional and intravenous transplantation. Spine. 2013;38(17):E1065-1074.doi: 10.1097/BRS.0b013e31829839fa.

17. Boido M, Garbossa D, Fontanella M, Ducati A, Vercelli A. Mesenchymal stem cell transplantation reduces glial cyst and improves functional outcome after spinal cord compression. World neurosurg. 2014;81(1):183-190.doi: 10.1016/j.wneu.2012.08.014.

18. Park SI, Lim JY, Jeong CH, et al. Human umbilical cord blood-derived mesenchymal stem cell therapy promotes functional recovery of contused rat spinal cord through enhancement of endogenous cell proliferation and oligogenesis. J Biomed Biotechnol. 2012;2012:362473.doi: 10.1155/2012/362473.

19. Li J, Lepski G. Cell transplantation for spinal cord injury: a systematic review. Biomed Res Int.2013;2013:786475. doi: 10.1155/2013/786475.

20. Clínica Las Condes. LIT INNOVA CORFO. Autologous mesenchymal stem cells in spinal cord injury (SCI) patients (MSC-SCI). In: ClinicalTrials.gov [Internet]. Bethesda (MD): National Library of Medicine (US). 2000- [cited 2016 July]. Available from: https://clinicaltrials.gov/ct2/show/NCT01694927 NLM Identifier: NCT01694927.

21. Pharmicell Co, Ltd. Safety and efficacy of autologous mesenchymal stem cells in chronic spinal cord injury. In: ClinicalTrials.gov [Internet]. Bethesda (MD): National Library of Medicine (US). 2000- [cited 2016 July]. Available from: https://clinicaltrials.gov/ct2/show/NCT01676441 NLM Identifier: NCT01676441.

22. Limin Rong, Sun Yat-Sen University. Umbilical cord mesenchymal stem cells transplantation to patients with spinal cord injury. In: ClinicalTrials.gov [Internet]. Bethesda (MD): National Library of Medicine (US). 2000- [cited 2016 July]. Available from: https://clinicaltrials.gov/ct2/show/NCT0248144 NLM Identifier: NCT02481440.

23. Hospital Sao Rafael; Ricardo Ribeiro dos Santos. Evaluation of autologous mesenchymal stem cell transplantation in chronic spinal cord injury: a pilot study. In: ClinicalTrials.gov [Internet]. Bethesda (MD): National Library of Medicine (US). 2000- [cited 2016 July]. Available from:https://clinicaltrials.gov/ct2/show/NCT02152657 NLM Indentifier: NCT02152657.

24. Administration of Expanded Autologous Adult Bone Marrow Mesenchymal Cells in Established Chronic Spinal Cord Injuries. In: ClinicalTrials.gov [Internet]. Bethesda (MD): National Library of Medicine (US). 2000- [cited 2016 July]. Available from:https://clinicaltrials.gov/ct2/show/NCT02570932 NLM Identifier: NCT02570932.

25. Liu J, Han D, Wang Z, et al. Clinical analysis of the treatment of spinal cord injury with umbilical cord mesenchymal stem cells. Cytotherapy. 2013;15(2):185-191.

26. Mendonca MV, Larocca TF, de Freitas Souza BS, et al. Safety and neurological assessments after autologous transplantation of bone marrow mesenchymal stem cells in subjects with chronic spinal cord injury. Stem Cell Res Ther. 2014;5(6):126.doi: 10.1186/scrt516.

27. Jiang PC, Xiong WP, Wang G, et al. A clinical trial report of autologous bone marrow-derived mesenchymal stem cell transplantation in patients with spinal cord injury. Exp Ther Med. 2013;6(1):140-146.

28. Ichim TE, Solano F, Lara F, et al. Feasibility of combination allogeneic stem cell therapy for spinal cord injury: a case report. Int Arch Med. 2010;3:30.doi: 10.1186/1755-7682-3-30.

Additional References

Roussos I, Rodriguez M, Villan D, Ariza A, Rodriguez L, Garcia J. Development of a rat model of spinal cord injury and cellular transplantation. Transplant Proc. 2005;37(9):4127-30.

Mansilla E, Marin GH, Sturla F, et al. Human mesenchymal stem cells are tolerized by mice and improve skin and spinal cord injuries. Transplant Proc. 2005;37(1):292-4.

Bakshi A, Barshinger AL, Swanger SA, et al. Lumbar puncture delivery of bone marrow stromal cells in spinal cord contusion: a novel method for minimally invasive cell transplantation. J Neurotrauma. 2006;23(1):55-65.

Vaquero J, Zurita M, Oya S, Santos M. Cell therapy using bone marrow stromal cells in chronic paraplegic rats: systemic or local administration? Neurosci Lett. 2006;398(1-2):129-34.

Yano S, Kuroda S, Lee JB, et al. In vivo fluorescence tracking of bone marrow stromal cells transplanted into a pneumatic injury model of rat spinal cord. J Neurotrauma. 2005;22(8):907-18.

Park HC, Shim YS, Ha Y, et al. Treatment of complete spinal cord injury patients by autologous bone marrow cell transplantation and administration of granulocyte-macrophage colony stimulating factor. Tissue Eng. 2005;11(5-6):913-22.

Newman MB, Davis CD, Kuzmin-Nichols N, Sanberg PR. Human umbilical cord blood (HUCB) cells for central nervous system repair. Neurotox Res. 2003;5(5):355-68.

Lee J, Kuroda S, Shichinohe H, Ikeda J, et al. Migration and differentiation of nuclear fluorescence-labeled bone marrow stromal cells after transplantation into cerebral infarct and spinal cord injury in mice. Neuropathology. 2003;23(3):169-80.

Akiyama Y, Radtke C, Honmou O, Kocsis JD. Remyelination of the spinal cord following intravenous delivery of bone marrow cells. Glia. 2002;39(3):229-36.

Chapter Seven

Notes from Interview

1. Johnson SP, Catania JM, Harman RJ, Jensen ED. Adipose derived stem cell collection and characterization in bottlenose dolphins (Tursiops truncatus). Stem Cells Dev. 2012 Nov 1;21(16):2949-57. doi: 10.1089/scd.2012.0039.
2. Harman RJ. Stem cell therapy in veterinary dermatology. Vet Dermatol. 2013 Feb;24(1):90-6.e23-4. doi: 10.1111/vde.12000.
3. Harman RJ, Carlson K, Gaynor J, et al. A prospective, randomized, masked, and placebo-controlled efficacy study of intraarticular allogeneic adipose stem cells for the treatment of osteoarthritis in dogs. Front Vet Sci. 2016;3:81. doi: 10.3389/fvets.2016.00081.
4. Ichim T, Harman R, Ming W, et al. Autologous stromal vascular fraction cells: A tool for facilitating tolerance in rheumatic disease. Cell Imm. 2010;264:7-17.
5. Ichim T, Solano F, Lara F, Paris E, Ugalde F, Rodriguez J, Minev B, Bogin V, Ramos F, Woods E, Murphy M, Patel A, Harman R, Riordan N. Feasibility of combination allogeneic stem cell therapy for spinal cord injury: a case report. Int Arch Med, 3:30, 2010.
6. Riordan N, Ichim T, Harman R et al. Non-expanded adipose stromal vascular fraction cell therapy for multiple sclerosis. Journal of Translational Medicine, 7:29, 24 April, 2009.

7. Rodriguez J, Murphy M, Madrigal M, March K, Minev B, Harman R, Chen C, Berrocal R, Marleau A, Riordan N. Autologous stromal vascular fraction therapy for rheumatoid arthritis: rationale and clinical safety. Int Arch Med, 5:5, 2012.

8. Wood J, Chung D, Park S, et al. Periocular and intra-articular injection of canine adipose-derived mesenchymal stem cells: An in vivo imaging and migration study. *Journal of ocular pharmacology and therapeutics : the official journal of the Association for Ocular Pharmacology and Therapeutics.* 2011;28(3):307–17.

9. Arzi B, Mills-Ko E, Verstraete FJM, et al. Therapeutic efficacy of fresh, Autologous Mesenchymal stem cells for severe refractory Gingivostomatitis in cats. 2015;5(1).

10. Pérez-Merino E, Usón-Casaús J, Duque-Carrasco J, et al. Safety and efficacy of allogeneic adipose tissue-derived mesenchymal stem cells for treatment of dogs with inflammatory bowel disease: Endoscopic and histological outcomes. Veterinary journal (London, England : 1997). 2015;206(3):391–7.

11. Harman R, Carlson K, Gaynor J, et al. A prospective, Randomized, masked, and placebo-controlled efficacy study of Intraarticular Allogeneic Adipose stem cells for the treatment of osteoarthritis in dogs. 2016;3

Interview Aditional References: VetStem Peer-Reviewed Publications

Astor D, Hoelzler M, Harman R, Bastian R. Patient factors influencing the concentration of stromal vascular fraction (SVF) for adipose-derived stromal cell (ASC) therapy in dogs. Can J Vet Res, 77:177-182.

Black L, Gaynor J, Harman R, et al. Effect of adipose-derived mesenchymal stem and regenerative cells on lameness in dogs with chronic osteoarthritis of the coxofemoral joints: a randomized, double-blinded, multicenter controlled trial. Vet Ther, 8:4:272-284, Winter 2007.

Black L, Gaynor J, Harman R, et al. Effect of intraarticular injections of autologous adipose-derived mesenchymal stem and regenerative cells on clinical signs of chronic osteoarthritis of the elbow joint in dogs. Vet Ther, 9:3, Fall 2008.

Brown G, Harman R, Black L. Adipose-derived stem cell therapy for severe muscle tears in working german shepherds: Two case reports. Stem Cells Disc, 2(2):41-44, 2012.

Harman R, Carlson K, Gaynor J, et al. A prospective, randomized, masked, and placebo-controlled efficacy study of intraarticular allogeneic adipose stem cells for the treatment of osteoarthritis in dogs. Front Vet Sci, 3:81.

Harman R. One medicine: a development model for cellular therapy of diabetes. Clin Trans Med. 5(suppl 1):26.

Johnson S, Catania J, Harman R, Jensen E. Adipose-derived stem cell collection and characterization in bottlenose dophins (Tursiops truncates), Stem Cells Dev, 2012; Apr 24 Epub.

Meirelles L, Sand T, Harman R et al. MSC frequency correlates with blood vessel density in equine adipose tissue. Tis Eng, 15(2), 221-29, 2009.

Norbert K, Harman R. (2013) FDA's possible regulation of veterinary stem cell therapy, in FDA's Regulation of Veterinary Drug Products (Eds C Hughes-Coons and K Norbert), Food and Drug Law Institute, Washington, D.C., 82-85.

Harman R. (2015) The market for stem cell medicine for domestic and high value animals, in Stem Cells in Regenerative Medicine – Science, Regulation, and Business Strategies (Eds. A Vertes, N Qureshi, A Caplan, L Babiss), Wiley, Chichester, UK.

Harman R. (2015) Stem cell veterinary medicines, in Stem Cells in Regenerative Medicine – Science, Regulation, and Business Strategies (Eds. A Vertes, N Qureshi, A Caplan, L Babiss), Wiley, Chichester, UK.

Nixon A, Dahlgren L, Haupt J, et al. Effect of adipose-derived nucleated cell fractions on tendon repair in a collagenase-induced tendinitis model. Am J Vet Res, 69:526-37, 2008.

Rich FR. (2014) Single-center study of 83 horses with suspensory injuries treated with adipose-derived stem and regenerative cells. Stem Cell Disc 4:44-55.

Chapter Notes

1. Pluchino S, Quattrini A, Brambilla E, et al. Injection of adult neurospheres induces recovery in a chronic model of multiple sclerosis. Nature. 2003;422(6933):688-94.
2. van den Berg B, Walgaard C, Drenthen J, et al. Guillain-Barré syndrome: Pathogenesis, diagnosis, treatment and prognosis. Nat Rev Neurol. 2014 Aug;10(8):469-82. doi: 10.1038/nrneurol.2014.121.
3. Poloni G, Minagar A, Haacke EM, Zivadinov R, et al. Recent developments in imaging of multiple sclerosis. Neurologist. 2011 Jul;17(4):185-204. doi: 10.1097/NRL.0b013e31821a2643.
4. Burt RK, Traynor AE. Hematopoietic stem cell transplantation: A new therapy for autoimmune disease. Stem Cells. 1999;17(6):366-72.
5. Tanasescu R, Ionete C, Chou IJ, Constantinescu CS. Advances in the treatment of relapsing-remitting multiple sclerosis. Biomed J.2014;37(2):41-49.doi: 10.4103/2319-4170.130440.
6. Rodgers JM, Robinson AP, Miller SD. Strategies for protecting oligodendrocytes and enhancing remyelination in multiple sclerosis. Discov Med. 2013;16(86):53-63.
7. Caplan AI. Adult mesenchymal stem cells for tissue engineering versus regenerative medicine. J Cell Physiol. 2007;213(2):341-347.
8. Chamberlain G, Fox J, Ashton B, Middleton J. Concise review: mesenchymal stem cells: their phenotype, differentiation capacity, immunological features, and potential for homing. Stem Cells. 2007;25(11):2739-2749.
9. Xiao J, Yang R, Biswas S, Qin X, Zhang M, Deng W. Mesenchymal stem cells and induced pluripotent stem cells as therapies for multiple sclerosis. Int J Mol Sci. 2015;16(5):9283-9302.doi: 10.3390/ijms16059283.
10. Al Jumah MA, Abumaree MH. The immunomodulatory and neuroprotective effects of mesenchymal stem cells (MSCs) in experimental autoimmune encephalomyelitis (EAE): a model of multiple sclerosis (MS). Int J Mol Sci. 2012;13(7):9298-9331.doi: 10.3390/ijms13079298.
11. Payne NL, Sun G, McDonald C, et al. Distinct immunomodulatory and migratory mechanisms underpin the therapeutic potential of human mesenchymal stem cells in autoimmune demyelination. Cell Transplant. 2013;22(8):1409-1425.doi: 10.3727/096368912X657620.
12. Burt RK, Cohen BA, Russell E, et al. Hematopoietic stem cell transplantation for progressive multiple sclerosis: Failure of a total body irradiation–based conditioning regimen to prevent disease progression in patients with high disability scores. Blood. 2003 Oct 1;102(7):2373-8.
13. Connick P, Kolappan M, Patani R, et al. The mesenchymal stem cells in multiple sclerosis (MSCIMS) trial protocol and baseline cohort characteristics: An open-label pre-test: Post-test study with blinded outcome assessments. Trials. 2011 Mar 2;12:62. doi: 10.1186/1745-6215-12-62.
14. Ardeshiry Lajimi A, Hagh MF, Saki N, Mortaz E, Soleimani M, Rahim F. Feasibility of cell therapy in multiple sclerosis: a systematic review of 83 studies. Int J Hematol Oncol Stem Cell Res. 2013;7(1):15-33.

15. Bonab MM, Sahraian MA, Aghsaie A, et al. Autologous mesenchymal stem cell therapy in progressive multiple sclerosis: an open label study. Curr Stem Cell Res Ther. 2012;7(6):407-414.

16. Connick P, Kolappan M, Crawley C, et al. Autologous mesenchymal stem cells for the treatment of secondary progressive multiple sclerosis: an open-label phase 2a proof-of-concept study. Lancet Neurol. 2012;11(2):150-156.doi: 10.1016/S1474-4422(11)70305-2.

17. Yamout B, Hourani R, Salti H, et al. Bone marrow mesenchymal stem cell transplantation in patients with multiple sclerosis: a pilot study. J Neuroimmunol. 2010;227(1-2):185-189.doi: 10.1016/j.jneuroim.2010.07.013.

18. Northwestern University; Richard Burt, MD. Stem cell therapy for patients with multiple sclerosis failing alternate approved therapy- a randomized study. In: ClinicalTrials.gov [Internet]. Bethesda (MD): National Library of Medicine (US). 2000- [cited 2016 July]. Available from: https://clinicaltrials.gov/ct2/show/NCT00273364 NLM Identifier: NCT00273364.

19. Translational Biosciences. Feasibility study of human umbilical cord tissue-derived mesenchymal stem cells in patients with multiple sclerosis. In: ClinicalTrials.gov [Internet]. Bethesda (MD): National Library of Medicine (US). 2000- [cited 2016 July]. Available from: https://clinicaltrials.gov/ct2/show/NCT02034188 NLM Identifier: NCT02034188.

20. University of Louisville. Allogeneic stem cell transplantation for the treatment of multiple sclerosis. In: ClinicalTrials.gov [Internet]. Bethesda (MD): National Library of Medicine (US). 2000- [cited 2016 July]. Available from: https://clinicaltrials.gov/ct2/show/NCT00497952 NLM Identifier: NCT00497952.

21. Karolinska Institutet; Ellen Iacobaeus. Mesenchymal stem cells for multiple sclerosis. In: ClinicalTrials.gov [Internet]. Bethesda (MD): National Library of Medicine (US). 2000- [cited 2016 July]. Available from: https://clinicaltrials.gov/ct2/show/NCT01730547 NLM Identifier: NCT01730547.

22. University Hospital, Toulouse. MEsenchymal StEm Cells for Multiple Sclerosis (MESEMS). In: ClinicalTrials.gov [Internet]. Bethesda (MD): National Library of Medicine (US). 2000- [cited 2016 July]. Available from: https://clinicaltrials.gov/ct2/show/NCT02403947 NLM Identifier: NCT02403947.

23. The Cleveland Clinic. Autologous mesenchymal stem cell (msc) transplantation in MS. In: ClinicalTrials.gov [Internet]. Bethesda (MD): National Library of Medicine (US). 2000- [cited 2016 July]. Available from: https://clinicaltrials.gov/ct2/show/NCT00813969 NLM Identifier: NCT00813969.

24. Riordan NH, Ichim TE, Min WP, et al. Non-expanded adipose stromal vascular fraction cell therapy for multiple sclerosis. J Transl Med. 2009 Apr 24;7:29. doi: 10.1186/1479-5876-7-29.

25. Translational Biosciences. Feasibility study of human umbilical cord tissue-derived mesenchymal stem cells in patients with multiple sclerosis. In: ClinicalTrials.gov [Internet]. Bethesda (MD): National Library of Medicine (US). 2000- [cited 2016 July]. Available from: https://clinicaltrials.gov/ct2/show/NCT02034188 NLM Identifier: NCT02034188.

Chapter Eight

1. Yeh ET, Zhang S, Wu HD, Körbling M, Willerson JT, Estrov Z. Transdifferentiation of human peripheral blood CD34+-enriched cell population into cardiomyocytes, endothelial cells, and smooth muscle cells in vivo. Circulation. 2003;108(17):2070-3.

2. Zhang S, Wang D, Estrov Z, Raj S, Willerson JT, Yeh ET. Both cell fusion and transdifferentiation account for the transformation of human peripheral blood CD34-positive cells into cardiomyocytes in vivo. Circulation. 2004;110(25):3803-7.

3. Ma N, Stamm C, Kaminski A, et al. Human cord blood cells induce angiogenesis following myocardial infarction in NOD/scid-mice. Cardiovasc Res. 2005;66(1):45-54.
4. Takahashi T, Lord B, Schulze PC, et al. Ascorbic acid enhances differentiation of embryonic stem cells into cardiac myocytes. Circulation. 2003;107(14):1912-6.
5. Sánchez-Lázaro IJ, Almenar L, Reganon E, et al. Inflammatory markers in stable heart failure and their relationship with functional class. Int J Cardiol. 2008;129(3):388–393.
6. Alonso-Martínez JL, Llorente-Diez B, Echegaray-Agara M, Olaz-Preciado F, Urbieta-Echezarreta M, Gonzalez-Arencibia C. C-reactive protein as a predictor of improvement and readmission in heart failure. Eur J Heart Failure. 2002;4(3):331–336.
7. Satoh M, Minami Y, Takahashi Y, Nakamura M. Immune modulation: Role of the inflammatory cytokine cascade in the failing human heart. Curr Heart Fail Rep. 2008;5(2):69–74.
8. Le Blanc K, Ringdén O. Immunomodulation by mesenchymal stem cells and clinical experience. J Intern Med. 2007;262(5):509–525.
9. Keyser KA, Beagles KE, Kiem HP. Comparison of Mesenchymal stem cells from different tissues to suppress t-cell activation. Cell Transplant. 2007;16(5):555–562.
10. Ortiz LA, DuTreil M, Fattman C, et al. Interleukin 1 receptor antagonist mediates the antiinflammatory and antifibrotic effect of mesenchymal stem cells during lung injury. Proc Natl Acad Sci U S A. 2007;104(26):11002–11007.
11. Madrigal M, Rao KS, Riordan NH. A review of therapeutic effects of mesenchymal stem cell secretions and induction of secretory modification by different culture methods. J Transl Med. 2014;12(1):260. doi: 10.1186/s12967-014-0260-8.
12. Ryan JM, Barry F, Murphy JM, Mahon BP. Interferon-γ does not break, but promotes the immunosuppressive capacity of adult human mesenchymal stem cells. Clin Exp Immunol. 2007;149(2):353–363.
13. Nishiyama N, Miyoshi S, Hida N, et al. The significant Cardiomyogenic potential of human Umbilical cord blood-derived Mesenchymal stem cells in vitro. Stem Cells. 2007;25(8):2017–2024.
14. Itescu S, Kocher AA, Schuster MD. Adult bone marrow-derived angioblasts for improvement of cardiomyocyte function after myocardial ischemia. Gene Ther Reg. 2001;1(4):375–386. doi: 10.1163/156855801760107037.
15. Hare JM, Fishman JE, Gerstenblith G, et al. Comparison of allogeneic vs autologous bone marrow–derived mesenchymal stem cells delivered by transendocardial injection in patients with ischemic cardiomyopathy: the POSEIDON randomized trial. JAMA. 2012;308(22):2369.
16. Chin SP, Poey AC, Wong CY, et al. Intramyocardial and intracoronary autologous bone marrow-derived mesenchymal stromal cell treatment in chronic severe dilated cardiomyopathy. Cytotherapy. 2011;13(7):814–821.doi: 10.3109/14653249.2011.574118.
17. Du YY, Zhou SH, Zhou T, et al. Immuno-inflammatory regulation effect of mesenchymal stem cell transplantation in a rat model of myocardial infarction. Cytotherapy. 2008;10(5):469–478.doi: 10.1080/14653240802129893.
18. Narita T, Suzuki K. Bone marrow-derived mesenchymal stem cells for the treatment of heart failure. Heart Fail Rev. 2014;20(1):53–68.doi: 10.1007/s10741-014-9435-x.
19. Yannarelli G, Dayan V, Pacienza N, Lee CJ, Medin J, Keating A. human umbilical cord perivascular cells exhibit enhanced cardiomyocyte reprogramming and cardiac function after experimental acute myocardial infarction. Cell Transplant. 2013;22(9):1651–1666. doi: 10.3727/096368912X657675. Epub 2012 Oct 4.
20. López Y, Lutjemeier B, Seshareddy K, et al. Wharton's jelly or bone marrow Mesenchymal Stromal cells improve cardiac function following myocardial infarction for more than 32 weeks in a rat model: a preliminary report. Curr Stem Cell Res Ther. 2013;8(1):46–59.

21. Liao W, Xie J, Zhong J, et al. Therapeutic effect of human Umbilical cord Multipotent Mesenchymal Stromal cells in a rat model of stroke. Transplantation. 2009;87(3):350–359.doi: 10.1097/TP.0b013e318195742e.
22. Mathiasen AB, Qayyum AA, Jørgensen E, et al. Bone marrow-derived mesenchymal stromal cell treatment in patients with severe ischaemic heart failure: A randomized placebo-controlled trial (MSC-HF trial). Eur Heart J. 2015;36(27):1744–1753.doi: 10.1093/eurheartj/ehv136.
23. Perin EC, Borow KM, Silva GV, et al. A phase II dose-escalation study of allogeneic mesenchymal precursor cells in patients with ischemic or nonischemic heart failure. Circ Res. 2015;117(6):576–584.doi: 10.1161/CIRCRESAHA.115.306332.
24. Perin EC, Dohmann HF, Borojevic, et al. Transendocardial, autologous bone marrow cell transplantation for severe, chronic Ischemic heart failure. Circulation. 2003;107(18):2294–2302.
25. Fisher SA, Brunskill SJ, Doree C, Mathur A, Taggart DP, Martin-Rendon E. Stem cell therapy for chronic ischaemic heart disease and congestive heart failure. Cochrane Database Syst Rev. 2014;(4):CD007888. doi: 10.1002/14651858.CD007888.pub2.
26. Fisher SA, Doree C, Mathur A, Martin-Rendon E. Meta-Analysis of cell therapy trials for patients with heart failure. Circ Res. 2015;116(8):1361–1377.doi: 10.1161/CIRCRESAHA.116.304386.
27. Ichim TE, Solano F, Lara F, et al. Combination stem cell therapy for heart failure. Int Arch Med. 2010;3(1):5.doi: 10.1186/1755-7682-3-5.
28. Tuma J, Carrasco A, Castillo J, et al. RESCUE-HF trial: Retrograde delivery of Allogeneic Umbilical cord lining Sub-Epithelial cells in patients with heart failure. Cell Transplant. 2016; January. [Epub ahead of print]
29. Silvestre JS, Menasché P. The evolution of the stem cell theory for heart failure. EBioMedicine. 2015;2(12):1871–1879. doi: 10.1016/j.ebiom.2015.11.010.
30. Menasché P. Stem cells for the treatment of heart failure. Philos Trans R Soc Lond B Biol Sci. 2015;370(1680):20140373. doi: 10.1098/rstb.2014.0373.
31. Poglajen G, Vrtovec B. Stem cell therapy for chronic heart failure. Curr Opin Cardiol. 2015;30(3):301–310.doi: 10.1097/HCO.0000000000000167.
32. Winters AA, Bou-Ghannam S, Thorp H, et al. Evaluation of multiple biological therapies for ischemic cardiac disease. Cell Transplant. 2016;25(9):1591-1607.
33. Wang J, Zhang S, Rabinovich B, et al. Human CD34+ cells in experimental myocardial infarction: long-term survival, sustained functional improvement, and mechanism of action. Circ Res. 2010;106(12):1904-11.oi: 10.1161/CIRCRESAHA.110.221762.
34. Zhang S, Shpall E, Willerson JT, Yeh ET. Fusion of human hematopoietic progenitor cells and murine cardiomyocytes is mediated by alpha 4 beta 1 integrin/vascular cell adhesion molecule-1 interaction. Circ Res. 2007;100(5):693-702.
35. Shabbir A, Zisa D, Suzuki G, Lee T. Heart failure therapy mediated by the trophic activities of bone marrow mesenchymal stem cells: a noninvasive therapeutic regimen. Am J Physiol Heart Circ Physiol. 2009;296(6):H1888-97. doi: 10.1152/ajpheart.00186.2009.

Chapter Nine

1. Fried LP, Tangen CM, Watson J, et al. Cardiovascular Health Study Collaborative Research Group. Frailty in older adults: evidence for a phenotype. J Gerontol A Biol Sci Med Sci. 2001;56(3):M146-56.
2. Lally F, Crome P. Understanding frailty. Postgrad Med J. 2007;83(975):16-20. doi: 10.1136/pgmj.2006.048587.

3. Espinoza S, Walston JD. Frailty in older adults: insights and interventions. Cleve Clin J Med. 2005;72(12):1105-12.
4. Marcell TJ. Sarcopenia: causes, consequences, and preventions. J Gerontol A Biol Sci Med Sci. 2003;58(10):M911-M916.
5. Jensen GL. Inflammation: roles in aging and sarcopenia. JPEN J Parenter Enteral Nutr. 2008;32(6):656-9.
6. de Gonzalo-Calvo D, Neitzert K, Fernández M, et al. Differential inflammatory responses in aging and disease: TNF-alpha and IL-6 as possible biomarkers. Free Radic Biol Med. 2010;49(5):733-737. doi: 10.1016/j.freeradbiomed.2010.05.019.
7. Lepperdinger G. Inflammation and mesenchymal stem cell aging. Curr Op Immunol. 2011;23(4):518-524.doi: 10.1016/j.coi.2011.05.007.
8. Boyette LB, Tuan RS. Adult Stem Cells and Diseases of Aging. J Clin Med.2014;3(1):88-134.doi: 10.3390/jcm3010088.
9. Wong TY, Solis MA, Chen YH, Huang LL. Molecular mechanism of extrinsic factors affecting anti-aging of stem cells. World JStem Cells.2015;7(2):512-520.doi: 10.4252/wjsc.v7.i2.512.
10. Baxter MA, Wynn RF, Jowitt SN, Wraith JE, Fairbairn LJ, Bellantuono I. Study of telomere length reveals rapid aging of human marrow stromal cells following in vitro expansion. Stem Cells.2004;22(5):675-682.
11. Caplan AI. Adult mesenchymal stem cells for tissue engineering versus regenerative medicine. J Cell Physiol.2007;213(2):341-347.
12. Sethe S, Scutt A, Stolzing A. Aging of mesenchymal stem cells. Ageing Res Rev. 2006;5(1):91-116.
13. Sethe S, Scutt A, Stolzing A. Aging of mesenchymal stem cells. Ageing Res Rev. 2006;5(1):91-116.
14. Zhou S, Greenberger JS, Epperly MW, et al. Age-related intrinsic changes in human bone-marrow-derived mesenchymal stem cells and their differentiation to osteoblasts. Aging Cell.2008;7(3):335-343.
15. Stenderup K, Justesen J, Clausen C, Kassem M. Aging is associated with decreased maximal life span and accelerated senescence of bone marrow stromal cells. Bone.2003;33(6):919-926.
16. Sharpless NE, DePinho RA. How stem cells age and why this makes us grow old. Nat Rev Mol Cell Biol.2007;8(9):703-713.
17. Fan M, Chen W, Liu W, et al. The effect of age on the efficacy of human mesenchymal stem cell transplantation after a myocardial infarction. Rejuv Res.2010;13(4):429-438.doi: 10.1089/rej.2009.0986.
18. Golpanian S, DiFede DL, Pujol MV, et al. Rationale and design of the allogeneiC human mesenchymal stem cells (hMSC) in patients with aging fRAilTy via intravenoUS delivery (CRATUS) study: A phase I/II, randomized, blinded and placebo controlled trial to evaluate the safety and potential efficacy of allogeneic human mesenchymal stem cell infusion in patients with aging frailty. Oncotarget. 2016;7(11):11899-912. doi: 10.18632/oncotarget.7727.
19. Barja G, Herrero A. Oxidative damage to mitochondrial DNA is inversely related to maximum life span in the heart and brain of mammals. FASEB J. 2000;14(2):312-8.
20. Islam MN, Das SR, Emin MT, et al. Mitochondrial transfer from bone-marrow-derived stromal cells to pulmonary alveoli protects against acute lung injury. Nat Med. 2012;18(5):759-65. doi: 10.1038/nm.2736.
21. Sinha P, Islam MN, Bhattacharya S, Bhattacharya J. Intercellular mitochondrial transfer: bioenergetic crosstalk between cells. Curr Opin Genet Dev. 2016;38:97-101. doi: 10.1016/j.gde.2016.05.002.
22. Holstege H, Pfeiffer W, Sie D, et al. Somatic mutations found in the healthy blood compartment of a 115-yr-old woman demonstrate oligoclonal hematopoiesis. Genome Res. 2014 May;24(5):733-42. doi: 10.1101/gr.162131.113.

Chapter Ten

1. Erokhin VV, Vasil'eva IA, Konopliannikov AG, et al. [Systemic transplantation of autologous mesenchymal stem cells of the bone marrow in the treatment of patients with multidrug-resistant pulmonary tuberculosis]. Probl Tuberk Bolezn Legk. 2008;(10):3-6.
2. Elias JA, Zhu Z, Chupp G, Homer RJ. Airway remodeling in asthma. J Clin Invest. 1999;104(8):1001–1006.doi: 10.1172/JCI8124.
3. Maddox L, Schwartz DA. The pathophysiology of asthma. Annu Rev Med. 2002;53(1):477–498.
4. Iyer SS, Co C, Rojas M. Mesenchymal stem cells and inflammatory lung diseases. Panminerva Med. 2009;51(1):5–16.
5. Sueblinvong V, Weiss DJ. Stem cells and cell therapy approaches in lung biology and diseases. Transl Res. 2010;156(3):188–205. doi: 10.1016/j.trsl.2010.06.007.
6. Mora AL, Rojas M. Adult stem cells for chronic lung diseases. Respirology. 2013;18(7):1041–6. doi: 10.1111/resp.12112.
7. Stessuk T, Ruiz MA, Greco OT, Bilaqui A, Ribeiro-Paes MJ, Ribeiro-Paes JT. Phase I clinical trial of cell therapy in patients with advanced chronic obstructive pulmonary disease: Follow-up of up to 3 years. Rev Bras Hematol Hemoter. 2013;35(5):352-7. doi: 10.5581/1516-8484.20130113.
8. Jones CP, Rankin SM. Bone marrow-derived stem cells and respiratory disease. Chest. 2011;140(1):205-11. doi: 10.1378/chest.10-2348.
9. Cruz FF, Borg ZD, Goodwin M. Systemic administration of human bone marrow-derived mesenchymal stromal cell extracellular vesicles ameliorates Aspergillus hyphal extract-induced allergic airway inflammation in immunocompetent mice. Stem Cells Transl Med. 2015;4(11):1302-16. doi: 10.5966/sctm.2014-0280.
10. Braza F, Dirou S, Forest V, et al. Mesenchymal stem cells induce suppressive macrophages through phagocytosis in a mouse model of asthma. Stem Cells. 2016;34(7):1836-45. doi: 10.1002/stem.2344.
11. Bonfield T, Sutton M, Lennon D, Caplan A. Mesenchymal stem cells: New directions in treating asthma (THER2P.955). J Immunol. 2015;194(1 Supplement):6–67.
12. Ge X, Bai C, Yang J, Lou G, Li Q, Chen R. Effect of mesenchymal stem cells on inhibiting airway remodeling and airway inflammation in chronic asthma. J Cell Biochem. 2013;114(7):1595–1605. doi: 10.1002/jcb.24501.
13. Mohammadian M et al. Effect of bone marrow derived mesenchymal stem cells on lung pathology and inflammation in ovalbumin-induced asthma in mouse. Iranian journal of basic medical sciences. 2016;19(1):55–63.
14. Cho K-S et al. Adipose-Derived stem cells ameliorate allergic airway inflammation by inducing regulatory T cells in a mouse model of asthma. Mediators of Inflammation. 2014;2014:1–12.
15. Song X et al. Mesenchymal stem cells alleviate experimental asthma by inducing polarization of alveolar Macrophages. Inflammation. 2014;38(2):485–492.
16. Cho K-S et al. IFATS collection: Immunomodulatory effects of Adipose tissue-derived stem cells in an allergic Rhinitis mouse model. Stem Cells. 2009;27(1):259–265.
17. Mariñas-Pardo L et al. Mesenchymal stem cells regulate airway contractile tissue remodeling in murine experimental asthma. Allergy. 2014;69(6):730–740.
18. Trzil JE et al. Long-term evaluation of mesenchymal stem cell therapy in a feline model of chronic allergic asthma. Clinical & Experimental Allergy. 2014;44(12):1546–1557
19. Srour N et al. Stem cells in animal asthma models: A systematic review. Cytotherapy. 2014;16(12):1629–1642.

20. Blanchet M-R, McNagny KM. Stem cells, inflammation and allergy. Allergy, Asthma & Clinical Immunology. 2009;5(1):13.

21. Li J et al. Human mesenchymal stem cells elevate CD4+CD25+CD127low/- regulatory T cells of asthmatic patients via heme oxygenase-1. Iranian Journal of Allergy, Asthma and Immunology. 2015;12(3):228–235.

22. Cengiz Kirmaz, Celal Bayar University. Experimental Autologous Mesenchymal Stem Cell Therapy in Treatment of Chronic Autoimmune Urticaria. In: ClinicalTrials.gov [Internet]. Bethesda (MD): National Library of Medicine (US). 2000- [cited November 2016]. Available from: https://clinicaltrials.gov/ct2/show/NCT02824393. NLM Identifier:NCT02824393.

23. Translational Biosciences. Safety and Feasibility Study of Intranasal Mesenchymal Trophic Factor (MTF) for Treatment of Asthma. In: ClinicalTrials.gov [Internet]. Bethesda (MD): National Library of Medicine (US). 2000- [cited November 2016]. Available from: https://clinicaltrials.gov/ct2/show/NCT02192736. NLM Identifier: NCT02192736.

24. Tsyb AF et al. In vitro inhibitory effect of mesenchymal stem cells on zymosan-induced production of reactive oxygen species. Bull Exp Biol Med. 2008;146(1):158-64.

25. Tu Z et al. Mesenchymal stem cells inhibit complement activation by secreting factor H. Stem Cells Dev 2010;19(11):1803-9.

26. Kemp K et al. Mesenchymal stem cell-secreted superoxide dismutase promotes cerebellar neuronal survival. J Neurochem. 2010;114(6):1569-80.

27. Ortiz LA et al. Interleukin 1 receptor antagonist mediates the antiinflammatory and antifibrotic effect of mesenchymal stem cells during lung injury. Proc Natl Acad Sci U S A. 2007;104(26):11002-7.

28. Osugi M et al. Conditioned media from mesenchymal stem cells enhanced bone regeneration in rat calvarial bone defects. Tissue Eng Part A. 2012;18(13-14):1479-89

Chapter Eleven

1. Black LL, Gaynor J, Gahring D, et al. Effect of adipose-derived mesenchymal stem and regenerative cells on lameness in dogs with chronic osteoarthritis of the coxofemoral joints: a randomized, double-blinded, multicenter, controlled trial. Vet Ther. 2007 Winter;8(4):272-84.

2. Theis KA, Murphy L, Hootman JM, Helmick CG, Yelin E. Prevalence and correlates of arthritis-attributable work limitation in the US population among persons ages 18-64: 2002 National Health Interview Survey Data. Arthritis Rheum. 2007;57(3):355-363.

3. Liu-Bryan R, Terkeltaub R. Emerging regulators of the inflammatory process in osteoarthritis. Nat Rev Rheumatol. 2015;11(1):35-44.doi: 10.1038/nrrheum.2014.162.

4. Goldring MB, Otero M. Inflammation in osteoarthritis. Curr Opin Rheumatol. 2011;23(5):471-478.doi: 10.1097/BOR.0b013e328349c2b1.

5. Madrigal M, Rao KS, Riordan NH. A review of therapeutic effects of mesenchymal stem cell secretions and induction of secretory modification by different culture methods. J Transl Med. 2014;12(1):260.doi: 10.1186/s12967-014-0260-8.

6. Caplan AI. Adult mesenchymal stem cells for tissue engineering versus regenerative medicine. J Cell Physiol. 2007;213(2):341-347.

7. Gupta PK, Das AK, Chullikana A, Majumdar AS. Mesenchymal stem cells for cartilage repair in osteoarthritis. Stem Cell Res Ther. 2012;3(4):25.doi: 10.1186/scrt116.

8. Arufe MC, De la Fuente A, Fuentes I, De Toro FJ, Blanco FJ. Umbilical cord as a mesenchymal stem cell source for treating joint pathologies. World J Orthop. 2011;2(6):43-50.doi: 10.5312/wjo.v2.i6.43.

9. Murphy JM, Fink DJ, Hunziker EB, Barry FP. Stem cell therapy in a caprine model of osteoarthritis. Arthritis Rheum. 2003;48(12):3464-3474.

10. Horie M, Sekiya I, Muneta T, et al. Intra-articular Injected synovial stem cells differentiate into meniscal cells directly and promote meniscal regeneration without mobilization to distant organs in rat massive meniscal defect. Stem Cells. 2009;27(4):878-887.doi: 10.1634/stemcells.2008-0616.

11. Grigolo B, Lisignoli G, Desando G, et al. Osteoarthritis treated with mesenchymal stem cells on hyaluronan-based scaffold in rabbit. Tissue Eng Part C Methods. 2009;15(4):647-658.doi: 10.1089/ten.TEC.2008.0569.

12. Al Faqeh H, Norhamdan MY, Chua KH, Chen HC, Aminuddin BS, Ruszymah BH. Cell based therapy for osteoarthritis in a sheep model: gross and histological assessment. Med J Malaysia. 2008;63 Suppl A:37-38.

13. Black LL, Gaynor J, Adams C, et al. Effect of intraarticular injection of autologous adipose-derived mesenchymal stem and regenerative cells on clinical signs of chronic osteoarthritis of the elbow joint in dogs. Vet Ther. 2008;9(3):192-200

14. Al Faqeh H, Nor Hamdan BM, Chen HC, Aminuddin BS, Ruszymah BH. The potential of intra-articular injection of chondrogenic-induced bone marrow stem cells to retard the progression of osteoarthritis in a sheep model. Exp Gerontol. 2012;47(6):458-464.doi: 10.1016/j.exger.2012.03.018.

15. Koh YG, Choi YJ. Infrapatellar fat pad-derived mesenchymal stem cell therapy for knee osteoarthritis. Knee. 2012;19(6):902-907.doi: 10.1016/j.knee.2012.04.001.

16. Davatchi F, Abdollahi BS, Mohyeddin M, Shahram F, Nikbin B. Mesenchymal stem cell therapy for knee osteoarthritis. Preliminary report of four patients. Int J Rheum Dis. 2011;14(2):211-215.doi: 10.1111/j.1756-185X.2011.01599.x.

17. Pers YM, Rackwitz L, Ferreira R, et al. Adipose mesenchymal stromal cell-based therapy for severe osteoarthritis of the knee: a phase I dose-escalation trial. Stem Cells Transl Med. 2016;5(7):847-56. doi: 10.5966/sctm.2015-0245.

18. Vega A, Martín-Ferrero MA, Del Canto F, et al. Treatment of knee osteoarthritis with allogeneic bone marrow mesenchymal stem cells: a randomized controlled trial. Transplantation. 2015;99(8):1681-1690.doi: 10.1097/TP.0000000000000678.

19. Orozco L, Munar A, Soler R, et al. Treatment of knee osteoarthritis with autologous mesenchymal stem cells: a pilot study. Transplantation. 2013;95(12):1535-1541.doi: 10.1097/TP.0b013e318291a2da.

20. Jo CH, Lee YG, Shin WH, et al. Intra-articular injection of mesenchymal stem cells for the treatment of osteoarthritis of the knee: a proof-of-concept clinical trial. Stem Cells. 2014;32(5):1254-1266.doi: 10.1002/stem.1634.

21. Emadedin M, Ghorbani Liastani M, Fazeli R, et al. Long-term follow-up of intra-articular injection of autologous mesenchymal stem cells in patients with knee, ankle, or hip osteoarthritis. Arch Iran Med. 2015;18(6):336-344.doi: 015186/AIM.003.

22. MEDIPOST | Stem Cell Drugs| Cartistem. http://www.medi-post.com/cartistem/ Accessed October 31st, 2016.

23. Park YB, Ha CW, Lee CH, Yoon YC, Park YG, et al. Cartilage regeneration in osteoarthritic patients by a composite of allogeneic umbilical cord blood-derived mesenchymal stem cells and hyaluronate hydrogel: results from a clinical trial for safety and proof-of-concept with 7 years of extended follow-up. Stem Cells Transl Med. September 2016.

24. Medipost Co Ltd. Evaluation of Safety and Exploratory Efficacy of CARTISTEM®, a Cell Therapy Product for Articular Cartilage Defects. In: ClinicalTrials.gov [Internet]. Bethesda (MD): National Library of Medicine (US). 2000- [cited 2016 November]. Available from:https://clinicaltrials.gov/ct2/show/NCT01733186. NLM Identifier: NCT01733186.

25. Regenerative Pain Center, Illinois. Outcomes data of bone marrow stem cells to treat hip and knee osteoarthritis. In: ClinicalTrials.gov [Internet]. Bethesda (MD): National Library of Medicine (US). 2000- [cited 2016 July]. Available from:https://clinicaltrials.gov/ct2/show/NCT01601951 NLM Identifier: NCT01601951.

26. Stempeutics Research Pvt Ltd. Allogeneic mesenchymal stem cells for osteoarthritis. In: ClinicalTrials.gov [Internet]. Bethesda (MD): National Library of Medicine (US). 2000- [cited 2016 July]. Available from:https://clinicaltrials.gov/ct2/show/NCT01448434 NLM Identifier: NCT01448434.

27. International Stemcell Services Limited. Safety and efficacy of autologous bone marrow stem cells for treating osteoarthritis. In: ClinicalTrials.gov [Internet]. Bethesda (MD): National Library of Medicine (US). 2000- [cited 2016 July]. Available from:https://clinicaltrials.gov/ct2/show/NCT01152125 NLM Identifier: NCT01152125.

28. South China Research Center for Stem Cell and Regenerative Medicine. UCMSC transplantation in the treatment of cartilage damage. In: ClinicalTrials.gov [Internet]. Bethesda (MD): National Library of Medicine (US). 2000- [cited 2016 July]. Available from:https://www.clinicaltrials.gov/ct2/show/NCT02776943 NLM Identifier: NCT02776943.

29. Translational Biosciences. Clinical Study of Umbilical Cord Tissue Mesenchymal Stem Cells (UC-MSC) for Treatment of Osteoarthritis. In: ClinicalTrials.gov [Internet]. Bethesda (MD): National Library of Medicine (US). 2000- [cited 2016 July]. Available from:https://clinicaltrials.gov/ct2/show/NCT02237846 NLM Identifier: NCT02237846.

30. Alamanos Y, Voulgari PV, Drosos AA. Incidence and prevalence of rheumatoid arthritis, based on the 1987 American College of Rheumatology criteria: a systematic review. Semin Arthritis Rheum.2006;36(3):182-8.

31. Carmona L, Cross M, Williams B, Lassere M, March L. Rheumatoid arthritis. Best Pract Res Clin Rheumatol. 2010;24(6):733-745.

32. Michaud K, Wolfe F. Comorbidities in rheumatoid arthritis. Best Pract Res Clin Rheumatol. 2007;21(5):885-906.

33. Bansard C, Lequerré T, Daveau M, et al. Can rheumatoid arthritis responsiveness to methotrexate and biologics be predicted? Rheumatology (Oxford). 2009;48(9):1021-1028.

34. Hoogduijn MJ, Crop MJ, Peeters AM, et al. Human heart, spleen, and perirenal fat-derived mesenchymal stem cells have immunomodulatory capacities. Stem Cells Dev. 2007;16(4):597-604.

35. English K, Barry FP, Mahon BP. Murine mesenchymal stem cells suppress dendritic cell migration, maturation and antigen presentation. Immunol Lett. 2008;115(1):50-8.

36. Caplan AI. Adult mesenchymal stem cells for tissue engineering versus regenerative medicine. J Cell Physiol. 2007;213(2):341-347.

37. La Rocca G, Lo Iacono M, Corsello T, Corrao S, Farina F, Anzalone R. Human Wharton's jelly mesenchymal stem cells maintain the expression of key immunomodulatory molecules when subjected to osteogenic, adipogenic and chondrogenic differentiation in vitro: new perspectives for cellular therapy. Curr Stem Cell Res Ther. 2013;8(1):100-13.

38. Liang J, Zhang H, Hua B, et al. Allogenic mesenchymal stem cells transplantation in refractory systemic lupus erythematosus: a pilot clinical study. Ann Rheum Dis. 2010;69(8):1423-9.

39. Sun L, Wang D, Liang J, et al. Umbilical cord mesenchymal stem cell transplantation in severe and refractory systemic lupus erythematosus. Arthritis Rheum. 2010;62(8):2467-75.

40. Hu J, Yu X, Wang Z, et al. Long term effects of the implantation of Wharton's jelly-derived mesenchymal stem cells from the umbilical cord for newly-onset type 1 diabetes mellitus. Endocr J. 2013;60(3):347-57.

41. Connick P, Kolappan M, Crawley C, et al. Autologous mesenchymal stem cells for the treatment of secondary progressive multiple sclerosis: an open-label phase 2a proof-of-concept study. Lancet Neurol. 2012;11(2):150-6.

42. Gupta PK, Das AK, Chullikana A, Majumdar AS, et al. Mesenchymal stem cells for cartilage repair in osteoarthritis. Stem Cell Res Ther. 2012;3(4):25.

43. Arufe MC, De la Fuente A, Fuentes I, De Toro FJ, Blanco FJ, et al. Umbilical cord as a mesenchymal stem cell source for treating joint pathologies. World J Orthop.2011;2(6):43-50.

44. Zhou B, Yuan J, Zhou Y, et al, Administering human adipose-derived mesenchymal stem cells to prevent and treat experimental arthritis. Clin Immunol. 2011;141(3):328-37.

45. Park MJ, Park HS, Cho ML, et al. Transforming growth factor beta-transduced mesenchymal stem cells ameliorate experimental autoimmune arthritis through reciprocal regulation of Treg/Th17 cells and osteoclastogenesis. Arthritis Rheum. 2011;63(6):1668-80.

46. González MA, Gonzalez-Rey E, Rico L, et al. Treatment of experimental arthritis by inducing immune tolerance with human adipose-derived mesenchymal stem cells. Arthritis Rheum. 2009;60(4):1006-19.

47. Augello A, Tasso R, Negrini SM, Cancedda R, Pennesi G, et al. Cell therapy using allogeneic bone marrow mesenchymal stem cells prevents tissue damage in collagen-induced arthritis. Arthritis Rheum. 2007;56(4):1175-86.

48. Wang Q, Li X, Luo J, et al. The allogeneic umbilical cord mesenchymal stem cells regulate the function of T helper 17 cells from patients with rheumatoid arthritis in an in vitro co-culture system. BMC Musculoskelet Disord. 2012;13:249.

49. Liu Y, Mu R, Wang S, et al. Therapeutic potential of human umbilical cord mesenchymal stem cells in the treatment of rheumatoid arthritis. Arthritis Res Ther. 2010;12(6):R210.

50. Ichim TE, Harman RJ, Min WP, et al. Autologous stromal vascular fraction cells: a tool for facilitating tolerance in rheumatic disease. Cell Immunol. 2010;264(1):7-17. doi: 10.1016/j.cellimm.2010.04.002.

51. Rodriguez JP, Murphy MP, Hong S, et al. Autologous stromal vascular fraction therapy for rheumatoid arthritis: rationale and clinical safety. Int Arch Med. 2012 Feb 8;5:5. doi: 10.1186/1755-7682-5-5.

52. Wang L, Wang L, Cong X, et al. Human umbilical cord mesenchymal stem cell therapy for patients with active rheumatoid arthritis: Safety and efficacy. Stem Cells Dev. 2013 Dec 15;22(24):3192-202. doi: 10.1089/scd.2013.0023.

53. Mesoblast, Ltd. A double-blind, randomized, placebo-controlled, dose-escalation, multi-center study a single intravenous infusion of allogeneic mesenchymal precursor cells (MPCs) in patients with rheumatoid arthritis and incomplete response to at least one TNF-alpha inhibitor. In: ClinicalTrials.gov [Internet]. Bethesda (MD): National Library of Medicine (US). 2000- [cited 2016 Jul 7]. Available from: https://clinicaltrials.gov/ct2/show/NCT01851070 NLM Identifier: NCT01851070.

54. Alliancells Bioscience Corporation Limited. Safety and efficacy study of umbilical cord-derived mesenchymal stem cells for rheumatoid arthritis (RA). In: ClinicalTrials.gov [Internet]. Bethesda (MD): National Library of Medicine (US). 2000- [cited 2016 Jul 7]. Available from: https://clinicaltrials.gov/ct2/show/NCT01547091 NLM Identifier: NCT01547091.

55. Shenzhen Hornetcorn Bio-technology Company, LTD. Human umbilical cord-mesenchymal stem cells for rheumatoid arthritis. In: ClinicalTrials.gov [Internet]. Available from: https://clinicaltrials.gov/ct2/show/NCT02643823. NLM Identifier: NCT02643823.

56. Translational Biosciences. Umbilical cord tissue-derived mesenchymal stem cells for rheumatoid arthritis. In: ClinicalTrials.gov [Internet]. Bethesda (MD): National Library of Medicine (US). 2000- [cited 2016 Jul 7]. Available from: https://clinicaltrials.gov/ct2/show/NCT01985464 NLM Identifier: NCT01985464.

Chapter Twelve

1. Nakazawa F, Matsuno H, Yudoh K, Watanabe Y, Katayama R, Kimura T. Corticosteroid treatment induces chondrocyte apoptosis in an experimental arthritis model and in chondrocyte cultures. Clin Exp Rheumatol. 2002;20(6):773-781.
2. Farkas B, Kvell K, Czömpöly T, Illés T, Bárdos T. Increased chondrocyte death after steroid and local anesthetic combination. Clin Orthop Relat Res. 2010;468(11):3112-3120.doi: 10.1007/s11999-010-1443-0.
3. Wernecke C, Braun HJ, Dragoo JL. The effect of intra-articular corticosteroids on articular cartilage: a systematic review. Orthop J Sports Med. 2015;3(5):2325967115581163.doi: 10.1177/2325967115581163. eCollection 2015.
4. Fubini SL, Todhunter RJ, Burton-Wurster N, Vernier-Singer M, MacLeod JN. Corticosteroids alter the differentiated phenotype of articular chondrocytes. J Orthop Res. 2001;19(4):688-695.
5. Céleste C, Ionescu M, Robin Poole A, Laverty S. Repeated intraarticular injections of triamcinolone acetonide alter cartilage matrix metabolism measured by biomarkers in synovial fluid. J Orthop Res. 2005;23(3):602-610.
6. Sherman SL, James C, Stoker AM, et al. In vivo toxicity of local anesthetics and corticosteroids on chondrocyte and synoviocyte viability and metabolism. Cartilage. Apr 2015;6(2):106-112.doi: 10.1177/1947603515571001.
7. Sherman SL, Khazai RS, James CH, Stoker AM, Flood DL, Cook JL. In vitro toxicity of local anesthetics and corticosteroids on chondrocyte and synoviocyte viability and metabolism. Cartilage. 2015;6(4):233-240.doi: 10.1177/1947603515594453.
8. Wada J, Koshino T, Morii T, Sugimoto K. Natural course of osteoarthritis of the knee treated with or without intraarticular corticosteroid injections. Bull Hosp Jt Dis. 1993;53(2):45-48.
9. Lewis M, Hay EM, Paterson SM, Croft P. Local steroid injections for tennis elbow: does the pain get worse before it gets better?: Results from a randomized controlled trial. Clin J Pain. 2005;21(4):330-334.
10. Olaussen M, Holmedal Ø, Mdala I, Brage S, Lindbæk M. Corticosteroid or placebo injection combined with deep transverse friction massage, Mills manipulation, stretching and eccentric exercise for acute lateral epicondylitis: a randomised, controlled trial. BMC Musculoskelet Disord. 2015;16:122.doi: 10.1186/s12891-015-0582-6.
11. Sayegh ET, Strauch RJ. Does nonsurgical treatment improve longitudinal outcomes of lateral epicondylitis over no treatment? A meta-analysis. Clin Orthop Relat Res. 2015;473(3):1093-1107. doi: 10.1007/s11999-014-4022-y.
12. Smidt N, Assendelft WJ, van der Windt DA, Hay EM, Buchbinder R, Bouter LM. Corticosteroid injections for lateral epicondylitis: a systematic review. Pain. 2002;96(1-2):23-40.
13. Smidt N, van der Windt DA, Assendelft WJ, Devillé WL, Korthals-de Bos IB, Bouter LM. Corticosteroid injections, physiotherapy, or a wait-and-see policy for lateral epicondylitis: a randomised controlled trial. Lancet. 2002;359(9307):657-662.
14. Rafols C, Monckeberg JE, Numair J, Botello J, Rosales J. Platelet-rich plasma augmentation of arthroscopic hip surgery for femoroacetabular impingement: a prospective study with 24-month follow-up. Arthroscopy. 2015;31(10):1886–1892.doi: 10.1016/j.arthro.2015.03.025.
15. Zhang Q, Ge H, Zhou J, Cheng B. Are platelet-rich products necessary during the arthroscopic repair of full-thickness rotator cuff tears: a meta-analysis. PLoS ONE. 2013;8(7):e69731.doi: 10.1371/journal.pone.0069731.

16. Duif C, Vogel T, Topcuoglu F, Spryou G, von Schulze Pellengahr C, Lahner M. Does intraoperative application of leukocyte-poor platelet-rich plasma during arthroscopy for knee degeneration affect postoperative pain, function and quality of life? A 12-month randomized controlled double-blind trial. Arch Orthop Trauma Surg. 2015;135(7):971–977.doi: 10.1007/s00402-015-2227-5.

17. Lopez-Vidriero E, Goulding KA, Simon DA, Sanchez M, Johnson DH. The use of platelet-rich plasma in arthroscopy and sports medicine: optimizing the healing environment. Arthroscopy. 2010;26(2):269-78. doi: 10.1016/j.arthro.2009.11.015.

18. DiBartola AC, Everhart JS, Magnussen RA, et al. Correlation between histological outcome and surgical cartilage repair technique in the knee: A meta-analysis. Knee. 2016;23(3):344–9. doi: 10.1016/j.knee.2016.01.017.

19. Mithoefer K, McAdams T, Williams RJ, Kreuz PC, Mandelbaum BR. Clinical efficacy of the microfracture technique for articular cartilage repair in the knee: an evidence-based systematic analysis. Am J Sports Med. 2009;37(10):2053-63.doi: 10.1177/0363546508328414.

20. Sophia Fox AJ, Bedi A, and Rodeo SA. The basic science of articular cartilage: structure, composition, and function. *Sports Health.* 2009;1(6):461-468. doi:10.1177/1941738109350438.

21. Fricker J, "Cartilage transplantation: an end to creaky knees?" *Lancet.* 1998;352(9135):1202.

22. Hattori K, Takakura Y, Ohgushi H, Habata, T, Uematsu K, Ikeuchi K. Novel ultrasonic evaluation of tissue-engineered cartilage for large osteochondral defects—non-invasive judgment of tissue-engineered cartilage. J Orthop Res. 2005;23(5):1179-83.

23. Briggs TW, Mahroof S, David LA, Flannelly J, Pringle J, Bayliss M. Histological evaluation of chondral defects after autologous chondrocyte implantation of the knee. J Bone Joint Surg Br. 2003; 85(7):1077-83.

24. Peterson L, Brittberg M, Kiviranta I, Akerlund EL, Lindahl A. Autologous chondrocyte transplantation. Biomechanics and long-term durability. Am J Sports Med. 2002; 30(1):2-12.

25. Henderson I, Tuy B, Oakes B. Reoperation after autologous chondrocyte implantation. Indications and findings. J Bone Joint Surg Br. 2004; 86(2):205-11.

26. Caplan AI. Adult mesenchymal stem cells for tissue engineering versus regenerative medicine. J Cell Physiol. 2007;213(2):341-347.

27. Madrigal M, Rao KS, Riordan NH. A review of therapeutic effects of mesenchymal stem cell secretions and induction of secretory modification by different culture methods. J Transl Med. 2014;12(1):260.doi: 10.1186/s12967-014-0260-8.

28. Arufe MC, De la Fuente A, Fuentes I, De Toro FJ, Blanco FJ. Umbilical cord as a mesenchymal stem cell source for treating joint pathologies. World J Orthop. 2011;2(6):43-50.doi: 10.5312/wjo.v2.i6.43.

29. Saw KY, Hussin P, Loke SC, et al. Articular cartilage regeneration with autologous marrow aspirate and hyaluronic Acid: an experimental study in a goat model. Arthroscopy. 2009;25(12):1391-1400. doi: 10.1016/j.arthro.2009.07.011.

30. Fortier LA, Potter HG, Rickey EJ, et al. Concentrated bone marrow aspirate improves full-thickness cartilage repair compared with microfracture in the equine model. J Bone Joint Surg Am. 2010;92(10):1927-1937.doi: 10.2106/JBJS.I.01284.

31. Ferris DJ, Frisbie DD, Kisiday JD, et al. Clinical outcome after intra-articular administration of bone marrow derived mesenchymal stem cells in 33 horses with stifle injury. Vet Surg. 2014;43(3):255–265.doi: 10.1111/j.1532-950X.2014.12100.x.

32. Degen RM, Carbone A, Carballo C, et al. The effect of purified human bone marrow–derived mesenchymal stem cells on rotator cuff tendon healing in an athymic rat. Arthroscopy. June 2016. [Epub ahead of print.]

33. Hendrich C, Franz E, Waertel G, Krebs R, Jäger M. Safety of autologous bone marrow aspiration concentrate transplantation: initial experiences in 101 patients. Orthop Rev. 2009;1(2):e32.doi: 10.4081/or.2009.e32.

34. Gobbi A, Karnatzikos G, Scotti C, Mahajan V, Mazzucco L, Grigolo B. One-step cartilage repair with bone marrow aspirate concentrated cells and collagen matrix in full-thickness knee cartilage lesions: results at 2-year follow-up. Cartilage. 2011;2(3):286-299.doi: 10.1177/1947603510392023.

35. Jäger M, Jelinek EM, Wess KM, et al. Bone marrow concentrate: a novel strategy for bone defect treatment. Curr Stem Cell Res Ther. 2009;4(1):34-43.

36. Pasquali PJ, Teixeira ML, de Oliveira TA, de Macedo LG, Aloise AC, Pelegrine AA. Maxillary sinus augmentation combining bio-oss with the bone marrow aspirate concentrate: a histomorphometric study in humans. Int J Biomater. 2015;2015:121286.doi: 10.1155/2015/121286.

37. Campbell KJ, Boykin RE, Wijdicks CA, Erik Giphart J, LaPrade RF, Philippon MJ. Treatment of a hip capsular injury in a professional soccer player with platelet-rich plasma and bone marrow aspirate concentrate therapy. Knee Surg Sports Traumatol Arthrosc. 2013;21(7):1684-1688.doi: 10.1007/s00167-012-2232-y.

38. Stein BE, Stroh DA, Schon LC. Outcomes of acute Achilles tendon rupture repair with bone marrow aspirate concentrate augmentation. Int Orthop. 2015;39(5):901-905.doi: 10.1007/s00264-015-2725-7.

39. Iafrati MD, Hallett JW, Geils G, et al. Early results and lessons learned from a multicenter, randomized, double-blind trial of bone marrow aspirate concentrate in critical limb ischemia. J Vasc Surg. 2011;54(6):1650-1658.doi: 10.1016/j.jvs.2011.06.118.

40. Chahla J, Dean CS, Moatshe G, Pascual-Garrido C, Serra Cruz R, LaPrade RF. Concentrated bone marrow aspirate for the treatment of chondral injuries and osteoarthritis of the knee: a systematic review of outcomes. Orthop J Sports Med. 2016;4(1):2325967115625481.doi: 10.1177/2325967115625481. eCollection 2016.

41. Campbell KJ, Boykin RE, Wijdicks CA, Erik Giphart J, LaPrade RF, Philippon MJ. Treatment of a hip capsular injury in a professional soccer player with platelet-rich plasma and bone marrow aspirate concentrate therapy. Knee Surg Sports Traumatol Arthrosc. 2013;21(7):1684-1688.doi: 10.1007/s00167-012-2232-y.

42. Ellera Gomes JL, da Silva RC, R Silla, LM, Abreu MR, Pellanda R. Conventional rotator cuff repair complemented by the aid of mononuclear autologous stem cells. Knee Surg Sports Traumatol Arthrosc. 2011;20(2):373–377.doi: 10.1007/s00167-011-1607-9

43. Hernigou P, Flouzat Lachaniette CH, Delambre J, et al. Biologic augmentation of rotator cuff repair with mesenchymal stem cells during arthroscopy improves healing and prevents further tears: A case-controlled study. Int Orthop. 2014 Sep;38(9):1811-8. doi: 10.1007/s00264-014-2391-1.

44. Samsung Medical Center. Development of novel strategy for treatment of anterior cruciate ligament (ACL) injury using stem cell. In: ClinicalTrials.gov [Internet]. Bethesda (MD): National Library of Medicine (US). 2000-[cited 2016 July] Available from: https://clinicaltrials.gov/ct2/show/NCT02755376 NLM Identifier: NCT02755376.

45. Rush University Medical Center. Mesenchymal stem cell augmentation in patients undergoing arthroscopic rotator cuff repair. In: ClinicalTrials.gov [Internet]. Bethesda (MD): National Library of Medicine (US). 2000-[cited 2016 July] Available from: https://clinicaltrials.gov/ct2/show/NCT02484950 NLM Identifier: NCT02484950.

46. Duke University. Bone marrow aspirate concentrate (BMAC) supplementation for osteochondral lesions (BMAC). In: ClinicalTrials.gov [Internet]. Bethesda (MD): National Library of Medicine (US). 2000-[cited 2016 July] Available from: https://clinicaltrials.gov/ct2/show/NCT02011295 NLM Identifier: NCT02011295.

47. McKenna RW, Riordan HN. Minimally invasive autologous bone marrow concentrate stem cells in the treatment of the chronically injured Achilles tendon: A case report. CellR4. 2014;2(4):e1100.

48. Hernigou P, Flouzat Lachaniette CH, Delambre J, et al. Biologic augmentation of rotator cuff repair with mesenchymal stem cells during arthroscopy improves healing and prevents further tears: A case-controlled study. Int Orthop. 2014 Sep;38(9):1811-8. doi: 10.1007/s00264-014-2391-1.

Additional References

Bark S, Piontek T, Behrens P, Mkalaluh S, Varoga D, Gille J. Enhanced microfracture techniques in cartilage knee surgery: Fact or fiction? World Journal of Orthopedics. Sep 18 2014;5(4):444-449.

Bert JM. Abandoning microfracture of the knee: has the time come? Arthroscopy. Mar 2015;31(3):501-505.

DiBartola AC, Everhart JS, Magnussen RA, et al. Correlation between histological outcome and surgical cartilage repair technique in the knee: A meta-analysis. The Knee. Jun 2016;23(3):344-349.

Goyal D, Keyhani S, Lee EH, Hui JH. Evidence-based status of microfracture technique: a systematic review of level I and II studies. Arthroscopy. Sep 2013;29(9):1579-1588.

Kon E, Filardo G, Berruto M, et al. Articular cartilage treatment in high-level male soccer players: a prospective comparative study of arthroscopic second-generation autologous chondrocyte implantation versus microfracture. The American Journal of Sports Medicine. Dec 2011;39(12):2549-2557.

McCormick F, Harris JD, Abrams GD, et al. Trends in the surgical treatment of articular cartilage lesions in the United States: an analysis of a large private-payer database over a period of 8 years. Arthroscopy. Feb 2014;30(2):222-226.

Oussedik S, Tsitskaris K, Parker D. Treatment of articular cartilage lesions of the knee by microfracture or autologous chondrocyte implantation: a systematic review. Arthroscopy. Apr 2015;31(4):732-744.

Chapter Thirteen

1. Vargas DL, Nascimbene C, Krishnan C, Zimmerman AW, Pardo CA. Neuroglial activation and neuroinflammation in the brain of patients with autism. Ann Neurol. 2005;57(1):67-81.

2. Stubbs G, Interferonemia and autism. J Autism Dev Disord. 1995;25(1):71-3.

3. Sweeten TL, Posey DJ, Shankar S, McDougle CJ. High nitric oxide production in autistic disorder: a possible role for interferon-gamma. Biol Psychiatry. 2004;55(4):434-7.

4. Ichim TE, Solano F, Glenn E, et al. Stem cell therapy for autism. J Transl Med. 2007;5:30.doi: 10.1186/1479-5876-5-30.

5. Ashwood P, Anthony A, Torrente F, Wakefield AJ. Spontaneous mucosal lymphocyte cytokine profiles in children with autism and gastrointestinal symptoms: mucosal immune activation and reduced counter regulatory interleukin-10. J Clin Immunol. 2004;24(6):664-73.

6. Okada K, Hashimoto K, Iwata Y, Nakamura K, Tsujii M, Tsuchiya KJ, et al. Decreased serum levels of transforming growth factor-beta1 in patients with autism. Prog Neuropsychopharmacol Biol Psychiatry. 2007;31(1):187-90.

7. Neuhaus E, Beauchaine TP, Bernier R. Neurobiological correlates of social functioning in autism. Clinical psychology review. 2010;30(6):733-748.doi: 10.1016/j.cpr.2010.05.007.

8. Park SY, Cervesi C, Galling B, et al. Antipsychotic use trends in youth with autism spectrum disorder and/or intellectual disability: a meta-analysis. J Am Acad Child Adolesc Psychiatry. 2016;55(6):456-468.e4. doi: 10.1016/j.jaac.2016.03.012.
9. Golnik AE and Ireland M. Complementary alternative medicine for children with autism: a physician survey. J Autism Dev Disord. 2009;39(7):996-1005.doi: 10.1007/s10803-009-0714-7.
10. Al-Ayadhi LY and Mostafa GA. Elevated serum levels of macrophage-derived chemokine and thymus and activation-regulated chemokine in autistic children. J Neuroinflammation. 2013;10:72. doi: 10.1186/1742-2094-10-72.
11. Ashwood P, Krakowiak P, Hertz-Picciotto I, Hansen R, Pessah IN, Van de Water J. Altered T cell responses in children with autism. Brain Behav Immun. 2011;25(5):840-9.doi: 10.1016/j.bbi.2010.09.002.
12. Şimşek Ş et al. Elevated levels of tissue plasminogen activator and E-selectin in male children with autism spectrum disorder. Autism Research. May 2016.
13. Tsilioni I et al. Translational psychiatry - children with autism spectrum disorders, who improved with a luteolin-containing dietary formulation, show reduced serum levels of TNF and IL-6. Translational Psychiatry. 2015;5(9):647.
14. Nikolov RN, Bearss KE, Lettinga J, et al. Gastrointestinal symptoms in a sample of children with pervasive developmental disorders. J Autism Dev Disord. 2009;39(3):405-413.doi: 10.1007/s10803-008-0637-8.
15. Mazurek MO, Vasa RA, Kalb LG, et al. Anxiety, sensory over-responsivity, and gastrointestinal problems in children with autism spectrum disorders. J Abnorm Child Psychol. 2013;41(1):165–176.doi: 10.1007/s10802-012-9668-x.
16. Horvath K and Perman JA. Autism and gastrointestinal symptoms. Curr Gastroenterol Rep. 2002;4(3):251-8.
17. Pramparo T, Pierce K, Lombardo MV, et al. Prediction of autism by translation and immune/inflammation coexpressed genes in toddlers from pediatric community practices. JAMA Psychiatry. 2015;72(4):386-394.doi: 10.1001/jamapsychiatry.2014.3008.
18. Herbert MR et al. Dissociations of cerebral cortex, subcortical and cerebral white matter volumes in autistic boys. Brain. 2003;126(5):1182–1192.
19. Herbert MR. Large brains in autism: The challenge of pervasive abnormality. The Neuroscientist. 2005;11(5):417–440.
20. Kern JK et al. Relevance of Neuroinflammation and encephalitis in autism. Frontiers in Cellular Neuroscience. 2016;9.
21. Di Marco B, Bonaccorso CM, Aloisi E, D'Antoni S, Catania MV. Neuro-Inflammatory mechanisms in developmental disorders associated with intellectual disability and autism spectrum disorder: A Neuro- immune perspective. CNS & Neurological Disorders - Drug Targets. 2016;15(4):448–463.
22. Ichim, TE et al. Stem cell therapy for autism. J Transl Med, 2007. 5: p. 30.
23. Madrigal M, Rao KS, and Riordan NH. A review of therapeutic effects of mesenchymal stem cell secretions and induction of secretory modification by different culture methods. J Transl Med. 2014;12(1):260.doi: 10.1186/s12967-014-0260-8.
24. Liang J, Zhang H, Hua B, et al. Allogeneic mesenchymal stem cells transplantation in treatment of multiple sclerosis. Mult Scler. 2009;15(5):644-6.doi: 10.1177/1352458509104590.
25. Sheikh AM, Nagai A, Wakabayashi K, et al. Mesenchymal stem cell transplantation modulates neuroinflammation in focal cerebral ischemia: contribution of fractalkine and IL-5. Neurobiol Dis. 2011;41(3):717-724.doi: 10.1016/j.nbd.2010.12.009.

26. Sun L, Wang D, Liang J, et al. Umbilical cord mesenchymal stem cell transplantation in severe and refractory systemic lupus erythematosus. Arthritis Rheum. 2010;62(8):2467-75.doi: 10.1002/art.27548.

27. Xu J, Wang D, Liu D, et al. Allogeneic mesenchymal stem cell treatment alleviates experimental and clinical Sjögren syndrome. Blood. 2012;120(15):3142-51.doi: 10.1182/blood-2011-11-391144.

28. Gesundheit B, Ashwood P, Keating A, Naor D, Melamed M, Rosenzweig JP. Therapeutic properties of mesenchymal stem cells for autism spectrum disorders. Med Hypotheses. 2015;84(3):169-77. doi: 10.1016/j.mehy.2014.12.016.

29. Lalu MM, McIntyre L, Pugliese C, et al. Safety of cell therapy with mesenchymal stromal cells (SafeCell): a systematic review and meta-analysis of clinical trials. PLoS One. 2012;7(10):e47559. doi: 10.1371/journal.pone.0047559.

30. Lv YT, Zhang Y, Liu M, et al. Transplantation of human cord blood mononuclear cells and umbilical cord-derived mesenchymal stem cells in autism. J Transl Med. 2013;11:196.doi: 10.1186/1479-5876-11-196.

31. Sharma A, Gokulchandran N, Sane H, et al. Autologous bone marrow mononuclear cell therapy for autism: an open label proof of concept study. Stem Cells Int. 2013;2013:623875.doi: 10.1155/2013/623875.

32. Hospital Universitario; Jose Gonzalez. autologous bone marrow stem cells for children with autism spectrum disorders. In: ClinicalTrials.gov [Internet]. Bethesda (MD): National Library of Medicine (US). 2000- [cited 2016 July]. Available from: https://clinicaltrials.gov/ct2/show/NCT01740869 NLM Identifier: NCT01740869.

33. Translational Biosciences. allogeneic umbilical cord mesenchymal stem cell therapy for autism. In: ClinicalTrials.gov [Internet]. Bethesda (MD): National Library of Medicine (US). 2000- [cited 2016 July]. Available from: https://clinicaltrials.gov/ct2/show/NCT02192749 NLM Identifier: NCT02192749.

34. Sutter Health; Michael Chez, MD. Autologous cord blood stem cells for autism. In: ClinicalTrials.gov [Internet]. Bethesda (MD): National Library of Medicine (US). 2000- [cited 2016 July]. Available from: https://clinicaltrials.gov/ct2/show/NCT01638819 NLM Identifier: NCT01638819.

35. NeuroGen Brain and Spine Institute. Stem Cell Therapy in Autism Spectrum Disorders. In: ClinicalTrials.gov [Internet]. Bethesda (MD): National Library of Medicine (US). 2000- [cited 2016 July]. Available from:https://clinicaltrials.gov/ct2/show/NCT01974973 NLM Identifier: NCT01974973.

36. Ageless Regenerative Institute. Adipose Derived Stem Cell Therapy for Autism. In: ClinicalTrials.gov [Internet]. Bethesda (MD): National Library of Medicine (US). 2000- [cited 2016 July]. Available from:https://clinicaltrials.gov/ct2/show/NCT01502488 NLM Identifier: NCT01502488.

Additional References

Germain B, Eppinger MA, Mostofsky SH, DiCicco-Bloom E, Maria BL. Recent advances in understanding and managing autism spectrum disorders. J Child Neurol. 2015;30(14):p. 1887-920. doi: 10.1177/0883073815601499.

Nikolov RN, Bearss KE, Lettinga J, et al. Gastrointestinal symptoms in a sample of children with pervasive developmental disorders. J Autism Dev Disord. 2009;39(3):405-13.doi: 10.1007/s10803-008-0637-8.

Sheikh AM, Nagai A, Wakabayashi K, et al. Mesenchymal stem cell transplantation modulates neuroinflammation in focal cerebral ischemia: contribution of fractalkine and IL-5. Neurobiol Dis. 2011;41(3):717-24.doi: 10.1016/j.nbd.2010.12.009.

Ichim TE, Solano F, Glenn E, et al. Stem cell therapy for autism. J Transl Med. 2007;5:30. doi: 10.1186/1479-5876-5-30.

Siniscalco D, Bradstreet JJ, and Antonucci N. Therapeutic role of hematopoietic stem cells in autism spectrum disorder-related inflammation. Front Immunol. 2013;4:140.doi: 10.3389/fimmu.2013.00140.

Sharma A, Gokulchandran N, Chopra G, et al. Administration of autologous bone marrow-derived mononuclear cells in children with incurable neurological disorders and injury is safe and improves their quality of life. Cell Transplant. 2012;21 Suppl 1:S79-90. doi: 10.3727/096368912X633798.

Simberlund J, Ferretti CJ, and Hollander E. Mesenchymal stem cells in autism spectrum and neurodevelopmental disorders: pitfalls and potential promises. World J Biol Psychiatry. 2015;1-8.

Chapter Fourteen

1. Lazebnik LB, Kniazev OV, Parfenov AI, et al. [Transplantation of allogeneic mesenchymal stem cells from the bone marrow increases duration of remission and reduces the risk of ulcerative colitis relapse]. Eksp Klin Gastroenterol. 2010;(3):5-10.
2. Lazebnik LB, Kniazev OV, Konoplyannikov AG, et al. [Allogeneic mesenchymal stromal cells in patients with ulcerative colitis: two years of observation]. Eksp Klin Gastroenterol. 2010;(11):3-15.
3. Knyazev OV, Parfenov AI, Konoplyannikov AG, Boldyreva ON. [Use of mesenchymal stem cells in the combination therapy of ulcerative colitis]. Ter Arkh. 2016;88(2):44-8.
4. Gonçalves Fda C, Schneider N, Pinto FO, et al. Intravenous vs intraperitoneal mesenchymal stem cells administration: what is the best route for treating experimental colitis? World J Gastroenterol. 2014;20(48):18228-39. doi: 10.3748/wjg.v20.i48.18228.
5. He XW, He XS, Lian L, Wu XJ, Lan P. Systemic infusion of bone marrow-derived mesenchymal stem cells for treatment of experimental colitis in mice. Dig Dis Sci. 2012 Dec;57(12):3136-44. doi: 10.1007/s10620-012-2290-5.
6. Lin Y, Lin L, Wang Q, et al. Transplantation of human umbilical mesenchymal stem cells attenuates dextran sulfate sodium-induced colitis in mice. Clin Exp Pharmacol Physiol. 2015 Jan;42(1):76-86. doi: 10.1111/1440-1681.12321.
7. Li L, Liu S, Xu Y, et al. Human umbilical cord-derived mesenchymal stem cells downregulate inflammatory responses by shifting the Treg/Th17 profile in experimental colitis. Pharmacology. 2013;92(5-6):257-64. doi: 10.1159/000354883.
8. Sun T, Gao GZ, Li RF, et al. Bone marrow-derived mesenchymal stem cell transplantation ameliorates oxidative stress and restores intestinal mucosal permeability in chemically induced colitis in mice. Am J Transl Res. 2015 15;7(5):891-901.
9. Affiliated Hospital to Academy of Military Medical Sciences. Human umbilical-cord-derived mesenchymal stem cell therapy in active ulcerative colitis (UCMSC-UC). In: ClinicalTrials.gov [Internet]. Bethesda (MD): National Library of Medicine (US). 2000- [cited 2016 July]. Available from: https://clinicaltrials.gov/ct2/show/NCT02442037?term=umbilical+cord+mesenchymal+stem+cells+ulcerative+colitis&rank=2 NLM Identifier: NCT02442037.

Chapter Fifteen

1. Centers for Disease Control and Prevention. National Diabetes Statistics Report: Estimates of Diabetes and Its Burden in the United States, 2014. Atlanta, GA: U.S. Department of Health and Human Services; 2014.

2. Hoyert DL and Xu J. Deaths: preliminary data for 2011. Natl Vital Stat Rep. 2012 Oct 10;61(6):1-51.
3. American Diabetes Association. Economic costs of diabetes in the U.S. in 2012. Diabetes Care. 2013 Apr;36(4):1033-46. doi: 10.2337/dc12-2625.
4. Centers for Disease Control and Prevention. National diabetes fact sheet: national estimates and general information on diabetes and prediabetes in the United States, 2011. Atlanta, GA: U.S. Department of Health and Human Services, Centers for Disease Control and Prevention, 2011.
5. Barker, JM, Goehrig SH, Barriga K, et al. Clinical characteristics of children diagnosed with type 1 diabetes through intensive screening and follow-up. Diabetes Care, 2004. 27(6):1399-404.
6. Pitkäniemi J, Onkamo P, Tuomilehto J, Arjas E. Increasing incidence of Type 1 diabetes--role for genes? BMC Genet. 2004 2;5:5.
7. Basta G, Montanucci P, Luca G, et al. Long-term metabolic and immunological follow-up of nonimmunosuppressed patients with type 1 diabetes treated with microencapsulated islet allografts: Four cases. Diabetes Care. 2011 Nov;34(11):2406-9. doi: 10.2337/dc11-0731.
8. Luca G, Fallarino F, Calvitti M, et al. Xenograft of microencapsulated Sertoli cells reverses T1DM in NOD mice by inducing neogenesis of beta-cells. Transplantation. 2011;90(12):1352–7.
9. Mital P, Kaur G, Dufour J. Immunoprotective Sertoli cells: Making allogeneic and xenogeneic transplantation feasible. Reproduction. 2010;139(3):495-504. doi: 10.1530/REP-09-0384.
10. Zhao Y, Jiang Z, Zhao T, et al. Reversal of type 1 diabetes via islet β cell regeneration following immune modulation by cord blood-derived multipotent stem cells. BMC Med. 2012 Jan 10;10:3. doi: 10.1186/1741-7015-10-3.
11. Hu J, Wang Y, Gong H, et al. Long term effect and safety of Wharton's jelly-derived mesenchymal stem cells on type 2 diabetes. Exp Ther Med. 2016 Sep;12(3):1857-1866. Epub 2016 Jul 26.
12. Carlsson PO, Schwarcz E, Korsgren O, Le Blanc K. Preserved β-cell function in type 1 diabetes by mesenchymal stromal cells. Diabetes. 2015 Feb;64(2):587-92. doi: 10.2337/db14-0656.
13. Bhansali A, Upreti V, Khandelwal N, et al. Efficacy of autologous bone marrow-derived stem cell transplantation in patients with type 2 diabetes mellitus. Stem Cells Dev. 2009 Dec;18(10):1407-16. doi: 10.1089/scd.2009.0164.
14. Skyler JS, Fonseca VA, Segal KR, Rosenstock J. Allogeneic mesenchymal precursor cells in type 2 diabetes: A Randomized, placebo-controlled, dose-escalation safety and tolerability pilot study. Diabetes Care. 2015 Sep;38(9):1742-9. doi: 10.2337/dc14-2830.
15. Wu H, Mahato RI. Mesenchymal stem cell-based therapy for type 1 diabetes. Discov Med. 2014 Mar;17(93):139-43.

Chapter Sixteen

1. Sun, L, Akiyama K, Zhang H, et al. Mesenchymal stem cell transplantation reverses multi-organ dysfunction in systemic lupus erythematosus mice and humans. Stem Cells. 2009; 27(6): 1421–1432. doi: 10.1002/stem.68.
2. Liang J, Zhang H, Wang H, et al. Allogenic mesenchymal stem cells transplantation in refractory systemic lupus erythematosus: a pilot clinical study. Ann Rheum Dis. 2010;69(8):1423-9. doi: 10.1136/ard.2009.123463.
3. Sun L, Wang D, Liang J, et al. Umbilical cord mesenchymal stem cell transplantation in severe and refractory systemic lupus erythematosus. Arthritis Rheum. 2010;62(8):2467-75. doi: 10.1002/art.27548.
4. Shi D, Wang D, Li X, et al. Allogeneic transplantation of umbilical cord-derived mesenchymal stem cells for diffuse alveolar hemorrhage in systemic lupus erythematosus. Clin Rheumatol. 2012;31(5):841-6. doi: 10.1007/s10067-012-1943-2.

5. Wang D, Zhang H, Liang J, et al. Allogeneic mesenchymal stem cell transplantation in severe and refractory systemic lupus erythematosus: 4 years of experience. Cell Transplant. 2013;22(12):2267-77. doi: 10.3727/096368911X582769.
6. Medical University of South Carolina. MsciSLE: MSCs in SLE trial. In: ClinicalTrials.gov [Internet]. Bethesda (MD): National Library of Medicine (US). 2000- [cited 2016 July]. Available from: https://clinicaltrials.gov/ct2/show/NCT02633163 NLM Identifier: NCT02633163.

Chapter Seventeen

1. Baglio SR, Pegtel DM, Baldini N. Mesenchymal stem cell secreted vesicles provide novel opportunities in (stem) cell-free therapy. Front Physiol. 2012;3:359. doi: 10.3389/fphys.2012.00359.

Chapter Eighteen

1. Hill JM, Zalos G, Halcox JP, et al. Circulating endothelial progenitor cells, vascular function, and cardiovascular risk. N Engl J Med. 2003 Feb 13;348(7):593-600.
2. Van Craenenbroeck EM, Conraads VM. Endothelial progenitor cells in vascular health: focus on lifestyle. Microvasc Res. 2010;79(3):184-92. doi: 10.1016/j.mvr.2009.12.009.
3. Dunac A, Frelin C, Popolo-Blondeau M, Mahagne MH, Philip PJ. Neurological and functional recovery in human stroke are associated with peripheral blood CD34+ cell mobilization. J Neurol. 2007;254(3):327-32.
4. Leone AM, Galiuto L, Garramone B, et al. Usefulness of granulocyte colony-stimulating factor in patients with a large anterior wall acute myocardial infarction to prevent left ventricular remodeling (the rigenera study). Am J Cardiol. 2007;100(3):397-403.
5. Shintani S, Murohara T, Ikeda H, et al. Mobilization of endothelial progenitor cells in patients with acute myocardial infarction. Circulation. 2001;103(23):2776-9.
6. Lee ST, Chu K, Jung KH, et al. Reduced circulating angiogenic cells in Alzheimer disease. Neurology. 2009 May 26;72(21):1858-63. doi: 10.1212/WNL.0b013e3181a711f4.
7. Lee ST, Chu K, Jung KH, et al. Decreased number and function of endothelial progenitor cells in patients with migraine. Neurology. 2008;70(17):1510-7. doi: 10.1212/01.wnl.0000294329.93565.94.
8. Esposito K, Ciotola M, Maiorino MI, et al. Circulating CD34+ KDR+ endothelial progenitor cells correlate with erectile function and endothelial function in overweight men. J Sex Med. 2009;6(1):107-14. doi: 10.1111/j.1743-6109.2008.01042.x.
9. Hoetzer GL, Van Guilder GP, Irmiger HM, Keith RS, Stauffer BL, DeSouza CA. Aging, exercise, and endothelial progenitor cell clonogenic and migratory capacity in men. J Appl Physiol (1985). 2007;102(3):847-52.
10. Yang Z, Xia WH, Su C, et al. Regular exercise-induced increased number and activity of circulating endothelial progenitor cells attenuates age-related decline in arterial elasticity in healthy men. Int J Cardiol. 2013;165(2):247-54. doi: 10.1016/j.ijcard.2011.08.055.
11. Walther C, Gaede L, Adams V, et al. Effect of increased exercise in school children on physical fitness and endothelial progenitor cells: a prospective randomized trial. Circulation. 2009;120(22):2251-9. doi: 10.1161/CIRCULATIONAHA.109.865808.
12. Mano R, Ishida A, Ohya Y, Todoriki H, Takishita S. Dietary intervention with Okinawan vegetables increased circulating endothelial progenitor cells in healthy young women. Atherosclerosis. 2009;204(2):544-8. doi: 10.1016/j.atherosclerosis.2008.09.035.

13. Chaudhari SN, Mukherjee M, Vagasi AS, et al. Bacterial folates provide an exogenous signal for C. elegans germline stem cell proliferation. Develop Cell. 2016; 38(1):33-46. doi: http://dx.doi.org/10.1016/j.devcel.2016.06.013.
14. Mikirova NA, Jackson JA, Hunninghake R, et al. Circulating endothelial progenitor cells: a new approach to anti-aging medicine? J Transl Med. 2009;7:106. doi: 10.1186/1479-5876-7-106.
15. Mikirova NA, Jackson JA, Hunninghake R, et al. Nutraceutical augmentation of circulating endothelial progenitor cells and hematopoietic stem cells in human subjects. J Transl Med. 2010;8:34. doi: 10.1186/1479-5876-8-34.
16. Ichim TE, Zhong Z, Mikirova NA, et al. Circulating endothelial progenitor cells and erectile dysfunction: possibility of nutritional intervention? Panminerva Med. 2010;52(2 Suppl 1):75-80.
17. Wolf NS, Penn PE, Jiang D, Fei RG, Pendergrass WR. Caloric restriction: conservation of in vivo cellular replicative capacity accompanies life-span extension in mice. Exp Cell Res. 1995 Apr;217(2):317-23.
18. Rickman AD, Williamson DA, Martin CK, et al. The CALERIE Study: design and methods of an innovative 25% caloric restriction intervention. Contemp Clin Trials. 2011;32(6):874-81. doi: 10.1016/j.cct.2011.07.002.
19. Taya Y, Ota Y, Wilkinson AC, et al. Depleting dietary valine permits nonmyeloablative mouse hematopoietic stem cell transplantation. Science. 2016. doi: 10.1126/science.aag3145.
20. Kondo T, Hayashi M, Takeshita K, et al. Smoking cessation rapidly increases circulating progenitor cells in peripheral blood in chronic smokers. Arterioscler Thromb Vasc Biol. 2004;24(8):1442-7.
21. Theiss HD, Adam M, Greie S, Schobersberger W, Humpeler E, Franz WM. Increased levels of circulating progenitor cells after 1-week sojourn at moderate altitude (Austrian Moderate Altitude Study II, AMAS II). Respir Physiol Neurobiol. 2008;160(2):232-8.
22. Murray CJL, Kulkarni SC, Michaud C, et al. Eight Americas: Investigating mortality disparities across races, counties, and race-counties in the United States. PLoS Medicine. 2006;3(9):e260. doi:10.1371/journal.pmed.0030260.
23. Thom SR, Bhopale VM, Velazquez OC, Goldstein LJ, Thom LH, Buerk DG. Stem cell mobilization by hyperbaric oxygen. Am J Physiol Heart Circ Physiol. 2006;290(4):H1378-86.
24. Heyboer M 3rd, Milovanova TN, Wojcik S, et al. CD34+/CD45-dim stem cell mobilization by hyperbaric oxygen - changes with oxygen dosage. Stem Cell Res. 2014;12(3):638-45. doi: 10.1016/j.scr.2014.02.005.
25. Vasa M, Fichtlscherer S, Adler K, et al. Increase in circulating endothelial progenitor cells by statin therapy in patients with stable coronary artery disease. Circulation. 2001;103(24):2885-90.

Chapter Nineteen

1. Sheyn D, Shapiro G, Tawackoli W, et al. PTH induces systemically administered mesenchymal stem cells to migrate to and regenerate spine injuries. Mol Ther. 2016;24(2):318-30. doi: 10.1038/mt.2015.211.

Conclusion

1. American Diabetes Association. Economic costs of diabetes in the U.S. in 2012. Diabetes Care. 2013 Apr;36(4):1033-46. doi: 10.2337/dc12-2625.
2. Wikinvest. Arthritis Drug Market. http://www.wikinvest.com/wiki/Arthritis_Drug_Market. Accessed Dec 2016.

ACKNOWLEDGMENTS

Perhaps there's a little poetic justice here—it took nine months to complete this book, which is essentially about afterbirth. Unlike making a baby, it took more than just two people to bring it into the world! I have many people to thank.

This book wouldn't have been possible without the many patients and their family members who enthusiastically volunteered personal details about, very often, distressing medical conditions. I extend a heartfelt thank you to them for their generous contributions to this book. Hearing how stem cell treatment has changed their lives for the better is the most rewarding part of this journey for me.

Secondly, I would like to thank all my colleagues and friends with whom I've had so many fascinating conversations, meetings, and collaborative scientific ventures, in the order we met: James Jackson, PhD, Joseph Casciari, PhD, Ron Hunninghake, MD, Michael Rodriguez, PhD, DSc, Jorge Miranda-Massari, PhD, Nina Mikirova, PhD, Fabio Solano, MD, Leonard Smith, MD, John Clement, MD, Thomas Ichim, PhD, Roger Nocera, MD, Marialaura Madrigal, PhD, Bob Harman DVM, Amit Patel, MS, MD, Keith March, MD, PhD, Boris Minev, MD, Jorge Paz Rodriguez, MD, Lic. Rodolfo Fernandez, Professor Arnold Caplan, PhD, Eduardo Mansilla, MD, Robert Hariri, MD, PhD, and Peter Diamandis, MD. Your insightful and stimulating out-of-the-box approaches have been invaluable and constantly pushed me to strive for that proverbial next step in regenerative medicine.

I would also like to thank my team and staff at Medistem Panama and at the Riordan Medical Institute for their outstanding dedication and hard work all of these years, particularly Jay Lenner, Cindy Cunningham, and Silvia Molina.

I owe my children Chloe, Michaela, Brinn, and Tierney a big THANK YOU for not only doing without some time with their father, but for also having to endure countless hours of conversation about stem cells.

Last but not least, a big thank you to those who've been directly involved in the production of this book. It's been a long road, and it's been worth it through and through! Thank you Jamey Jones, Michael Black, Dorita Avila, and Pamela Sapio for helping me get my message out into the world.

CPSIA information can be obtained
at www.ICGtesting.com
Printed in the USA
LVHW051034211219
641338LV00011B/101